# THE DRAGON KEY

# The Dragon Key
## Book I: Memoirs of a Galactic Guardian

# Adam Apollo

# DEDICATION

*My deepest heartfelt thanks and gratitude to all those who experienced this journey of life with me. These stories are about real people and their memories, carried in the tales of my own personal self-discovery. This book contains explicit sexual content, deeply personal experiences, and reveals many of the private details of my lives. Many names have been altered in order to protect the identities of my closest loved ones in this series, except in some cases where I've been given explicit approval to use their real name. I'm honored to share these stories for the benefit of all those who seek to understand their own personal journey through time, across lives, and gain a better perspective on the context of our current evolutionary threshold on Earth.*

*The journey of life is not always easy, but blessings can be found even in our darkest hours. To all those who I have hurt along the way, I am sorry, please forgive me. I am always listening, learning, and growing with the intent on being a better and more integral person. If you hurt me, I forgive you. I understand that so many of our wounds come from traumas in this life or others. If we have loved each other deeply and fully in even a single moment of expression, thank you. Your love has made the whole journey as a Soul more than worth it. If we lived together, died together, held our children together, or found solace in each other, it has truly been an honor. May the emanation of this book restore your awareness, transform your pain to pleasure, awaken your Soul's Love, and bring you closer to your own experience of Divinity.*

*Love All Ways*
*Always Love,*

Adam Apollo

# CONTENT WARNING

This book is intended for adult audiences only. It contains explicit sexual content and dynamics with multiple partners, as well as graphic language that some may find offensive. All sexual activity covered in this work is consensual between adults. The content also contains non-sexually related violence, and death, as well as scenes depicting slavery, abuse, and controversial perspectives. The content may challenge religious beliefs, and stimulate spiritual insights and energetic experiences that may significantly shift readers' states of awareness and initiate substantial transformations in their lives. The reader, duly informed, may proceed at their own risk. Discretion, awareness, and care is advised.

PROLOGUE ------------------------------------------------------------------1

Reunion of Souls ----------------------------------------------------------3

The Red Road ------------------------------------------------------------23

Extraterrestrial Contact --------------------------------------------------35

Sword & Chalice----------------------------------------------------------44

Songs of the Desert ------------------------------------------------------55

INTRODUCTION ----------------------------------------------------------59

The Science of Past-Lives------------------------------------------------61

The Phenomenology of Time---------------------------------------------70

The Physics of Time & Entanglement ----------------------------------77

Experiencing Total Recall ------------------------------------------------91

Of Heaven & Hell, and the story of Good & Evil -------------------96

Soul Contracts & Soul Families --------------------------------------103

Archetypal Memory vs Individual Memory ---------------------------106

Notes on my Translations of this Journey----------------------------110

IN THE BEGINNING--------------------------------------------------------115

Before Incarnation -----------------------------------------------------116

DRAGON ANDROMEDA GALAXY----------------------------------------121

Birth ----------------------------------------------------------------------123

The Conclave ------------------------------------------------------------126

A Coalition of Care -----------------------------------------------------131

Exploring Worlds -------------------------------------------------------141

Epilogue: Dragons------------------------------------------------------157

SHIHAELEI BETELGEUSE REGION ORION SYSTEM---------------163

A Sudden Departure 熏 ------------------------------------------------165

Captivity 火 --------------------------------------------------------------171

Hackers 水 ---------------------------------------------------------------182

Escape 隘-------------------------------------------------------------------185

Rescue 濟 --------------------------------------------------------------------201

Into the Deep 墮------------------------------------------------------------208

Rebirth & Death 死-------------------------------------------------------220

Shihaeleio 沙 ---------------------------------------------------------------232

Oath of the Galactic Guardians 轟------------------------------250

Elf-Kin 家 -----------------------------------------------------------------259

the Ambassador 缘 -----------------------------------------------------262

Finding a Path 道 ----------------------------------------------------269

DarkMoon Station 冥 -----------------------------------------------282

Epilogue: Shihaelei -------------------------------------------------298

## TIARA DANAN VEGA SYSTEM--------------------------------305

Shiara -------------------------------------------------------------------------307

Receiving the Tiara ---------------------------------------------------312

Assault of the Valkrye ----------------------------------------------317

Once a Dragon------------------------------------------------------------325

Pleiadian Path -----------------------------------------------------------332

Into the Depths of Presence ---------------------------------------343

Gate of Goddessence-----------------------------------------------------350

Total Transformation-----------------------------------------------------365

Arcturian Halls------------------------------------------------------------373

Epilogue: Tiara Danan----------------------------------------------------393

## BOOK II: THE JOURNEY TO GAIA~TERRA PLEIADIAN MAIA STAR SYSTEM------------------------------------------------------403

The Becoming---------------------------------------------------------------405

Discovering Gaia-----------------------------------------------------------420

Glossary: --------------------------------------------------------------------433

About the Author----------------------------------------------------------445

# PROLOGUE

*Where the whispering winds of time*
*Brush the forces of Creation*
*The streams of pattern rhyme*
*Revealing a Trail of Elation*

*As the liberating fires of Passion*
*Birth forth the Intentional breath*
*Dancing in the vortex of Relation*
*Life emerges from every death*

*What tales pray tell of its journey*
*Through the growth and change of life*
*And every cycle of returning*
*Even through the challenge and strife*

*Finding the Way back to the Center*
*Heart of Being Becoming Itself*
*To the threshold of Sacred Surrender*
*Where the Soul knows Eternal Wealth*

# PROLOGUE - PART 1
# REUNION OF SOULS

My girlfriend's roommate always made coffee exactly the way I loved it. I sat in the chair we had taken from one of the dorm building's desolate "lounges," set next to the coffee maker and artistically drawn spreadsheet where Rastara had diagrammed the ways every one of her friends liked their coffee. The rich dark liquid was somewhat of a passion for her, along with many other mysterious things, embodied by the obscure quote taped word by word across the wall above her bed: "*where passion is not found no virtue ever dwelt.*"

I remembered the first time I had seen Rastara, catching a glimpse of each other's eyes as we passed in front of Founders Hall, our dormitory, at the University of North Carolina at Asheville. Some strange magic was in the air, though it passed just as swiftly as the shifting breeze that caught the long straight cascade of her blonde hair, rippling gold in the afternoon sun. Time slowed down for a moment, stretching out with every detail becoming vivid, as our eyes made contact. In the soft shared gaze, there was a spark of something impossible to define.

Now I was dating Shannon, her roommate. I'd been invited over to watch a movie with them, after seeing Shannon a few times out at parties. Trey, a tall handsome raver with earrings and occasionally multi-colored short brown hair was sitting next to Rastara, so I took the seat next to Shannon on Rastara's bed. That night Shannon and I ended up on an adventure together. Shannon was deeply interested in my energy work, metaphysics, and the discoveries I had made about the nature of reality. She wanted to hang out, play outside, and have sex. Being a freshman in college with few experiences, I was game, but

I also had some resistance. I didn't understand it at the time, but I enjoyed being around Shannon, Rastara, and Trey, and we all got closer.

One day I was sitting in a chair in their room, sipping a delicious cup of hazelnut coffee; "Light and creamy, soft and sweet, like the skin of a faerie's teat," was the description in Rastara's chart. She was sitting on her bed, talking to two of her lady friends standing, while I was chatting with two guys my age sitting on the floor. I looked over at her at one point, and while she was laughing, my whole world shifted…

*When this icon appears, it means we are jumping to another point in the timeline of the Soul Stream.*

I was suddenly standing in a large medieval ballroom, built of huge log posts and beams, with a high ceiling dripping with heavy metal oil lamp chandeliers. The walls were darkly draped with heavy tapestries depicting nature scenes, knights on horseback, and various other imagery in dark heavy cloth as thick as a rug. I could smell the burning oil from the lamps, and the light sweetness of the candles in alcoves around the room.

I could feel the weight of my ornamental armor, straps pressing into my collarbone and slightly chafing my armpits. A peace-bound sword hung at my side, a richly decorated ceremonial hilt tied with a small piece of white cloth that wrapped around the jeweled scabbard. A violet velvet cloak hung over one shoulder to the floor, while a small Dragon symbol on deep purple was stitched into the breastplate on the right side of my chest.

Yet all of this was taken in with the instantaneous synesthesia of physical embodiment; I was there. And so was she.

Rastara had her hair up in a gorgeous swirling bun decorated with small symbols hanging from fine chains, bound by a silver circlet, all revealing a long silky neck arching above a bare collarbone and a tease of her cleavage and shoulders. Her corset-bound dress stuffed her body into glorious slender curves, cascading to the ground in a way that made her appear to be floating above the many layers of fabric. Silver patterns decorated her bodice, and cascaded down her arms in tight filmy lace to her wrists.

As she laughed, her ladies laughed with her, and I noticed I was in a conversation.

Two lords stood before me with serious grimaces, though I knew their disgruntled manner had nothing to do with me. We were discussing ambushes happening in a particular valley between our lands. The isolated road along the valley floor was a perfect place for vandals and mercenaries to attack our convoys, trains of horse pulled wagons filled with grain, goods, money and other resources. In my mind, it immediately seemed clear that by placing scouting archers along a particular ridge above the valley floor, and sending scouts to different points in the valley, we could more easily spot potential attackers and catch them in a pincher from above and below. My fellow Lord was a bit concerned about the level of manpower needed, but I had the sense the problem was solved and my attention was drifting back to the woman with her hair up.

I caught her eye for a moment and a rush of ecstasy flowed through my body, an overwhelming deep sense of love and pride suffusing my entire being. Deep within, I knew that she was the love of my life and that I wanted to have a family with her, raise kids in my castle, and defend her with every breath. All at once.

::: ⌛ :::

And then, in a blink of an eye, I was back in the dorm room, and my mouth hung open as I saw Rastara on her bed talking to a couple college girls, two guy friends sitting looking at me with confused faces, and I almost dropped my coffee. One of the guys said, "Adam, are you okay?" I sat stunned for a moment as all I could think of was archers on ridges, protecting our trade, and the overwhelming feeling of connection I felt with Rastara...

"I think I need some water," I said as I put down my coffee and shakily rose to stumble out of the dorm room. In the hall, I went to the water fountain to drink, take a breath, and gather my wits. I had no idea what had just happened, but I had a pretty strong feeling it was something extraordinarily important.

Making my way back to the dorm room after a few deep circulations of breath and chi, grounding in my lower *Tan Tien*[1], I opened the door. Directly to my left, Rastara was in the bathroom washing her face in the sink a few steps away from me. She looked up at me with wide eyes that looked both surprised and intensely curious. "Did you..." she started.

"Oh my god, you did too...?" I asked. She nodded and took a deep breath, shuddering a bit. I nodded and was a bit dazed. At that moment, I was filled with excitement, concern, and a little bit of fear as my thoughts drifted to Shannon.

That was the beginning. Then we had dreams of this other time begin to come in, each seeing different moments, and

---

[1] From the ancient Chinese term for the "lower crucible," a point on the Haric Line (vertical pillar or Djed) in the pelvis, approximately three finger widths below the belly button. This point stores *Chi* in the body, allowing the cultivation of a reservoir that can be accessed at any time.

even having an awareness of two names that we may have used. At one point we had a private conversation to discuss these things and shared the names we had dreamed about... *Kaylan & Tara.*

Days later, I was walking across the Quad, a big grassy field with patterns of walkways between some of the main UNCA campus buildings. As I was crossing from one side, I saw Rastara walking on the far side towards the Library. Suddenly, I was no longer on the open lawn in the sunshine...

Though I was cloaked in the shadows behind leaves at the edge of the forest, I could see her easily, carrying a basket behind her head, hair dark and skin copper, with eyes as peaceful as the last slit of sunset. She walked towards the simple village, towards her home at the edge of the glade that separated us. My heart pounded, sweat threatening to bead on my forehead behind my mask and helm.

Would her husband beat her again today when she arrived home? Everything inside me screamed and I knew I could end it in an instant. I felt so angry. She was going home to a man who beat her regularly. Something about her pulled on my *Shen*[2] in a way that was both exciting and a bit destabilizing. I could not stand the idea of her being hurt by this man, and I was ready to end his life...

Katana and Wakizashi both strapped tightly to my body, along with snuggly fitting plated armor, I held the reins of my horse behind me, not moving a muscle, but every line of me tense. Even the most well trained warriors would

---

[2] From the ancient Chinese term for "spirit" or mind, often seen as one of the three Treasures of the Body (San Bao), along with Jing (or Ching, sexual energy), and Qi (or Chi, vital energy).

struggle to get past my blade, but with my Ancestral Armor, I had shields on my Shoulders, deflecting plates on my chest and stomach, large thigh guards, and even shin armor and sharp boots. Fighting some fool from a village would not be an honorable battle. It would be a slaughter.

But I couldn't take it anymore. She had caught my heart in Geisha form, before she was banished away to this village and sold to this horrible man. I couldn't see her suffer anymore, and that was that.

He would die at sunset...

...was my last thought as Rastara disappeared behind the library, heading for the Art Department at UNCA.

Someone walking by me on the Quad shifted me out of the flashback, and I was back on the University Campus and definitely not wearing Samurai armor. Still, the feeling lingered, along with a well of physical signals reminding me of what it felt like to wield a Katana, all the martial arts practices that had come naturally to me, my recent discoveries in tai-chi, and I could still feel the aura of danger around me, as though I was ready to kill in an instant. It was so vivid even in the afterburn...so real... What was happening to me?

There were a few other moments like this between Rastara and I, and I began seriously strategizing about how to end my brief relationship dance with Shannon. We had also discovered that Rastara and Shannon were born on the same exact day of the same year, within an hour of each other. Trey, who had become a close friend, was queer, and a fantastic party buddy, had exactly the same birthday as me, in the same year, within a couple hours. There was something profound going on here, and somehow there was some kind of Astrological pairing mismatch that night watching a movie in Rastara's room. In any case my curiosity was on fire to understand all these flashbacks, while another part of me was deeply concerned that I was somehow embroiled in a some kind of deep inner fantasy. Were we imagining all of this, and just telepathically connected in some way to share in these fantasies?

On Halloween that year, shortly after all this had begun to accelerate, I got my answer. A guy that I had only met briefly, who was apparently interested in one of Rastara's girlfriends, came with us as a group to a Halloween party. I discovered Rastara knew it was Samhain, and that she celebrated the old ways…which was yet another interesting point of synergy between us. Yet at this event, it was Jon who changed my life.

It seemed like only a short time after we arrived, Jon came careening outside to where I was standing with a few others, Rastara nearby and Shannon nowhere to be seen. Jon was boring his eyes into me intensely, babbling what I thought at first was nonsense, and then he was overcome with emotion. As he began to cry openly, his words became very clear and serious.

"I'm so sorry man. I'm sorry I took her Kaylan. She wanted to come with me on the ship, she wanted me! But I know I fucked up, I seduced her, man. And then what I did…"

As he began to cry harder, I felt pain searing in my gut, my heart exploding with fear and anger and pain. The wave of physical feelings was quick and shocking, but then subsided into a hardened strength. I felt acceptance, as I began to see all the things he described. I felt hurt, and sad, but I also felt my commitment and love for the woman he was speaking of…

"Tara was so perfect man, and I couldn't help myself." He was wracked with grief as he struggled to continue, "All those villages man...and then you. You and I. God we were great weren't we man? Fucking shit we KILLED each other... Fuck man... I'm so sorry..."

::: ⌛ :::

I saw the villages burning, riding as fast as I could back to my castle. I brought in everyone I could and closed the gate. Archers manned the walls, and his army came calling. They assaulted the castle at first, losing men and occasionally getting some of ours. In the height of midday, knowing that this siege would result in countless deaths, I came to the bridge above the portcullis.

I remembered calling him forth from his army, and inviting him to a single dual. Him and me. "This is not about any of them. This is about us. You and I. If you want her, you'll have to face me in combat. Now. In my courtyard. Just you and me, you have my word."

We allowed him in along with an honor guard, and he and I quickly dropped layers of our armor as people gathered along the walls, and safely behind many of my brothers, my warriors. We began to circle each other like ancient dragons analyzing each others footsteps, movements, and sword postures.

Our battle ensued, a long and exhausting series of assaults and parries, each connection of our swords ringing echoing through the courtyard. I'd rise like a tide, he'd crash down and step aside in fluid form. He'd jab at me to gain distance, then charge and strike repeatedly with mad fervor, and I would dance aside from his momentum and use it to destabilize him for split seconds, before he'd regain his position and stance.

We went on for what seemed like forever, our arms hanging more, swords held lower as our bodies took the beating of each resonating note of steel on steel. Sweat dripped in my eyes, and soaked my body under the chainmail and leather I wore. My forearms screamed with fatigue and pain. Each moment became deeper, more focused, more ominous, more dangerous.

I finally knew how to end it, in a flash of desperate inspiration. My sword swept upward in a fluid arc, and I opened myself up to a strike from his sword just above my waist and feigned a surprised look on my face. With his teeth gritted he took the bait and jumped forward to pierce my guts deep with his blade…but as it slid into my skin, my sword fell on his neck like lightning, cutting straight through his collarbone and deep into his chest. His eyes were shocked for a moment, and then he fell backwards to his death.

I stumbled backwards, then exhaustion and pain overtook me and I fell to the hard stones, grueling pain overwhelming me as the stones pushed the sword back through my body, and a last jolt of energy let me shakily pull it out the rest of the way to let the bloody blade drop beside me.

Her face was above me, beautiful and radiant. She looked like an Angel, tears streaming down her cheeks and dripping on me like a soft rain. Things felt warmer, brighter, easier, and as I spoke words of love always, all ways, I felt a different kind of sensation vibrate through my entire being, and I drifted out of my body. Her grief filled protests held my heart as I looked down at the scene of carnage, now a serene and peaceful moment of release.

That was the first time I remembered dying, leaving my body, and seeing myself lifeless on the courtyard stones, next to the gory mangled form of my opponent. It was

Rastara crying over me, *Tara* was her name in that time, overwhelmed with grief and love that was also subtly stained by a bitter anger at the stupidity of men.

It was difficult to leave, and I felt myself slip through moments in time with her that were sliding by like memories, being there with her through her grief, through her prayers, and through her process of reclaiming our people's strength.

Too soon, but perhaps just in time, I found myself crossing through curtains of light that beckoned me onward, and I entered the Spirit World. I remember reunions, powerful waves of realization and deeper understanding about my life, and many lifetimes, and experienced a growing state of deep surrender to the Divine Love and the Eternal Bliss that forms the Symphony underlying all of our experience.

I also remember glimpses of other things in the Spirit World, from shared cities of light to gardens of delightful essences, and moments with circles of Souls sharing deep and profound love and promises to show up for each other again and again. Then in one memory I'm standing with a few close guides and beloveds around a "portal" in the shape of a round table, similar to the "*scrying* pools" spoken of in the occult mystery traditions. Yet this round mirror like surface rendered a holographic view of people and places in the physical world, and from there I watched the journeys of incarnated Souls I loved until I found the two people I wanted to have as my next parents, and began exploring the moment of my next incarnation.

And here we were, hundreds of years later, many lifetimes later, at a College Keg Party on Halloween. Jon had too much to drink, certainly, but the visceral memories his words evoked in me were no hallucination. He knew me by name from that life in the Middle Ages, and he knew Rastara's name as well... Those were names we had never revealed to anyone. The scientist in me knew this was irrefutable data; a third-party verification of a specific lifetime, with no prior knowledge, that evoked a direct visceral and psychological response in me, matching data points and specific details from my prior memories and dreams.

As for Rastara and I, our journey had just begun. The whirlwind of moments of synchronous memory with each other and others would lead to great revelations about ourselves and our lives in the years to come.

It had taken many moons to come together, after I had broken Shannon's heart by breaking up with her, not long after that fateful All Hallows Eve with Jon. There were so many adventures, crossings with other Souls who we shared memory with, and deep healings and blissful reunions. Many of the stories I'll share throughout these tomes, particularly from lifetimes on Earth, come from the endless waterfall of memories and reconnections from this time.

So many of these moments revealed deeper truths to life, reality, and myself. Every experience was like an initiation, and I began to realize that my memories were like keys to aspects of my consciousness. These keys could open doors of possibility, expand my awareness, and restore skills and powerful energetic artifacts within my Being... I discovered that sexual connection was one of the most potent ways for me to access and retain full recall, due to the depth of Soul connection possible in states of orgasmic bliss.

One night, Rastara and I returned to her bed wearing masks, after a finely-dressed night of adventures. As she let her red velvet dress fall to the floor, revealing her stunningly perfect body, the air in the room seemed to shimmer. She climbed into bed and I watched her hungrily, pulling my shirt over my head and suddenly feeling my whole body shift and transform...

The skin covered lodge was very warm inside, metal braziers lit with fresh coals and burning subtle sweet smells into the air. My body still glistened with sweat from hauling the Great Stag all the way back to our camp with my brothers. I should have been exhausted from hunting all evening, but I felt intensely alive, my heart racing as I took in the view before me.

Her upper face mostly hidden by a decorative leather mask made to look like the Goddess, the rest of her body was bare in the firelight, as she laid in an almost relaxed way on the soft bedding and pillows in the heart of the small chamber. Her light skin looked like white gold in subtle burnished shimmers, as anointing oils had clearly been massaged into her entire body. Light caught the shimmer of wet pink nipples standing at attention on breasts slightly larger than my hands, down a muscled torso to cradling hips. My eyes fell between her thighs, to the soft folds delicately decorated with a fuzz of glittering blonde hairs that were finely trimmed.

Her fingertips gently stroked her own stomach, probably to give her a sense of ease. After all, I was also wearing a mask. To her, I was some beast of a man, the Stag God, emerging from the forest to take her, to merge with her, and give our union to the Goddess and God for the blessing of all.

I felt blood swelling into my loins, my body eager to fulfill that promise, and to sanctify this prayer. But who was she? Was she afraid of me?

Almost in response she slid a hand between her legs, spreading her thighs apart slightly, and reached out her other hand towards me. I moved to the edge of the bed, and she sat up, her lithe body even more beautiful as she leaned towards my waist to grab at the ties of the skins which covered my waist and legs.

My hard member burst forth from those confines as soon as she unlaced them, and my pelts and weapons buckles fell away as quickly as my leggings. She seemed to be getting even more interested now, as she pulled me towards her, and kneeled on the bed between her legs, my feet still bound by boots and pants. Kicking them off me, I became more primal, gazing into her eyes as I slowly drove her backwards without touching her, just getting as close as slowly as possible until we were both fully on the bed. I hovered over her like a four-legged wolf, smelling her scent, the nectary floral sweetness of honeysuckle. My mouth watered, and a bead of clear moisture dripped from my swollen member.

I reached out a hand to touch her heart, as she inhaled deeply, keeping her hands at either side of her head in passive surrender. I touched her skin, and the electrical pulse of life coursed through me and her at the same time. Ever so gently, I caressed her with my fingertips, her entire body uncharted terrain, and I was the explorer.

I watched her respond as my hands moved around her body slowly. I was a hunter, finding the spots that opened her breath, made her squirm, spread her thighs even further. The mask of the King Stag I wore left my mouth uncovered, so I began to satiate my hunger by tasting her skin. I nibbled my way to her pink parts, biting her nipples, kissing her gasping lips, and finally made my way down to her Sacred Rose.

Her closely trimmed skin prickled, goosebumps rolling up her finely muscled stomach, and her exposed nipples couldn't seem to get any harder. The room was warm, very warm, or the fire in me was consuming my skin. I breathed deeply, the swell of desire roaring inside me like a volcano. I felt the weight of my body, grounding myself into the Heart of the Great Mother, and felt like a forged sword capable of penetrating to the center of the most torrential love...

Then I dove between her thighs, and devoured her whole. My mouth took in the layers of lips and succulent nectar that already started to ooze from inside her. She was like a fully blooming rose, whole in my mouth, petals pressing against every sense and sending trickles of lightning through my body.

Her deep sudden moan rumbled through her pelvis, and I focused in on her pubic bone, my tongue pressed against her pearl, and slowly, succulently, hummed back into her. Breathy whispers became a soft somber song, her raspy voice holding a resonance that strummed the strings of my heart... I knew her... I didn't know how... And though she felt a bit familiar with those lips and that voice, I felt like I knew her much more deeply, and we had shared these moments a thousand times.

Suddenly everything lit up, and I felt like a God in a Great Game: to Hunt the Spring of Eternal Life, and bring forth the gush of Living Nectar, the Golden Honey from the heart of the Goddess Queen's Hive.

My Soul suddenly lit with a calling to serve this woman with everything I had inside me, every single essence of my being, from sweat to tears to prayers to...love.

I plunged my tongue inside her ravenously, then began to eat her body with my mouth, sometimes softly, sometimes biting her in ways that made her giggle and gasp. I pounced her, held her down, roared at her, and gently bit her lip. One of her hands had slipped away, and suddenly she was grasping at my throbbing sword, pulling it between petals soaked with our shared sweetness. She gasped as my head entered her, and I held very still, letting her breathe.

She arched her back and stretched open her jaw, breathing deep into her pelvis, and her wet folds opened like a long sheen of curtains. She flexed once, squeezing wet lubricating juices all over me, and pulling wetness out of my own pulsing member. Her hand was now on my neck, pulling her body up towards me as I held myself above her, driving her hips down onto me, stretching yet taking me like she owned me. Perhaps I was not the Hunter here, but the Hunted.

I met her fierceness with my own, pulling back just a little, then driving forward slowly and intently. She drove back towards me a little, opening more, and smoothing the way for deeper motion. I pressed on, pushing our masks together as my lips brushed hers, my breath tickling passion. She suddenly sang loudly, her voice ringing in a high lilt that felt like Sun shining through the trees. I let my deep bass rumble with her, groaning but singing it out. It was effortless.

I was now plunged deep inside her, united in her pleasure, linked in a state of synchronous telepathic co-meditation, and we were the Great God & Goddess as One.

We danced, and I rode her like a horse, she mounted me like a Dragonrider, and then she had me. She drove her hips into me like she was riding the shaft of the Sun itself...and she was. I was a blazing torrent of Light erupting from the Sacred Center of All That Is, and she was the birth of All Life, All Experience, All Love, and All

Growth. I was the Beginning and End of the Story, but she was the Journey through it All. Together we were each other.

I was roaring at the top of my lungs, the waves of ecstasy rumbling through me like earthquakes, or perhaps a stampede of great warriors riding into battle, or perhaps a great blooming of seeds, abundant harvests, joy and health for all my people. Suddenly the light surged brighter, as the Goddess bloomed in a wave of orgasmic bliss. It felt like winds were blowing around us, rain was falling upon us, flowers were blooming all around us, and the fires of the Sacred Center were within us... We were Creation itself, and a New Universe was blooming through us.

Suddenly I could feel this new Energy, and it was a Being. He was masculine, yet beautiful and delicate in some ways. His eyes were hard as they looked at me, challenging me to be better. But we loved each other, so deeply and in such an ancient way. This was...my Son to be?

After that memorable lovemaking (in which I did not get Rastara pregnant in our time, as we chose our timing wisely), I knew what Sacred Ceremonial sex really was. I knew that it was a way to access the direct and visceral experience of the Divine. If we ask ourselves what moments in our lives are really truly peak experiences, it is almost always the trail of profound moments of deep Spiritual Communion that stand out. They shape and define us, revealing the sacred crystalline pattern of our Soul's Purpose.

One day at sunset on a snowy day a couple years later, Rastara unfolded a bundle of rich blue fabric, its sturdy weave heavy in her hands. "It's fireproof...and waterproof… Mostly." She grinned at me. Then with a flourish, she stood and opened the cloak, turning it so that it's shimmering silk lining caught the light, and the golden dragons on black that lined the trim would shine. She flipped back the large hood, revealing a hand stitched emblem on the inner heart of the cloak:

**Alban Arthuan** it read, decorated lettering inside a Star design.

"It means Light of Arthur," she said carefully, eyes glimmering with unshed tears. My heart tumbled in a thousand ways, whirling into love and spinning on the edge of pain. After all these memories, all these moments, it was so clear. We had come so far, my Partner Lover Past-Life Explorer Friend…and in some times, my Sister…and I had somehow found each other again and again, weaving love through some fabric of cosmic destiny…

The years deepening our relationship had been full of memories and magic beyond anything I had dreamed.

We had somehow pulled Souls out of the woodworks, drawing those to us who had shared so many adventures with us across the arc of our journey through time. Marianne, who sat with me by the lake, remembering our training in archery together. Mikayla, who had taken me in from the snowy tundra of Russia along with Marianne and Rastara, and danced with me in St. Petersburg for the Czar of the time and his wife, now named Wu and Hera. The three women had also been there in India when I made my way down from my monastery in the Himalayas, and had synchronistically ended up defending their bellydancing troupe from a group of horny mercenaries who couldn't keep their hands to themselves.

I had danced and loved and adventured with so many Souls, and without this powerful field between Rastara and I, part of me wondered if I would ever have had so many opportunities to reconnect with my Soul Family. Was she my Soul Mate? Twin Flame? And if so, why did we constantly struggle to give each other more freedom out of love, and yet continue to feel more separate, while the Universe seemed to bind us together forever?

Why did she often feel more like my Sister, though my attraction to her was undeniably strong, and why was there some hidden secret shame or pain inside of us, some part of our journey marred by traumas that we had not yet remembered?

I was forced to dive into these Mysteries suddenly, when Rastara shattered our covenant in a single day, taking me to a cemetery where we sat in an open field overlooking the tombstones, under the wary gaze of great oaks. She seemed shaky, and I soon understood why.

There was no amount of framing that could brace me for the final words of her brief expression. She told me flat out that she was not in love with me, and was not sure she ever had been.

For me, it shook the very foundations of my sense of sanity, after all that we had experienced together in over four years of deep and profound relationship. In my little room in a house on Chestnut Street that I shared with a master Astrologer, I was surrounded by all the emblems of our bond. From the two-handed Celtic broadsword leaning in the corner and the fireproof cloak hanging beside it, to the wooden box full of rose petals and the copper grail etched with "Willow" on the bottom, her gifts in honor of our shared memories suddenly felt lifeless and hollow.

I found myself spiraling into a pit of pain, a torrential whirlwind of anger and hate and sadness, until I wanted nothing more than death. An echo across time of taking my own life, a fearful uprising even during my childhood in this life, surged like fire and ice through my system. Yet I screamed into the face of my own destruction: "What if it all means NOTHING! What if I am NOTHING! What if I have NOTHING! There is NOTHING left...what do I have?"

I tumbled down the rabbit hole of my own sanity and psyche and found nothing. A vast empty void of Eternity...but it had a *feeling*... Omnipresent through the void of darkness was a warm sensation that tingled through my being and began to surge from my Core... I felt it hold me from within, from without, in every possible way, and I finally recognized the feeling as a flitting lightning bolt of mental recognition returned...

It was Love.

As I grasped this Truth, my whole being began to bloom into a geyser of Love, pouring from my eyes and lighting up my tears like diamonds. It came out of me in every direction, and I saw the threads of light that wove me with Rastara. I loved her in a way that was beyond words, and I knew that she loved me the same, because I could feel our bond, ancient and current. But more importantly, I LOVED. I LOVE. I Am Love.

And I knew in that moment, with an *adamantium* certainty, that I could never lose Love, no matter what else I might lose. It was a wellspring of life-force, and it was a Sacred Gift. Just to have the opportunity to give love is one of the greatest gifts of all existence.

I also realized that no amount of words, ideas, or concepts could take away my Identity. The past-life memories I had recovered had forged a deeper sense of Identity and Purpose within me than I had ever known in my life. It didn't make letting go of Rastara any easier, as the bond between us was still somehow ever-present.

And so, life spun us right back into the weave, our Soul Bonds steering the threads of our destinies to reconcile our pasts and truly move forward… We met at a coffee shop and she quickly acknowledged that she had lied to me that day, apologized profusely, and shared so many things that she had been going through, and all the ways it wasn't working to hold on to each other.

She told me that she believed this was her only way of finding liberation, but to do so she thought she needed to construct a lie that would slice deep and clean all the way through our connection. Yet this very act was intended to provide what we had been trying to give each other for years: *Freedom*.

I didn't understand this paradox entirely at the time, or why we held this bond that both gave us such a bounty of wisdom and memory, and yet also chafed at our Souls. We stayed in connection after that, and that is all I could have asked for at the time. Yet in the eventual dawning of this great paradox's final resolution, what I ended up getting was so much more than I ever dreamed, and for that, I will always be thankful to Rastara Amarisa.

# PROLOGUE - PART 2
# THE RED ROAD

It was a dark night in the deep desert on September 2nd 2005 that changed everything for me, and her, again. In the year before that adventure, a series of things happened in my life that opened my eyes to many new realities, a cascade of transformation initiated by the sometimes painful and always liberating ending of many other cycles... Graduation from Massage School, my partnership with Rastara ending, leaving my long time job at Bridgestone Firestone as a Sales Manager for three stores, having a $1M investment into my company Access Granted fall through, the slow dying of my venue Tribes Club I had co-created with Knowa and Orellana, and many more things...

This storm of events will be chronicled in detail elsewhere in these Tomes, but these thresholds must be acknowledged here. We find ourselves skipping like a stone through connected ripples in time, as moments in the past converge in resonance and entanglement with the Present.

The real wave began in 2004, when I was at a grocery store in Asheville and a man walked up to me. "Are you Adam?" He asked, and I got a look at him. A tall gangly guy with a strongly integrated feminine peered at me with bright, disarming eyes. I decided to ignore the yogurts and give him my full attention.

"Yeah." I said.

"I'm Paul, they call me the Hulaman. I know your Grandparents, and I met you when you were a little guy. You probably don't remember me but I recognize you."

"My grandparents?" I asked, "They certainly know a lot of people. Are you in the Meher Baba community?"

"Yeah, I know them through Baba, and Florida. I'm a famous Hula-hooper there." He went on to tell me various things about his Hulaman super-heroic status, and then suddenly changed subject. "Do you want to come up to Boone and cook for a bunch of Indigenous Elders with me?"

It was a surprising request to say the least. I wasn't a chef, though I did love to cook. A bunch of Elders? I asked him to tell me more.

"They are fulfilling a Hawaiian Prophecy: 'When the Tribes of the World meet in the Land of the Two Twins in the Eastern Mountains, the Sacred Hoop will begin to be re-woven.' The property in Boone is 500 acres owned by two twins. There's epic temples there built originally for Maharishi, but now it's mostly deserted except for one campus of them. This place is amazing, and I just feel like you're supposed to be there."

I couldn't argue with that, and this certainly sounded like an intriguing adventure. I love adventures.

So, that's how I found myself representing the Youth of All Nations in a council of Indigenous Elders from everywhere around the world, totaling nearly 150 in number. I held fire ceremonies and learned from Mayan Daykeeper Tata Apolonario, and was honored with a whale bone hook by Pu'uhonua Keiki Kanahele leader of the Hawaiian Sovereign Movement. I smoked the White Buffalo Peace Pipe passed down from Crazy Horse, and honored the White Buffalo Calf Bundle given to the Lakota Dakota Nakota-Sioux from the White Buffalo Calf Woman, both carried by Chief Arvol Looking Horse. Arvol's son had recently been in a car accident, and he asked me to help his daughter Gracie organize a Prayer Run for World Peace.

In 2005, we organized runners from the four corners of North America to converge in the Black Hills of South Dakota. With Gracie and a small group of kids from different reservations from South Dakota across the North and East, we started the run in New York State. We covered around 100 miles a day, scaling across the Adirondacks and then traveling south of the Great Lakes, across the vast plains to the badlands, and finally into the heart of Turtle Island, the Black Hills.

We converged for the Tenth Annual World Peace Prayer Day Ceremonies, and arrived into town in concert with runners from the West Coast, from deep in Mexico who had passed through New Mexico and Colorado, and both runners and riders on horseback in traditional Lakota gear who came down from Canada. The whirling vortex of energies we experienced running together and uniting our four Eagle Staffs from the four directions in a vast circular field on Sacred Lands was truly indescribable, but I can tell you that I saw White Animals of nearly every kind swarming the hills around the fields and shining in the sunlight in my peripheral vision. It was an Astral Gathering of epic proportions, not to mention the hundreds of Elders, Tribal Representatives, Youth, and various leaders of environmental projects who came together for those days.

The Prayer Run and my time with the indigenous families had anchored me solidly in this lifetime, grounded me in my body, and challenged me to stay fully present in my guidance in the moment. There is so much more to tell about these adventures, but I will save the in-depth version of these stories for a later Tome in this series.

Instead of traveling back to my home in Asheville North Carolina after the World Peace Prayer Day Ceremonies in the Black Hills, I found myself traveling to Los Angeles with Alison, the coordinator of the West Coast Runners. Synchronicities interconnected me with many amazing people, and led me to San Francisco, where I heard about a place called Burning Man.

One night at a beach party near the city on the Bay, I ended up dancing in Swordforms and losing myself in the embodiment of the art of flow. Suddenly I noticed someone was staring at me, wide eyed, as she sat on an art piece nearby. I completed one of my forms, then turned and strode straight towards her. I recognized her as Kellie, who was close to one of my performer friends from Asheville, and whom I had just met briefly earlier that night. As I came to sit with her, she seemed to struggle with what to say. "I remember you...moving like that... But on a Battlefield."

Her words took me by surprise for a split second, as it had been a long while since I had any sudden memory with anyone. She peered at me, trying to see if it was okay to proceed. I began to feel a current of energy arising inside me, a string of memory being strummed by her words, and I nodded at her to proceed.

"You just twirled and cut them down... It was glorious... and horrible that we had to...but it was so fluid and peaceful. Oh gods...that was a gnarly battle." She looked sick, but then her face melted as something else dawned on her. "But we won, and I remember sitting at this great table with you, and many others raising our mugs to our victory!" She smiled suddenly, grinning from ear to ear, then looked at me seriously. "And we raised our mugs to you."

The hall rang with laughter, and the grizzled knight struggling to keep a lady on each knee while raising his mug stared at me with a twinkle in his eyes. "Thank the Dragon, ye wielded well today An Dragan." His laughter rang through the chamber, and cheers followed in a roar. Firelight glinted off the mirrored plates on the table, and turned our polished copper goblets to golden fire.

I laughed heartily and felt the hand of my Lady on my thigh, taking in the rich sweet bouquet of the honey mead that warmed my belly, and my loins. I looked around the shining host of Lords and Ladies, Warlocks and Witches, Knights and Priestesses, my Soul Family, and let my words ring in with the notes of the Great Chamber, quieting the room.

"Any man can be a spear, harnessing the light of intention to pierce even the most vast of veils. Yet only when standing together do we become a star, blazing like an unquenchable fire, illuminating the shadows and restoring sight.

"What good is a sword, without the chalice which waters our lips? No stave laid cause for a flag, without the stones which found a Kingdom. We have built this together, and that which we have made will sing for all time, for ours is the Way of the Whispering Wind, the Song of the Sirens, the Dance of the Dragons. They will know us as the Roses bloom, as the Sun Rises, and the Stars Fall. As before, We Come Again!

"Sword and Chalice, Staff and Stone.
May the Eternal Goddess bless us all.
For the Rose and Round Table,
For All Life, For All Time! For Avalon!"

The roar was deafening, and the field seemed to quiver in a ripple through time…

::: ⌛ :::

Kellie and I had other memories too, moments connected to times as both lovers and friends. She had reignited something in me, a recognition of the deep and profound desire to quest deeper into my self-knowing. These glimpses also ignited fears, and a queasy feeling that surrounded the idea of accepting some of these new memories. They strongly reinforced some of the memories I'd had with Rastara, and pointed to a lifetime that seemed lost in the mists of history and legend.

That alone would not have been a problem, but the trail of memories, along with this one, seemed to have some pretty clear implications about who and where I was in that lifetime…

By this time in my journey, it had become pretty clear that people who had past life memories often tried to associate themselves with an important person in history. As I looked into this more, I found that most people had some memories of specific things around a particular famous person, but didn't necessarily have the direct visceral memories of that person themselves. I started to recognize that there were two types of memory:

First, there is the individual personal memory of an incarnation, in which intense physical, emotional, and mental experiences are recorded in the Soul Genome.

Second, there is collective non-personal Archetypal memory, which is connected to the stories, histories, and energetic imprint left by an individual or group who strongly embodied a particular Archetype.

We'll discuss these in detail later, but for now it is important to know that when one has a lot of very visceral individual memories, and those memories start to overlap with Archetypal stories in profound and undeniable ways, it forces one to begin a deep investigation.

I found myself rejecting the idea that I was a particular figure whose name was baked into the mythos of our time, but I could not deny that my memories and experiences were pushing me further and further into recognition of my Self. My entire journey through time was the Story of my own Soul's Song, and I had chosen particular incarnations which would in turn reveal more to me of who I Truly Am.

For the time being, I determined not to make any definitive decisions on my own identity in other lifetimes. Ah, the folly of youth. I never had to decide at all.

When I finally returned to Asheville, I was handed a Burning Man ticket by my dear friend and Elven Sister Amber at Transformus Festival. As I sat on a dock above a pure lake fed by a gushing creek that cascaded out of the lush temperate rainforest of North Carolina, she strode over to me and simply said, "Do you want my Burning Man ticket?" Then Pandoor and Ilsa told me they were driving out, and had room in their Van. They'd also be towing a beautiful wooden camper trailer, where I could stay during the Burn. Everything simply fell into my lap, and I was swept into an adventure that would change my life in every way imaginable.

After an arduous journey in which our trailer axle broke twice, we had a flat tire, the alternator died, and I lost my only debit card, we seemed to barely make it…out into the middle of nowhere. When I was a Samurai, my older brother was the Shogun. In this lifetime, he went by Knowa, and we had owned Tribes Club with Orellana, and threw tons of epic parties for various communities. We discovered our Samurai familial connections then, and he had tried to get me to read the *Book of Five Rings* many times. It would be many years before I fully confirmed who we were in that life through historical references and Theta Healing, and then many more before I read the Book of Five Rings, and rediscovered these sacred scrolls written by my Sword Master between 1614 and 1621. Yet that too, is a story for another time...

At Burning Man, Knowa shared that really cool wooden two-bedroom camper with me. Like an old ship inside, it was our stronghold in the desert storms and crazy chaos of Burning Man. I witnessed his ancient Mastery come alive one night, when we were dealing with some very intense energetics from a group of Russians who were in our camp. The danger felt very real, and for the first time, I felt fear sweep through Black Rock City itself. There was some evil force settling on the land, and it seemed to be distorting everything, twisting things into delusions of distrust, and the stinging wind felt violent.

Knowa looked at me calmly, sitting back in his camping chair and said simply, "It's just Wind on the Mountain."

His energy dropped into a Mountain, relaxed and fully comfortable with everything that was happening. I immediately followed his lead, grounding my energy in the Earth and feeling only the gentle breeze of changes all around me. It was powerful Magic, the stuff I had been learning to wield in so many ways since I was a teenager. His methods were elegant, to say the least.

My experience of Burning Man is worth of a book of its own, and much of that story will be told at the end of this great journey through time... Yet to take the clock far enough back to provide context for the content of this first Book, I will tell you a few details about the night the Man Burned, on September 2nd 2005.

On this fated night, I would meet my half-elven father from the Age of Atlantis in person, and work through deep and painful karma with him in relation to my mother from that Age. In the wake of this torrential healing and clearing work, it was as if a massive dam blocking the energy of my past had been released, and massive amounts of energy suddenly poured into me. I was swept into a journey through my past-lives by this wave, using the momentum of trust, acceptance, and forgiveness that I had built up in the healing process to clear *Sanskaras*[3] and karmic entanglements in a series of eight lifetimes following the Age of Atlantis. Each of the major clearings were related in subtle ways to the original wound I had retained from Atlantis with my parents, and many of them were also related to Rastara, whom I had been traveling with through all of these lives on Earth.

The roles often shifted, but as each of these clearings of past-lifetimes were completed, the many lessons and opportunities my Soul partner Rastara and I had given each other became more and more illuminated. It was as though I was undergoing some kind of unlocking sequence within my being, reconnecting points in time and experience and memory to find...more...of myself.

Finally, when I came into the present lifetime again in my consciousness, I found her fully present with me, nearly visible in her dream body. Although she was a thousand miles away, she was very much aware of me, and what we had just processed with each other, while Dreaming. In my physical form, out in the middle of the desert in the middle of the night, I began to run with her. Running with me in her dream, we finally slowed and came to a stop where a spectral rainbow leapt from the surface of the desert, contained in some kind of cylinder. In front of it

---

[3] Indian Philosophy: mental impressions, recollections, or psychological imprints, often seen as binding energy vortices.

was a simple glowing white triangle, seemingly floating above the ground, representing a prism. I knelt, put my head into the triangle intuitively, and suddenly found myself, and her, transported to another place entirely…

I sat down, and was aware of a smooth floor with inlaid metal geometries. She sat down directly across from me, under a dome ceiling through which the stars could be seen.

Immediately recognizing this place, it also began to dawn on me what we were doing. There were two vertical pillars of light floating between us, with each color in the spectrum highlighted in a certain position along the pillar, much like a spectrometer reading from a star or chemical. I knew that one of these pillars represented her energy body, and the other was mine, with the exact frequency of each of our *chakras* being displayed as a color line in the pillars. We were weaving these two pillars together, pulling the colors from each of the pillars into an energy form in the center that looked very much like DNA. I knew that we were creating a Soul-Bond, and that we were doing this so that we could leave our current physical bodies, and our Souls could travel to Gaia-Terra…Earth… This Soul-Bond would enable us to constantly feel an attraction to each other, so that we could find each other wherever we incarnated on this new planet, and help to trigger each other's memories of who we were before we made the interplanetary journey.

As my awareness bridged back to the present, sitting on the Desert floor, I also knew in that moment that this was our opportunity to unweave this Bond, and complete the circle we had traversed for over 13,000 years. Immediately, and in perfect sync, we began to unweave the fields again, bringing all the information in the DNA light-pillar back into our independent chakric pillars. It was completed quickly, with her and I working in perfect union, and as soon as it was done, we chanted to each other to finish bringing the magic into the present. "I Free You... I Free You... I Free You..." We called out each other's names across lives with the chant of freedom, knowing that this was the final gift we had been working for so long to give each other.

Then, in an instant, it was done, and a blinding flash of energy surged through my whole body, roaring with images of being a priestess, geisha, bellydancer, princess, wisdom, queen, medicine woman, and more. I felt as though the entire archetype of Woman poured through me in a split second, and I knew that this was a gift of having shared so many lives with each other, each of us holding only one polarity of male or female bodies through all of these time periods. I had been a male as long as I had been on Earth, so to suddenly be filled with this deep feminine awareness and memory was both startling and exhilarating. As her dream body responded to the massive energy influx in masculine form, I knew she was going to wake up, and said farewell, feeling a surge of love and respect for this incredible Soul that I had made this long journey with. A moment later, she was gone, and I found myself standing in the middle of the desert in the middle of the night, more complete as a Soul and Being than I had ever felt...ever.

In that moment, I also knew why I had made the journey to Earth. I had come as part of a family of Souls who were dedicated to helping the human population make its transition from being a Planetary species to a Galactic species. Even though I didn't know all the names and details at the time, so much information was immediately available to me in that moment, systematically filling in huge gaps of data in my memories of Atlantis...and of being from another world. I was Elven... Sirian...

It was suddenly obvious why all my memories of Atlantis and those of so many others in my Soul family are of an "Elven" race, as I had been of this species, nearly exactly as J.R.R. Tolkien describes them, as I'll discuss later. I had always known that my body-type in Atlantis had also been similar to that of the elegant Elves described in *The Silmarillion*, *The Hobbit*, and *The Lord of the Rings*. So many of his descriptions of cities in the forest seemed overwhelmingly familiar to me, and to many of my friends. When the movies were released, witnessing the citadel of Rivendell, and the tree-top architecture of Lothlorien, would bring tears to my eyes.

Yet this deep recognition that I was not from this planet was only the beginning of my journey that night. I tell the full story in two episodes of *Interviews with E.D.* by Reuben Langdon on Gaia Television through Amazon Prime, and Gaia's Online Platform. I'll also retell the story in full in a later book in this series, but this is perhaps the most important context setting for your entire experience of this Series.

# PROLOGUE - PART 3
# EXTRATERRESTRIAL CONTACT

My journey into the desert led me to meeting an extraterrestrial being, in physical form. She wore shimmering velvet robes that fell all the way to the floor, and a cloak that fell open from the front of her shoulders, trimmed with symbols that glittered with a golden light. They looked like constellations, but many were more geometric and fluidly connected, like crop-circles. It was at that moment that I was struck by the appearance of her face. The cowl of her hood was pulled back to the crown of her head, and did not shadow her pale skin or the finely chiseled bone structure that was unlike any human face I had ever seen. In fact, it was clearly not human.

Beautiful, radiating composure and elegance, her deep eyes pierced through my body, emotions, and mind. Her cheekbones were high, and had subtle angular points along their edges. Her eyebrows arched intensely across her forehead, which had what appeared to be a subtle ridge of bone up the center. And instead of her eyebrow bone ending in the distinctive point that every human has just above and outside their eyes, her bone extended further back, slightly hollowing out the space and giving her eyes a mysterious beauty that was both elvish and other-worldly. I could not help but step closer to her, until we stood about five feet apart. Reaching that distance, I felt an almost magnetic force settle into place, as if our energy fields engaged with each other, and a doorway was suddenly open between our minds.

"I know who you are," she said into my mind. Yet, they were not words, but a strobe of images and memories as intense and visceral as if someone had just dropped me into a VR headset and full-body haptic suit.

::: ⧗ :::

I saw a massive egg-shaped meeting room with many layers and levels... Outside, I glimpsed a city that stretched forever, and three towers overlooking gardens and endless skyscrapers. I saw flashes from different locations, and then looking into the sky, I was suddenly walking along an arched steel hallway looking out huge windows at this city covered planet from very high orbit. I wore a symbol on the right side of my chest...three Stars... 5-6-7 connected. On my right, there she was, walking with me. She looked different, but it was definitely her.

::: ⧗ :::

Then I saw deep forests filled with floating lights and long stairways that wound up trees with trunks hundreds of feet wide. Endless days and groves of night, elves dancing in the twinkles of golden light spilling upon the edges of fields. Purple mountains and towers like spears of white light shining up into the sky. Arched silver architecture woven into ice and mountains in the darkest area of the polar region, with starships coming and going, guided by telepathic interplanetary navigators. A moment standing in a beautiful garden, and there she was, smiling at me with a friendly smirk, in another body.

::: ⧗ :::

Next, a city of light, white stone, with gold and silver lacing running through its walls. Visions of the forests I had left, and the half-elven peoples who had come to this world. Gaia-Terra. I was wearing Purple robes and coordinating focused chanting in sacred geometry and sonic patterns, building intelligent crystal lattices and star-linked runes that could be used for communication between cities across the Atlantian civilization. As I stood

teaching on one of the high pavilions on this rocky
peninsula stretching out like a finger surrounded by
sapphire ocean and turquoise bays, she looked up at me
with young eager eyes.

I stood in the center of a stone circle, my arms vibrating as
I held up a sword, and light suddenly blinded me from
above, and reflected back at me in a thousand glints
around me off of swords and armor around me. I felt her,
acknowledging me from above. I walked the halls of a
massive castle set into a mountainside, looked out across a
beautiful lake, kissed beautiful priestesses, drank cups of
blood red wine and frothy honey mead, and celebrated
around a round-mirrored table.

As a child in this life, I looked up and saw a brilliant light
in the sky that hovered overhead for a moment, before
shooting over the horizon in a flash. Was she there too?
Then I had a flash of another triangular ship I saw with my
father and step-brother at nine years old. Then finally I
saw flashes of holding council with Indigenous Elders
from around the world, running the Prayer Run for World
Peace, holding Ceremony on the Summer Solstice, and
arriving at Burning Man and facing each and every trial so
that I might stand here in this moment full of Trust and
Truth.

The streaming memories of the past and present
converged in a flash. I'd seen it all in an instant, but each of
the moments stretched out in my mind and I could feel

their depth, importance, and connection to her words. She did know who I was...who I am.

Perhaps she knew me better than I did... Were these advanced extraterrestrial beings capable of accessing Akashic Memory, and did they have the capability of storing and recovering records of actual events into the distant past? In any case, her nonchalant way of showing me many lifetimes in a few seconds was...impressive.

At that moment, a couple guys wearing chainsaw hats, who looked like they had just jumped out of the back of a pickup truck in the mountains of western North Carolina, walked up to an art piece next to her. One of them glanced at her, saying "Whoa man, this shit is crazy." They both looked like they were drunk, while also on some form of psychedelics. They got lost in the art piece's lights, and the Extraterrestrial Ambassador glanced at them before looking at me seriously.

"Not all of you are ready," she then said into my mind.

The cascade of images led me on a journey from a young man in the mountains being beaten by his father, to escaping his fate as a farmer and the FFA through juvenile violence, then having his head shaved as he was forced into the military. From listening to sad country and shooting shotguns to losing himself in heavy metal while firing machine guns, I saw him come to accept his fate and anger as a harbinger of death, driving a tank and killing on sight somewhere in the Middle East. The flashes of images reminded me of *"The Fifth Element"* movie, when Leeloo is studying human history and looks up the word "War."

As painful as this was to see, I felt full understanding and acknowledgement. Yet I also understood the journey of this man in the images all too well. In fact, the two guys with chainsaw hats were a perfect representation, just like so many of the guys I grew up with in High School. Thanks to a few years of "redneck keg parties," I understood exactly where this human shadow originates from: trauma, loss of sovereignty, and loss of sense of purpose...all resulting in the overcompensation of the ego through domination, competition, and destruction. When abuse is combined with complete lack of freedom of choice, a nice kid can end up fighting his way out of his family's cages through any means necessary. If those wounds aren't healed, the pattern of trauma and violence is repeated over and over again, leaving one feeling the shame and guilt of believing one is evil, and experiencing total worthlessness.

When we lose our sense of worth within, we constantly attempt to prove it through external means. When there is no judgement but failure, regardless of our choice, the battle that rages inside is even greater than all the violence inflicted on others.

Yet in that moment I was so thankful for those two guys in flannels, trucker hats, and cheap gas station t-shirts. They *anchored* my reality, a constant reminder that I was not having some sort of hallucination. She was real, and we were having this conversation.

I felt huge gratitude for the guys, and for all the things I'd learned in my life about trauma, and its potential for healing. I also thought about all the people I knew who were more than ready for a new world to come...for Galactic Contact... People who were ready for whatever this woman from the stars was referring to... I consciously sent all that appreciation and acknowledgment to her, with the words, "Yes, but enough of us are."

Her serious face melted into a soft smile, her eyes twinkling. "Thank you for honoring your people," she said to me, and it felt like a wave of love cascaded into every cell of my body. It was...overwhelmingly powerful.

In that moment, I knew it was some kind of test. She wanted to know if I truly accepted humanity for their current state of being, challenges and horrors included. Thank God for those mountain men...because of them I passed with flying colors.

So much love was moving inside me, I bowed deeply to her, my body gushing gratitude for the opportunity to have all my doubts about extraterrestrials laid to rest. I took a deep breath in that bow, my eyes closing for only a moment as I felt a tremendous sense of peace and completion settling on my shoulders.

When I came up from my bow, she was gone. Just...gone.

The two guys were still there, and one of them glanced up in her direction, then looked startled. Whew. Shared reality. Good.

I couldn't help myself from looking for her, but the first light of the desert morning was in the sky as I exited what I would come to call the Stargate Temple in the middle of the deep playa, and she was nowhere to be found. Yet again, this was far from the end of my journey. It was the beginning of a path that would change my life forever.

My feet began to run beneath me, and I flew across the open desert towards the 2:00 line of Black Rock City in the distance. A sound began to grow inside and around me, a low bass tone vibrating my legs beginning to rise up into my loins and belly, growing higher pitched and louder moment by moment. The energy field around me began to spin faster and faster, and suddenly I felt a Merkaba forming around me, twin tetrahedral vortices counter-rotating around my body, matching the frequency of the sound as it continued ascending higher, and higher.

As the tone entered my head and neared my crown, it became piercingly high, then just as it crossed beyond hearing (and somehow thinking) range, I felt as though my entire body became light as a feather, and I was running effortlessly…or flying…or something…

A light exploded in the city directly ahead of me, and my voice shouted "ONE!" Then, my body was turning, and I was angling towards Center Camp far in the distance beyond the Temple and the smoke clouds of the Burned-down Man.

Another light exploded: "TWO!" Then another light near Center Camp, "THREE!" Then another light near 8:00 on the city, "FOUR!" Then another light at the edge of the city on 10:00, "FIVE." I was circling back the way I came, shooting across the desert floor like a meteorite, and then I was pointed directly at the StarGate Temple I had run so far from already. The light on top of the conic structure flashed, and my voice shouted, "SIX!"

I spiraled inward from there, curling in a circle tighter and tighter until I found myself looking upward and spinning on my feet shouting "SEVEN!"

Everything shifted and I was hurtling through an energy tunnel curving between star systems, a wormhole stretching my consciousness across the Galaxy, until suddenly everything became still, and I was in what seemed like a massive endless void at first. Yet the black space was not empty, it was full of brilliant star points… Not like the night sky, but still significant in number and large… *Seventy-three present*, my mind said.

As I put my attention on each of those star points, a vision of one or more beings would come into view. Each of the stars was a different species, with so many different qualities and variations. Many of them were humanoid, and some of them were not. I could spend an entire book just describing all the qualities of the beings I saw in that moment, and the experience in Galactic Council which unfolded afterwards.

However, for now, I will simply explain that I ended up bilocating into an Astral Galactic Council Chamber, and meeting Ambassadors of 73 different species from across the Galaxy. It's generally tough for anyone to read a sentence like that and not balk... Indeed, my experiences that night took me years to integrate enough to have the courage to tell the whole truth about my journey. For now, if laying such direct personal truth from my life experience on the table gives you pause, I'd like to ask you to simply consider my story as a data point, one piece of information that will either be validated by my work in this series and through your own direct experiences, or remain an unproven theory. Whether it holds value is ultimately up to you.

As a scientist and philosopher, I believe that it is critically important for us to ask questions, investigate our experiences, and study data points. We live in a time where people postulate fairly wild theories in reaction to the amount of lies and distortions that have dominated our modern media narrative. Some people feel so confused and uncertain about the state of the world, that they don't even trust that we know the shape of our own planet. Many have been confused by all the tales of lost civilizations like Atlantis, and without any training in engineering or architecture, assume buildings built in the 1800s were remnants of an advanced civilization that somehow was kept out of all of our history.

All people seek to understand what's really going on in the world, to have their own little "crack in the Matrix" to see through to the deeper reality. Some people might think this book series is my "crack," or maybe a fantastic hallucination mixed with science fiction. If I had not had these kinds of experiences over two and a half decades, and did not know hundreds of people who shared past-life memories with me, I would probably think that too.

So, knowing the conundrum the reader faces in embarking on this epic adventure that may stretch their beliefs, challenge their assumptions, and potentially provide counterpoints to other stories, I offer an open-hearted invitation. Embark upon this journey with me, and I will prepare you with some logic, tools, and practical approaches to find the truth for yourself.

In fact, that is the only way Truth is ever really found.

# PROLOGUE - PART 4
# SWORD & CHALICE

In the following chapters, we will explore the science and philosophy of Time and Memory. Yet there are a few more glimpses of moments to share here, as my experience of Galactic Contact was really a formative transition where integrating my ancient galactic past, lifetimes on Earth, and present life became the foundation for my personal spiritual journey. Within these memories lie keys of the codex of consciousness I have developed along my Travels, and each of the stories of my lifetimes will pass these keys to you, the reader, the Adventurer.

The glimpses I'd had of moments shared with the Ambassadors of the Galactic Council in the desert were emblazoned in my memory with a clarity that resounded through my head. Whenever I turned my attention to those flashes, I would see more of the moments around them, gathering a series of memorable events. I began to be able to stitch together some of these threads, often with the help of Soul Family showing up in just the right moments. One lifetime in particular didn't require my inner attention, as it pounded its way forth into my full awareness by a cascade of life events.

Standing in that stone circle...light from above...Sword ringing in my hands piercing the sky...

Life has a way of calling us forth towards our destiny, and before the Summer Solstice of the following year I found myself driving across the country in a dark blue hybrid Honda Civic that belonged to my Soul Brother Orellana, with an amazing young woman I had just met named Juniper. We were headed to Vancouver, British Columbia, to join in on my second Prayer Run for World Peace, where we would run with a group of indigenous youth of various tribes (mostly Lakota from Pine Ridge and Rosebud) all the way to Eklutna, Alaska. I'll tell that story in full another time...

Juniper was a young indigenous woman of Gaia's own heart, and she felt like a creature of the deep forest and swamps, but from the Pueblo Acoma lineage in the high deserts of New Mexico. She was already trained in Midwifery, with skills as Herbalist, Healer, and Medicine Keeper. She was a powerhouse Earth wielder and intuitive oracle, often wearing a moonstone on her forehead, dark hair pulled back and shoulders covered in Central and South American weaves and ponchos. Her adventures had taken her to Peru, and she held wisdom of Lake Titicaca and had her own experiences of Galactic Contact.

We had powerful life-changing events happen in every place we stopped along the way, from a weave with her beautiful friend Raven in Albuquerque to Galactic Adventures in Chaco Canyon, to synchronicities and connections with Soul Family in Phoenix, Venice Beach, and finally the great city of San Francisco and the Bay Area, what I would eventually come to call the "hub of the Rebel Alliance."

And so we found ourselves on a very interesting journey with an Asian Geisha, amplifying our awareness with Psilocybin. After navigating some Japanese karmic threads, we ended up in the city's great forested heart, the Golden Gate Park, alone in the trees and moonlight.

I brought my finest sword, once gifted to me by Rastara: a Carolingian Viking Longsword with leather scabbard bound in bands of steel. The blade's temper lines were visible, its lenticular blade smoothly hardened with a concave channel running down the center on each side. The sword just wanted to flow tonight, snaking through the soft breeze in arcs that set off flashes of moonlight in the dark, my feet just following along in the dance that followed the spinning blade.

Finally, after she had clearly been making some offerings and doing some witchy arcana to protect our space and create a palpable energy circle around our area, she came up to me, stretching out a hand. "Diki," she would say often for various purposes. In this moment, her desire for the sword was obvious, so I flipped around the blade and handed her the grip, keeping the scabbard.

She took it in hand and moved it around a bit, letting it bite towards me like a snake. I smiled at her, and said, "Let yourself feel the weight, and how it wants to move. Like this." I held the scabbard in my right hand, pointing straight up, as though I held the sword. I let it swing down and forward, then spin up behind me back to upward.

Mirroring me, Juniper let the sword fall and tried to relax her wrist enough to let it swing back up in a circle as I had done. She didn't quite get it, but gave an approving "mmm" and I knew she was onto my tip. She swung it again and again, and finally her eyes were bright and sharp and she started to actually look dangerous. As she began to move it around her in more of a dance, she let the sword lead more, and found herself nearly squealing in glee as she got deeper into the flow. She was remembering…

Suddenly, she brought the sword straight up in front of her with one hand, her other palm pressed against the blade. She walked towards me slowly and deliberately, her eyes deep and serious.

"I want you to Knight me."

She held out the sword to me like a sacred offering, as though she had passed a blade like this a thousand times.

I took the sword, and trusted that I knew exactly how to Knight someone… "Kneel," I said. She got on her knees on the Earth, placing two palms down in gratitude for the grass, then looked up at me and held her body as erect as a stone pillar.

"By the Sacred Power of The Goddess," I tapped her left shoulder with the blade.
"By the Infinite Wisdom of The God," I tapped her right shoulder.
"By the Divine Will within Me," I raised the Sword in front of my body.
"I Bless and Consecrate Thee by the Transformation of Fire," sword to her right shoulder.
"By the Healing Powers of Water," sword to left shoulder.
"By the Life-Giving Breath of Air," right shoulder.
"By the Loving Wisdom of Earth," left shoulder.
"By the Sacred Spirit within All Beings," I raised the sword high for the forest to see.
"I acknowledge the Divine Will within You," and touched sword to her right shoulder, letting it rest there as I could feel a massive channel of energy growing through me and the sword.
"Will you Dedicate your Life in Service to All Life?" I asked?

"I Will," she said with a soft inner strength.

"Will you Guard and Protect those who cannot protect themselves?"

"I Will," she said, resolve and intensity growing in her voice.

"Will you Stand for the Truth, for Love, and for Peace, in All Ways?"

"I Will, Always." Her eyes were shining.

"Then rise, and Stand for your Self, and fulfill your Great Purpose, Lady Juniper." I raised the sword high again.

Juniper stood, and I lowered the blade to hold it across my two hands, outstretched in offering to her, a warm smile on my face and my body literally glowing with chi. Everything felt like it was tingling, and the whole area seemed so much brighter. The park's lamps seemed more golden, the shadows of the leaves of trees more vivid.

"I knew it. It was YOU who held that sword. Ha," she barked, looking at me with narrowed eyes, and taking the sword from me. She held it in one hand, tapping the blade on her other palm. "Diki diki. Hmph. Want to know how I know?" A deeper twinkle now lit up her gaze, as she asked me playfully. I just waited for her response, the tingles in my body now becoming waves of vibration.

"It's because I'm the one who gave that sword back to you," Juniper said with a grin. "Diki-diki!" At that moment I had no doubt what she meant. The whole area seemed to warp and shift with her words. She suddenly looked like she walked out of a lake covered in seaweed and algae, carrying a box that shone in the moonlight where the sword. We still stood in the Golden Gate Park of San Francisco, deep in the trees late at night, but the field was reverberating through time, and she was no longer Juniper...

We were in shallow waters at the edge of a beautiful lake under the full moonlight. I knelt in the water as she strode towards me like a creature from the deep, eyes burning with a fire of intensity that seared into my Soul.

"The Dragon has Spoken…Haaaashsaaaaa…" she hissed, the kelp on her body enforcing the intensity of her words, an ancient priestess from another Realm dressed only in the living tattered drapes of the waters… "The Sword once Lost is Found Again…"

Murmurs arose behind me, but her words were so powerful they commanded my attention. And something began to happen to my body… The water was cold, but I was not shivering from the lake. My whole body began to vibrate in rhythmic waves, speeding up with my breaths inward, and purring through my entire frame with each breath out. My skin became alive with electricity, tingling threatening to consume my head as it grew in every direction like roots extending from my spine.

She was almost to me when two priestesses waded into the water to flank me on either side. They had weapons at their waists, but there was an air of confidence and trust that overtook the wariness in their eyes as they watched me carefully.

The case opened and the vibration in my body got stronger. She held out the case and I took in the glorious Sword before me.

The blade had the long wide expanse of an ancient Celtic Broadsword, but thinner and lighter, comparable to the length of an East Anglian Longsword. Its crossbar guard held a central disc that was emblazoned with the metal design of a Dragon, while the bars themselves extended into small points and branches like tongues of fire, some of the finest metalwork I had ever seen.

The sword grip was an elegant design of something that looked like white leather, bound by thin strips of gold. The pommel held the design of the Triscalion, the divine feminine Trinity. The sword was said to be ancient, but it looked as though it was forged this morning.

But no, I remembered the morning when it was completed…

::: ⧖ :::

Sunrise poured through the large arched window, the white stone walls and floor gleaming in the morning light. The colors were spectacular, as our little Sister Sun was also setting out the windows on the other side, dipping between the mountains and painting them in spectral fireworks. Yet even with the stunning natural beauty of this world and its twin suns, nothing quite outshone the Sword on the black stone table. It emanated energy, subtle ripples of light visible against the onyx surface.

"It will bond with you, to ensure the Spells we have cast upon it together are maintained through your journey to Gaia-Terra." My dear old friend, and master smith, gazed into my eyes with a subtle sadness. "I only wish I was going with you." His pointed ears twitched once, and his face relaxed into a smile.

Smiling back at him, I looked down at the sword and reached out my right hand, moving to take it by the grip up near the hilt…

::: ⧖ :::

I reached out my right hand, looking up into the eyes of the Lady in the lake, and my hand made contact with the sword grip… Immediately my whole body lit up even more, the vibrations spreading even more intensely across my face, my eyes, my lips…everything… I almost couldn't see straight anymore as it seemed my vision was vibrating, but I pressed on and closed my hand around the grip to take the Sword fully in hand.

As my hand closed around it, the muscles in my arm contracted, seemingly frozen and locked in place, waves of the ever present vibration now feeling like a vise around my right arm.

Ah, I remember this initiation…

My whole body relaxed into my breath, and my energy expanded from my body outward in swirls, picking up the sand and moving the desert in a vortex around me… I let myself become the spinning wind, surrendering all resistance into a state of communion and trust. The middle pyramid dais was just ahead up the temple path, and people were clearing the way for my duststorm…

I let myself become one with the desert, my steps carried on the winds and my breath spinning them around me, earth and air, stirred from the fusion of fire and water within. The Great Pyramid loomed to my right, and I felt as though it was dancing with me, amplifying the flow of energy in and around me…

And some part of me surrendered even deeper, feeling as though I was coming home…

…I surrendered to the Sword…then I surrendered to Everything. I relaxed every muscle in a deep breath that rolled through my body. The frequency of the vibration raised even higher, but became more fine at the same time. I slowly rose to standing, my knee coming out of the water that now felt like it was an extension of my body around me, and the sword moved with me. It turned to vertical as I rose to a balanced stance, and I reached down deep into the Earth to ground me as the electrical charge threatened to explode from my cells.

I let the top of my head extend upwards, and I felt a rushing tingle like the stars were now pouring into the crown of my head. A wave of energy began pulsing up from my roots, the response from the Great Mother from my call, and I felt it roar up through my loins, up into my belly, through my lungs and what felt like energetic wings out my back, through my arms and hands, into the sword and into my head at the same time.

As the energy moved up, the frequency moved with it, and at the moment it merged with the Heavenly Light above, it became Infinite, and everything came into perfect clarity and stillness.

I held the Sword of Light of Nuada, the Great Caliburn, the Blade of Integrity, the Sword from the Eye of the Mighty Wolf of the Heavens, Treasure of the Tuatha De Danann.

"Once yours, so it is Again, Keeper of the Treasure." The Lady in the lake said, her voice becoming like a song. "And so it is time, we go to the Circle of Stones." And so we would rise from the waters, leaving wet robes behind on rooms along the pathway up the cliffs, gathering armor and sacred tools, and awakening all those who had camped on the plateau above the cliffs, and took the path to the great Circle of Stones...

:::

I rose from my knees again, at the center of the great Circle, surrounded by knights in gleaming armor and priestesses in shining white. The light of the moon was still bright, though it cast considerable shadows from the stones by this late hour. It had taken long for all to be called from their beds and prepare in full regalia for this moment under the stars.

I'd never asked for this, nor did I want it most days. But what I wanted wasn't as important as what these people needed. They were my friends, my family, my beloveds. I would do anything for them, and since I could wield Caliburn…they would follow me to the end.

With a deep breath, eyes stinging from tears and body aching from the immense efforts of the initiations on this night, I raised the Sword to the sky.

Light suddenly beamed down from directly above, as though a new Star had just bloomed directly above our circle. The rays hit all the gleaming armor of the knights encircling me, and nearly blinded me as I was immersed in the light.

The total stillness I felt holding the Sword suddenly melted into the torrent of fire and water that was a hurricane inside of me, and I felt my body ringing with the stones, with the Sword, and with the waves of sound that now bathed us all in a multi-harmonic resonance. I felt the bass vibrations matching the rumble in my cells, sounds harmonizing with my heart, high notes shining inside my head, and I felt more alive than I had ever felt in my life.

I didn't need them all to accept me. I didn't need to be perfect. I just needed to Trust My Self. To surrender to just being my Self.

The sudden roar around me of cheers of joy and ecstasy came as a shock, but it just rolled into  and through me along with all the other waves, magnifying and growing into my own voice, as I threw back my head and roared with all my might into the sky… Like a Dragon…

And they chanted,
*"An Dragan...An Dragan...An Dragan..."*

::: ⌛ :::

That night with Juniper brought a lot up for me. Parts of me were getting stronger, while other parts felt like there was an even more imminent reconciliation coming. As the past was integrating, I could also feel great moments of pain and karma arising that I needed to face.

The journey to Alaska and back brought even more revelations, and so many more moments where I had to face the reality of my past-lifetimes. From clearing curses on the Sirian Elven family in Elfinstone British Columbia, to learning of the extraterrestrial roots in so many of the tribes at the World Peace Prayer Day Ceremonies in Alaska, to facing the karmic pains of Avalon as we found ourselves driving back to the Rainbow Gathering in Colorado after the Summer Solstice, to discovering deep and profound connections with Jessica at that gathering.

All these memories swirled like a fleet of Dragons in my heart, glittering scales mirroring experiences in this lifetime that were obviously connected to these moments in my past-lives. I felt overwhelming waves of intense emotions, and would cry my way through the grief around some of my visions. Yet other vibrations from my past integrated in more ecstatic ways, symphonies of love and reconnection as my life began to sweep me into a cascade of Soul Family reunions.

# PROLOGUE - PART 5
# SONGS OF THE DESERT

Visiting Mendocino in my journeys, I found the lady Jessica again, who I knew from moments in community in Asheville, and who was previously dating one of my dear friends Corey. In the first hour we spent together, we were visited by two Pleiadian beings, who were joyfully celebrating our reunion. As the night unfolded, I could feel massive waves of relief wash over me, as though we were reconciling Ages of missing each other and having lost each other quite a few times. In one of those times I remembered that night, I was making love to her in a stone room overlooking a fire-lit city in the desert...

Guards stormed into the room, and I nearly leapt away from her, scrambling off the bed naked. Shouting, they charged towards me with weapons drawn, and she screamed at them to stop. I turned and ran towards the window as fast as I could, my eyes glancing for a split moment at the beautiful girl, now a woman, who I had served my whole life. Love clutched at my heart, but my attention had to focus on this jump... Oh man, what had I done...?

With two strides I jumped straight out the open window and landed on a cloth overhang that was strung up on posts around an entry below. The wood cracked and the whole thing came with me, but this allowed me to ride its momentum and land on the streets at a run. I was naked, so I silently whispered prayers that some clothes would be hanging somewhere outside that I could grab.

I could hear the guards shouting down, and knew they would be hot on my tail. As I ran, my life spun through my mind: a flash of being whisked out of some grand building as a swaddled small child, glimpses of childhood serving her tea, traveling through the desert and camping at an oasis, hours of conversations by candlelight laughing and gazing at each other... Years of connection and love and friendship, now destroyed in one night.

The Gods were with me, as I pulled on a long robe and loose britches that were hanging just outside a window, only slightly cool and damp in the night air. They helped relieve my burning muscles, and a few streets later I found myself at the edge of open desert. Looking back, I could hear shouts in many different areas of the city behind me, and I knew there was only one way to go... Into the open desert.

I ended up moving to the San Francisco Bay Area not long after that, and shortly after began training in Theta Healing with my brother Dove. Our first classes were packed with Soul Family, some of whom I'd already dove in deep with and others I was just meeting for the first time, as though we were all called together to do this work in total synchronicity. In one session, we had a cascade of past-life healings come up around Egypt, and we found ourselves navigating painful reconciliations as a family.

It didn't take long for me to realize that these memories of a lifetime in Egypt directly intersected with the time in the desert I spent as Jessica's servant and protector. I had been taken away from my family, the family of Amenhotep III, as a child. His many children were under threat from rising militaristic forces, and in order to keep my identity secret, I was placed as the servant of a young high-born female being raised as a Great Royal Wife to bear children for the Pharaoh. My name was Ay...

I'll tell these stories in full later, but these experiences and my memories with the Sword of Light pushed me further into reconciliation, sorting out archetypal information from the direct visceral memories in order to face my karma and Sanskaras directly, and discover so many more details about my journey across lifetimes. I wanted to know who I was, the truth of it all, without the noise created by collective impressions, media, and even historical distortions caused by ethnocentric colonizers or religious evangelists.

The work I have done to pierce cultural bias, cross-reference memories with archeological evidence, complete transpersonal studies with the direct memories of others, and stitch together my own personal memories and experiences is the purpose of these Tomes.

As my memories of the past became clearer, more sequenced and defined, so did the weight of their implications. What did it really mean, to my life now, that I was a being from other worlds who had traversed this planet through so many intense times, some historical, and others lost to mythology? Why had my life become a tapestry that wove in memories from other times? Why was it that so many of my closest beloveds were having experiences like these, and yet I rarely heard stories like these from the masses? Perhaps most importantly, why was this journey of self-discovery both tremendously empowering, and horrifyingly painful? Would I ever be free from all these past karmas and times of pain? And what did being free from all that really mean? After all, there was so much beauty in all of it too…

Enlightenment is not a simple linear journey that only exists in its destination… Enlightenment is the journey itself, a multifaceted fractal path of Self Discovery that continuously challenges us to love, let go, and integrate all that we are.

# INTRODUCTION

# Introduction - Part i
# The Science of Past-Lives

Most people have had those eerie and seemingly unexplainable moments of *deja vu*, or the sensation of knowing someone for a long time, even when they just met. Yet, while these kinds of experiences are extremely common, the tendency in modern Western civilization is to simply assume that these moments are just fragments of random coincidence, a trick of the mind making meaning where none exists.

For millennia, the concept of past lives has captivated human imagination around the world, sparking endless debates between skeptics and believers. However, in cultures like Tibetan Buddhism, reincarnation is a staple for their entire societal structure, where the Dalai Lama is found through his ability as a child to recognize favored objects from his former life. This is also true for Tibetan Thangkha Master Arniko, who was identified in this lifetime as Romio Shrestha. Over the many years that I personally worked with Romio, his quirky personality and playful spirituality were the only things that could match his deep inherent wisdom.

Still, without the approval of modern scientific academia, these ideas are often discussed from the standpoint of sociocultural fascination with legacy belief systems, rather than addressed with serious inquiry.

That is all changing.

For the skeptical western mind, there is now considerable scientific research showing that reincarnation and past lives are far more likely to be fact, than fiction.

Dr. Ian Stevenson is a pioneering researcher whose three decades of meticulous investigation into past-life claims have shaken the foundations of our understanding of life, death, and consciousness. His work doesn't just entertain the possibility of reincarnation—it presents compelling evidence that challenges the very core of modern biological thinking.

At the heart of Stevenson's research lies a startling discovery: individuals claiming to remember past lives often bear birthmarks or birth defects that correspond to fatal wounds on the deceased persons whose lives they recall. This finding opens Pandora's box of questions that have long puzzled scientists and philosophers alike.

- Why are some children born with specific birth defects rather than others?
- What explains the inexplicable phobias that manifest in early infancy, absent any traumatic experiences or familial influences?
- How can we account for stark differences between identical twins who share the same genetic makeup?
- What drives the early emergence of gender-nonconforming behavior in some children, long before societal influences could take hold?

Stevenson's work offers tantalizing answers to these questions, suggesting a continuity of consciousness that transcends the boundaries of a single lifetime. As a respected scientist and Western medical professional, Stevenson approaches his subject with rigorous methodology and a healthy dose of skepticism.

Aware of the controversial nature of his findings, Stevenson has taken the bold step of publishing his entire corpus of cases. His evidence includes detailed photographs of birthmarks and illustrations of weapons, creating a compelling tapestry of data that demands serious consideration.

This groundbreaking research doesn't just challenge our current biological paradigms—it forces us to reconsider the very nature of human consciousness and identity. It beckons us to explore the possibility that our physical forms may carry imprints of past experiences, bridging the gap between lives in ways we're only beginning to understand.

As we stand on the precipice of potentially rewriting our understanding of life and death, Stevenson's work serves as a beacon, illuminating a path forward in our quest to solve one of humanity's greatest mysteries. Whether you're a physician, psychiatrist, biologist, anthropologist, or simply a curious mind grappling with the enigma of existence, this research offers a thrilling journey into the unknown—and perhaps a glimpse into the true nature of our eternal selves.

Imagine a toddler, barely past his second birthday, suddenly plagued by nightmares so vivid and terrifying that they shake the very foundations of reality. This is the story of James Leininger, a young boy whose nocturnal terrors would lead his family on an incredible journey through time, challenging everything they thought they knew about life, death, and the persistence of the human soul.

It began with blood-curdling screams in the dead of night. "Plane on fire! Little man can't get out!" These weren't the typical monsters-under-the-bed fears of a child. James Leininger was reliving something far more harrowing—something that, by all rational explanations, he should have had no knowledge of.

As days turned into weeks, and weeks into months, James' parents, Bruce and Andrea Leininger, found themselves facing a reality they could no longer ignore. Their son, barely old enough to form complete sentences, was recounting vivid details of planes, war, and tragedy — information that no toddler should possess. But this wasn't just a child's fantastical imagination running wild. The specificity and consistency of James' recollections pointed to something far more extraordinary.

What followed was a relentless quest for answers that deeply challenged the Leiningers' personal beliefs. As they pieced together the fragments of James' memories, a startling picture began to emerge: their young son appeared to be reliving the past life of James Huston, a World War II fighter pilot who had died decades before James Leininger was born.

The book "Soul Survivor" chronicles this family's extraordinary journey, taking readers on a gripping ride through skepticism, disbelief, and ultimately, acceptance. As James' father Bruce Leininger dug deeper, uncovering details of James Huston's life and death that would captivate military historians, he found himself on a collision course with his own belief system, rooted in Christianity, which generally does not account for past-lifetimes… However, it is worth mentioning that most Christians await the "return of Jesus Christ," which might subtly suggest that reincarnation has been a hidden part of Christian beliefs all along.

In a world that often dismisses the inexplicable, James Leininger's story stands as a compelling challenge to the common Westernized understanding of reality. It forces us to consider the possibility that our existence isn't limited to a single lifetime — that perhaps, against all odds and rational explanation, the echoes of past lives can reverberate through time, finding voice in the most unlikely of vessels: an innocent child.

As the story of James Leininger captivated the public imagination, it also caught the attention of the scientific community. Enter Dr. Jim B. Tucker, a renowned psychiatrist at the University of Virginia's Division of Perceptual Studies. Dr. Tucker, following in the footsteps of the pioneering Dr. Ian Stevenson, has dedicated his career to the rigorous investigation of children's claims of past-life memories. In James Leininger, he found a case that would push the boundaries of his research and challenge our understanding of consciousness itself.

Dr. Tucker's involvement brought a new level of scientific scrutiny to James' extraordinary story. In his paper, "The Case of James Leininger: An American Case of the Reincarnation Type," Tucker meticulously documented and analyzed the young boy's claims, applying the same rigorous methodology that has made the University of Virginia's research on this subject respected worldwide.

What sets Tucker's investigation apart is its commitment to objectivity. Rather than seeking to prove or disprove reincarnation, Tucker's approach focuses on documenting the phenomena and exploring possible explanations. His research into James' case involved extensive interviews with the Leininger family, verification of historical details mentioned by James, analysis of James' behaviors and phobias, and comparison with other cases of children claiming past-life memories.

One of the most striking aspects of Tucker's findings was the sheer volume and accuracy of James' recollections. The young boy provided over 50 specific details about the life of James Huston, including:

- The name of the aircraft carrier he flew from (Natoma)
- The name of his fellow pilot (Jack Larsen)
- Specific details about the Corsair planes he flew

These details were later verified through historical records, adding weight to the inexplicable nature of James' knowledge.

Tucker's research also explored James' behaviors that seemed consistent with a pilot from the 1940s. The boy's nightmares, his preoccupation with airplanes, and even his manner of speech at times seemed to reflect the personality of a man who had lived decades before.

Perhaps most intriguing was Tucker's analysis of James' phobias. The young boy's intense fear of airplane crashes and his aversion to certain loud noises aligned eerily with the experiences of a World War II pilot, raising fascinating questions about the potential for trauma to transcend a single lifetime.

As a scientist, Tucker approaches these cases with a healthy skepticism. Yet, the depth and consistency of James' recollections, combined with the family's credibility and the verifiable nature of many claims, led Tucker to conclude that this case represents one of the most compelling in the annals of reincarnation research.

While cases like James Leininger's have captured attention in the Western world, the phenomenon of children claiming past-life memories is not limited to any single culture or region. Dr. Erlendur Haraldsson, a professor emeritus of psychology at the University of Iceland, has conducted extensive research on this subject in Lebanon, providing a valuable cross-cultural perspective on the phenomenon of past-life memories.

Dr. Haraldsson's work, published in various peer-reviewed journals and his book "Children Who Remember Previous Lives: A Question of Reincarnation," presents a compelling collection of cases that share striking similarities with those documented in other parts of the world, while also reflecting unique cultural aspects.

Key findings from Haraldsson's research paint a fascinating picture of past-life memories in Lebanese children. A striking feature of these cases is the prevalence of violent deaths in the remembered lives. Many children recalled past lives that ended abruptly and traumatically, often mirroring Lebanon's tumultuous history. This pattern aligns with observations from other cultures, hinting at a possible universal tendency for traumatic deaths to leave more lasting imprints on consciousness.

The age at which these memories surface and fade follows a consistent pattern. Lebanese children, much like their counterparts in other parts of the world, typically began speaking about past lives between the ages of 2 and 4. These vivid recollections often started to dim as the children approached 7 or 8 years old, gradually fading into the background of their developing personalities.

Perhaps most intriguing are the behavioral traits and phobias exhibited by these children. Many displayed preferences, skills, and fears that seemed jarringly consistent with their claimed past-life identities. Imagine a young child, barely old enough to hold a wrench, showing an uncanny interest in and aptitude for machinery, all while insisting they were once a mechanic in a previous life. Such cases challenge our understanding of how personalities and skills develop.

Adding another layer of complexity to these cases, Haraldsson observed instances where children bore birthmarks or birth defects that corresponded to wounds or injuries from their purported past lives. This physical evidence echoes the groundbreaking findings of researchers like Ian Stevenson, suggesting a possible link between physical and metaphysical realms that defies our current scientific understanding.

These key findings, woven together, create a tapestry of evidence that pushes the boundaries of our comprehension of consciousness, memory, and the very nature of human identity. While each element is fascinating in its own right, it's the consistent pattern across numerous cases that elevates Haraldsson's research from mere anecdote to a compelling body of evidence worthy of serious scientific inquiry.

One particularly striking case from Haraldsson's research is that of Nazih Al-Danaf. At a young age, Nazih began speaking about a previous life as a man named Fuad, who had been killed in a car accident. Nazih provided numerous specific details about Fuad's life, family, and death, many of which were later verified.

Nazih's case stands out as particularly compelling due to its multi-faceted nature. The child provided strikingly accurate and verifiable information about his purported past life, exhibited behaviors and personality traits recognizable to the deceased's family, and bore a prominent birthmark corresponding to the fatal injury from his previous life. This convergence of mental, behavioral, and physical evidence creates a powerful narrative that challenges conventional explanations and demands serious consideration.

Haraldsson's thorough investigation of this case, including interviews with multiple witnesses and examination of relevant documents, provides a robust example of the phenomenon in a non-Western context.

Haraldsson's Lebanese cases offer profound insights. They suggest past-life memories might be a universal human experience, transcending cultural boundaries. These cases challenge our understanding of consciousness, hinting at its potential persistence beyond death. Haraldsson's rigorous methodology underscores the importance of scientific approach in such investigations. Moreover, these findings may have therapeutic applications, potentially aiding in treating certain childhood phobias and behavioral issues linked to past-life traumas.

When viewed alongside research from other parts of the world, including the work of Tucker in the United States and Stevenson's global studies, Haraldsson's findings in Lebanon contribute to a growing body of evidence that demands serious scientific consideration.

As we continue to explore these frontiers of consciousness, these studies serve as beacons, illuminating the vast unknown territories of the human mind and spirit. They remind us that in the quest to understand our existence, there are many mysteries yet to unfold.

# INTRODUCTION - PART 2
# THE PHENOMENOLOGY OF TIME

On my journey of reunion with so many Souls, I found deep value in honoring the deepest singular Soul Stream moving through an individual from their oldest incarnations, through the weave of lifetimes, cultures, experiences and connections, and into the present moment. These sovereign experiential journeys that each of us embark upon is very special: only we individually can have the complete information of visceral sensory events, the entirety of emotion involved with them, and the full mental realization of the purpose of the event in its grand sequence. It is this combination of physical, emotional, and mental experiences that *define* us as individuals.

Many Spiritual Paths provide teachings that help us Transcend these experiences so that we may merge back into our Awareness of All that Is. This experience of the Divine through the Totality of the Infinite can be extraordinarily liberating. This driving move towards liberation is similar to the masculine polarity of relational behavior detailed through countless works of modern authors including Mantak Chia, Margo Anand, David Deida, Jane Lyle and many more. In this spiritual context, this force is often referred to as the Divine Masculine. Through this path of liberation, we come to understand that we are Divinity in its very essence...

The masculine force focuses everything it is into a single direction, a powerful phalanx of consciousness uniting each of its faculties into a unified front. This focused intention is a geometric lens, amplifying and directing energy in a particular directional vector. The practice of awakening the Divine Masculine happens through reorienting outward direction to the center of the Self. The Center is the place of no-direction, and thus from this void of course state, becomes the radiant emanating Star shining in All-Directions, Omnidirectional Emanation. The focus on this Nucleus of Self allows consciousness to enter the Singularity of Being, where one truly becomes the Experience of Oneness, the state of God Realization. Our identity is then the Infinite Eternal Source of All that Is, and we come to the great end result of all experiences: unlimited Love, Power, and Bliss. It is Done. And the Symphony of All is concluded.

Then Time moves. We return to some semblance of Self experiencing the Divine, having been in the Eternal Now and then reflecting on that moment in a new and insightful pattern of experience. We feel gravity. We have a body, separate and distinct from all the objects around us. We might feel pain, pleasure, joy, grief, or anything in the spectrum of feeling. Our feelings are more distinct, more separate. Our toes are separate, as well as our fingers, which are all separate from our faces with which we hear and see, taste and smell. We see others, and they are different from us. We see everything in its infinitely complex individuation. Separation is what we think we are experiencing, while in some reality we know everything is completely interconnected. Yet somehow, we trick ourselves into thinking that this individuated experience is somehow "less good" and "limited" compared to the ease of the God State…

Why do we slip back into the individual lens, if it is so limited? Why not just stay in the Infinite Eternal Bliss and as they say, *just chill* in Samadhi?

Having made this journey to the Eternal and back to the edge countless times in my life and along my Soul's trail through many incarnations, I remembered exactly why… I choose to *experience*. I choose to be in *relationship*. I choose to live and feel, succeed and fail, celebrate and die, and rise from the ashes. I choose to witness the glorious dance of individuated Souls swirling in the rainbow spectral laser light show of the Divine in the Many. Many ancient peoples would say that if GOD is the ONE, then GODDESS is the ALL, in various tongues covering vastly diverse legends and traditions. The Male and Female aspects of Divine expression across cultures share this deeply profound synergy.

So a Spiritual Path that focuses on the Returning, the Integration of experience from our Divine Avatar State to the wild and crazy adventure of human life on Earth, is best defined as a Goddess Path. To fall in love with One's True Self can lead to a taste of the sweetness of the Divine, yet to fall in Love with an Others is to experience the multi-orgasmic rapture of discovery, growth, healing, transformation, realization, evolution, and inevitably Bliss.

Just as the often ascetic path to Oneness through the Masculine Spiritual Path can be difficult, painful, and full of trials where we must extract ourselves from attachments and *Sanskaras*, the path of sensual integration to Divine Love through the Feminine Spiritual Path is also not always easy. As we engage in the study of Relationship like others study Holy Books, we realize the many ways we have hurt and damaged the fabric of our society, families, and cultures through intense traumas and judgements.

In an attempt to deal with these experiences, we attempt to control more of reality around us, including others. As one attempts to control other people, they either unconsciously practice manipulation of other people's energy, or worse, they do this with full conscious awareness of their actions. These actions are referred to by Barbara Ann Brennan, NASA Astrophysicist turned founder of a School of Energy Healing, as "control dramas," and involve four major archetypes of energetic behavior where one individual is attempting to take energy from another individual. In modern psychology, these exact same patterns are referred to in the archetypes of "Borderline Personality Disorder," or BPD. The NLP Marin psychology group commonly teaches "there are two types of people in this world: borderline people, and borderline borderline people." The term borderline in BPD generally means "close to or on the edge of psychotic behavior." It might not be surprising for you to realize that what they're suggesting is that *everyone* has some level of BPD. Consider this from your own experiences, either mild or extreme:

We experience a moment of such profound pain we have no idea how to process it. We do everything we can to numb the pain, we can't stop thinking about it, we feel like we're stuck in a vortex, trapped in a moment that won't leave us alone. Our energy lashes out to grab on, shield, defend, attack, or otherwise react to others in order to save ourselves from experiencing the pain of that trauma again. We judge anything that even remotely reminds us of the trauma. All of these reactions arise because we have not allowed ourself to fully feel and integrate the painful experience in the past. As we resent it, regret it, reject it, hate it, fear it, and eventually ignore it, we build an energetic shield inside our own beings, constricting and collapsing energy flow within a specific region of our bodies and auric field (the human energy field around the body, which we will explore in more depth throughout this journey through time). This shielding causes us to lose some of the current moving through our bodies, and it becomes a tangled vortex of frozen memories that the Hindu call a "*Sanskara.*"

As fortune would have it, all people have done this in many lifetimes. All people, because even the greatest Spiritual Teachers and Avatars tell tales of their journey of Divine Awakening, which always involves the liberation and transmutation of these unimaginably painful moments. Accepting that we all have Sanskaras is one of the first steps to true and continuous Liberation and Bliss. With this Wisdom in mind, we can now begin to understand the energy dynamics that drive our journey across lifetimes, and the Infinite yet archetypal expressions of our Relationships. After all, if the end result of existence is Infinite Love, Power, and Bliss, these Sanskaras must serve a profound purpose in our Awakening to the Truth.

In each lifetime, we go through huge experiences of pleasure and pain. Some of the more painful experiences are hard to process, so we reject our memory of them. The actual memory and information in the experience is stored in our Energy Bodies, and down through our Cells, our DNA, and even our Protons (see my paper and presentations on Protons as Universal Data Storage). So what we're actually doing is *ignoring* our memory, because even if our minds are not accessing it, the memories still exist within the energy of the fabric of spacetime, the matter in the location of our experience, and in our bodies.

When we reject memories in our Past, it becomes harder to see memories prior to that moment in time. It is my assessment that this is the reason why many people lose their past life recall, when they may have had it as young children. Often children talk about being other kinds of people, in other places, and even other worlds. As we grow up and go through intense experiences, we often lose touch with those memories within us, as they are shielded by our rejection of experiences in this life. However, if we can open ourselves back up to those intense experiences and unwind these shields, or Sanskaras, we suddenly allow the flow of information from our past to come back into our conscious awareness.

From my own work in doing this throughout my life, and into and across every one of my past lifetimes, I have come to the profound conclusion that Time is experienced as a flowing stream of energy moving into us. We are either building dams against that flow of energy, resisting and restricting its flow which will ultimately create a massive intense breakthrough, or we are consciously dismantling the dams and enabling sustainable and regenerative flow that steadily increases our memory and skills.

Most people have so many dams put up they cannot even reach the stream of their prior lives and memories, and those dams are often built during childhood in this life. Once some of those are cleared, other information begins coming in, and we either face the painful and glorious realizations they guide us towards, or we resist them further. Unfortunately our modern academic narrative does not account for this past-life information, so common education suggests this information is "not real" and thus probably should be ignored as imagination.

There are many powerful psychic individuals in the world who have been able to access full clairaudience, clairvision, claircognizance, etc, but who were told by frightened parents that the things they are hearing/seeing/knowing are "not real," and the parents fear influences the child into being terrified of their own insights and gifts. This framing creates an internal conflict for psychic children, and along with the pressures of the status quo in school and social circles, the psychic abilities (and often past-life memories already present in the child) begin to be isolated internally, and dams are built to keep the energy within this part of the psyche from flowing.

Fortunately, there are also many children who either grew up in a supportive household, or had a massive identity breakthrough later in life, and are able to start tapping into their time-stream and accessing their inherent gifts. From my perspective, every individual has an array of Divine Gifts, or what Vedic traditions refer to as Siddhis. As these gifts are uncovered and integrated, each person steps through a Portal of Passage, and begins to become the

Superhero Avatar that is actually their true nature. As Richard Rudd illustrates in the Gene Keys, this often requires deep work on our Shadow, facing the information and memory that is most difficult for us, and alchemizing it through practicing its Gifts, and eventually Mastering the Siddhi.

Wherever you currently are on the path of self-integration, it is important to deeply embrace, accept, and love yourself through each challenging moment of this life that you can invoke in memory. Each of these healing links open up energy that can flow from your prior life-times, and increase the amount of information that will begin flowing into your life from those prior incarnations.

This is not just a metaphysical postulation. My theories on the physics of time and entanglement reveal that this may simply reflect the nature of the Universe.

While the next section might be difficult for some readers, I invite you to explore it with the same courage as might need to gather in adventuring into a new area of discovery. I've written out these ideas with as many simple translations as possible, and by the time you get to the end, the Big Picture of life and the memory of our experiences will start to really make sense...

# Introduction - Part 3
# The Physics of Time & Entanglement

The Universe is full of energy, moving all together, spinning in the form of Protons at the heart of atomic nuclei, rotating in electrical fields we call Electrons around them, vibrating in molecular crystal matrices, forming all the matter we experience all around us...and in us. We are matter and energy which forms spinning Planets or the swirling evolution of Stars. Those Stars rotate around the Galaxy, which dances in rotations with other Galaxies in a living, spinning, dynamic Universe.

Yet what are Protons? Studies have shown that positively charged Protons have a half-life equal to approximately four-times the lifetime of our entire Universe... In other words, as far as we know, Protons NEVER decay, never break down, never stop spinning, and are the most sustainable objects in the entire Universe. They better be, because ALL mass, matter, and EVERY material object you can see is made of Protons.

Protons bond and spin together in the nuclei of atoms (what we used to think were the primary building blocks of matter as you learned in school). We say that around half the Protons in the nucleus of atoms are neutrons (with no charge), however as soon as a neutron is separated from an atomic nucleus it decays nearly instantaneously into a Proton. In my theory of nuclear physics and the Weak Force, there are no neutrons. There are simply Protons conserving charge through conserving spin; in other words, they spin together and share the energy. They also share influence on the surrounding field of spacetime, causing it to move in a whirlpool of electrical charge we call the "Electron field."

Particle accelerator experiments attempting to understand the Proton suggest that Protons are made of a trilogy of subatomic and "more fundamental" particles called quarks. However, when we smash two Protons together at near the speed of light and take pictures of the energy scattering in all directions, the three lines we attempt to identify as quarks dissolve in fractions of a second. This is based on the physics rule commonly called "color confinement" in the Standard Model of Quantum Mechanics, which declares that quarks (and gluons) cannot be isolated, and therefore can never be directly observed!

Stop and think about that for a second. Our most prominent physics theory has a major problem here. Their most "fundamental" so-called particles that make up protons can never actually be studied in isolation. Basically these bundles of energy are either in a Proton and totally stable (seemingly forever), or they simply dissolve back into the energy of spacetime.

There is a better solution than these flighty abstractions: the energy lines we call quarks are actually layers of the spinning spherical Proton "cake," where the top hemisphere, bottom hemisphere, and central equatorial regions all break apart during a near-light-speed collision as the primary energy "blobs" ejected from the Proton structure.

The Proton structure must follow the first principles of spacetime curvature to be as sustainable and long-lived as they are. If we simply consider the Proton to be a spherically curved region of spacetime, and thus contain a singularity like a miniature black hole (The Schwarzschild Proton - Haramein), we begin to understand why it is so powerful and special as a building block for the Universe.

If spacetime is a structural light-lattice (think of a geometric network at a scale much smaller than the smallest particles that forms the "fabric of spacetime" itself and everything in the Universe) as many quantum gravity theories and my own work have ascertained, then a Proton is a spherical form of that light lattice. While Haramein is correct in that spacetime is generally triangulated and tetrahedral in its lattice (which allows massive amounts of energy to be stable and apparently dormant within it), in order to identify the curvature structure that can enable a Proton we must look to Buckminster Fuller.

I extrapolated Fuller's ideas around the Geodesic Dome, and came to the conclusion that Protons are layered *geodesic* spherical lattices. They are also toroidal vortices in superfluid crystalline form, as the lattice itself is made of Planck-length bundles of light (PSUs - Haramein), and the entire structure is spinning. According to Haramein, the whole structure spins at the speed-of-light. However, I corrected this assessment through geometry and addressing the spherical structure of the Proton, identifying that it is only the equator at the event horizon (Proton boundary condition) that is moving at C (light-speed), and that the rest of the Proton MUST by nature of it's spherical form be moving at less than C.

This accomplishes two amazing feats:

1) Since the equator is spinning at the speed of light it *shears* spacetime, operating as if it has *zero* mass-energy effect on the surrounding spacetime. In other words, the Proton acts like a little "anti-gravity" spaceship, eradicating it's own mass-dilation and enabling it to be perceived as an extremely light object when its normal "black hole" mass would be gargantuan.

2) As torsion increases on the surrounding spacetime as the speed of the surface horizon of the Proton spins at

less than the speed of light moving slower towards the poles, greater electrical charge is built by the co-moving spacetime field being pulled. In simple terms, the Proton has a vortex on the top and bottom which is pulling the structure of spacetime around it, making two big whirlpools we call the "Electron field" locations. In more complex atoms, there are various spinning whirlpool fields that form different whirlpool shapes (see Electron Orbital Configurations).

In summary, the Proton is like a little spaceship made of a spherically curved light lattice which is pulling other light around it, and exchanging information through the fabric of spacetime itself. That fabric is literally the light-lattice, and according to the most recent ER/EPR theories (Wheeler), the entire thing is made of entangled wormhole networks. Yes, spacetime is not only a structural lattice of light, but also an information exchanging network of connected threads. It's a holographic network. And every single moment, the whole thing is growing as the Universe grows...

Every moment that passes, the Universe grows, and every Proton grows with it. A moment in time is like a freeze frame where the Universe has generated an infinitely complex lattice of light in every position throughout spacetime, which is then imprinted into every Proton throughout the Universe. As this happens, each Proton grows by one quantum oscillating node: "PSU" (or Planck Spherical Unit - Haramein), similar to a 1 or 0 bit in computing, but in the complex lattice of spacetime each is an intersection of up to twelve vectors interconnecting them to other PSU. You can visualize this by seeing six rays, one of each color of the rainbow (red, orange, yellow, green, blue, purple), along with six opposite rays representing the reverse of that color. Each ray can be in a state of input, output, or superposition, which is similar to quantum bits as modern science currently defines them. So each PSU essentially acts as a dodecahedral quantum byte, a holographic data storage unit... I'll coin it a "PSU Holobyte."

Just so you can understand just how magical the Universe actually is, and why it organizes so intelligently, I just ran the calculation for how many combinations each of these "PSU Holobytes" (as I'd like to call them) can produce, as this gives us a sense of their data storage power. Twelve rays interacting with twelve rays (12 x 12) gives us 144 combinations. Yet each of these combinations also has three states (144 x 3) which gives us 432 total combinations. Is it a coincidence then, that the Sun's equatorial diameter in miles is 432 x 2000, or that the Moon's orbital speed in km/day is 432 x 200, or that the Earth's circumference in nautical miles is 43200 / 2, or that the number of seconds in a day is 432 x 200!? And of course the big one: the number of seconds in the estimated age of the Universe is **4.32 x 10$^{17}$!!!**

As each moment of data is stored, that information is radiated out in every direction from each Proton geodesic, traveling through the quantum wormhole networks which compose the actual fabric of spacetime in its tetrahedral woven lattice. Haramein proposes that there are around 10^40 wormhole connections on the surface of every Proton, which is the number of quantum node oscillations on the surface or *event horizon* of the Proton. So each Proton is communicating data back and forth with as many as 10,000,000,000,000,000,000,000,000,000,000,000,000,000 other Protons instantaneously. If we consider that in the moment of a full body experience, each of our Protons would store memory and also propagate information to 10^40 other Protons, we must also consider that we have 10,000,000,000,000,000,000,000,000,000 Protons in our body. Together, that is 10^68 entangled Proton communications every Planck second, or 10^111 Proton communications per second, directly from the Protons inside our body to each other and out into the Universe!

## OUR BODY POTENTIALLY PRODUCES:

1,000,000,000,000,000,000,000,000,000,000,000,000,000,000
,000,000,000,000,000,000,000,000,000,000,000,000,000,
000,000,000,000,000,000,000,000,000,000,000

## ENTANGLED PROTON COMMUNICATIONS

## PER SECOND.

That number is far beyond comprehension for most of us, but as a note of comparison, it's estimated that there are 200,000,000,000,000,000,000,000 stars in the entire Universe, widely estimating approximately 100 billion stars in each of two trillion galaxies. For a couple other quick references, we have about 70,000,000,000,000 cells in our body. Even if our bodies simultaneously entangled every star in the Universe with every cell in our body, this would encompass less of our total energy than a single grain of sand in comparison to the Sun! So where is all this information radiating from us going?

When we have an experience, we are both encoding the memory of that experience within us, and propagating the energy of the experience into the Universe all around us. Since many of the Protons we entangle with are outside of our immediate physiological or vibratory energetic experience around us, and because this information can propagate faster than light due to entanglement, we must logically acknowledge that this entangled radiation is influencing our *future*. Wait what?

In order to truly understand how Time works throughout this book, it is essential to understand not only the Past, but the Future. Let's take a closer look at the Future, and then we will take a step back to integrate the bigger picture of Spacetime itself.

It is extremely likely that if you are reading this, at some amount of time in the future, you will eat food. This food already exists, its atoms are assembled and awaiting you in the fridge or pantry or restaurant cold storage. That location is somewhere outside of you, distant from your body. Even if that distance is not far, it still takes time for light to travel from that location to you, which means that there is spacetime fabric between you and that food. If you want to physically experience that food, you will likely have to travel to its location (or have it travel to you). This food is essentially in your *future*.

If the same food is also in your past at some point (you took a bite of something, have leftovers in the fridge, or ate part of a bag of chips), you may have already entangled with this food in a feedback loop, storing the memory or information of it inside you. Now, when you think of this food, some of your Protons which are already entangled with this food send a communication "ping" to the food again, often checking to verify its existence, flavor profile, or other ideas we have in relationship to it. After all, part of that food is inside you if you ate it. Even if you simply touched it, you probably exchanged Protons through atomic or molecular exchange on contact. This why we have such widespread and constant quantum entangled messaging with so much of the world around us, and it happens every time we think about anything we have experienced, because our brain signaling involves both complex Proton masses (neurons) and those neurological structures have electromagnetic (light) exchanges between them.

This doesn't mean that we are suddenly going to exchange a huge amount of information with that food, and this is particularly important because we also think about other people all the time. Just because you have a reference point of information entangled to someone else doesn't mean that when you ping them, they will be aware of that information exchange. Perhaps even more importantly, we also tend to craft our own mental holograms of individual people and things based upon various other people and things, so in our minds we're interacting with more of a collective Astral *chimera* rather than an actual individual person. However, when we share a strong and significant memory with someone, bringing a lot of attention and feeling to that memory may very well stimulate enough connection to spontaneously trigger the surfacing of that memory or information in another person, if they are open and receptive to that memory. Returning to our food example, we can certainly always magnify our current energetic and forthcoming physical experience of that food through appreciation and *anticipation*.

In addition, while we may have entanglement with something, this doesn't necessarily mean data is being exchanged through that entanglement all the time. Theoretically, a quantum wormhole network could have series of states between two points, and if our point of reference is one of those points, the entangled pathway could: transmit, receive, do both simultaneously, or be neutral. Think of a computer network like the internet; we access websites, store some data, and then if we don't interact with that website or browser tab, it could be said that we have an "open pipe" to that address with no data exchange. When we do something on the site, we transmit, then receive new data, and sometimes do both as we both download information while uploading commands, data, and more to the server we are interacting with.

If we extend this analogy, we can look at interactions on the internet similarly to how we interact with the structure of Spacetime.

We enter a website "environment," then we issue some command in order to achieve a desired action, such as "load a game." We send a signal out into the servers on the network to download data back to us, so we can run the game locally for speed and efficiency on our computer. We essentially *intend* to play, signaling a network extending from us, and returning the programs and data necessary to *experience* that game play. We are commanding that a future experience come into our present experience through intentionality.

Now we are playing the game on our computer, and as we go along, we're both uploading new information from our progress to the game server, and we may also be saving data to our local hard-drive memory. Data in our hard-drive is the actual information of *past* events, frozen moments in time saved in a specific binary pattern. In the Proton data storage in our bodies, the information is not stored in binary, but in a quantum oscillating wavelength of Planck length with potentially infinite amplitudes. Patterns of quantum data storage inside a Proton are also theoretically holographic, meaning that data is also stored across larger standing light wavelengths, a spectral rainbow network illuminating the very essence of a moment's memory.

Here's where things get really interesting:

What if our personal "hard-drive" of memory is actually networked through our DNA, and through all the matter we entangled with in our lifetime? Our DNA is not just the genetic code of our parents, and the data storage of our ancestry all the way back into the basic shared codices of all forms of life, but it also includes *environmentally* interactive codes that modern biology has yet to fully understand. It is believed that this code is critical to evolution and the new codes established each generation to pass to the next, but these areas of our DNA are often considered to be "non-coding regions." We also know that much of this DNA changes, and yet also is not necessarily *new*. There is a gargantuan amount of genetic code that doesn't specifically seem to have some function from our ancestral coding, but influences gene expression and may *evolve*, with some estimates suggesting 80% of our DNA falls in this area.

Dr. Sonia Contera, a physicist and professor of biological physics at the University of Oxford, has been quoted as saying, "98% of DNA is a mystery. We know only 2% is coding for proteins." This statement refers to the fact that the vast majority of our DNA, often referred to as non-coding DNA, does not contain the instructions for building proteins, and its function is still not well understood by scientists.

This suggests that we have genetic data that is maternal (from the mother), paternal (from the father), and from some other unknown source with unknown function. It is my theory that this DNA is actually data stored from all of our Soul's experience across time, in every lifetime. We bring in this encoding when we incarnate into a body, and it carries data about everything we've ever experienced.

If you had a life in Egypt, touching stones inside the King's Chamber of the Great Pyramid at Giza, entangling with the land and sites and sacred relics, all of that information would essentially be there forever. A part of you has been "saved" in stone, literally. Of all forms of matter, dense solids like granite, crystals, metals, and other heavy elements are the most stable storage mechanisms because their Protons are well protected and networked in a larger molecular crystal structure. While Protons in air and water distribute information around the planet, stones and trees store that information in particular locations.

When you die, since energy cannot be destroyed, part of that stone's data is preserved in you as well. Like many others before me, I propose that this data is holographically preserved across several higher "planes" within the Universe, from the Astral to the Causal and the Akashic Plane, all part of your Soul's many layers of bodies. Your physical body keeps the Proton information intact and distributes it into the land where you were buried, or your ashes scattered.

Thousands of years later, you return to those sites and stones in Egypt with a new physical body, and suddenly all the ancient information you entangled with in the site lights up inside the matching codes in your DNA. The DNA radiates those codes throughout your cellular Proton matrix, informing your cellular structures and causing chemical actions that provide energy, gland secretions, and many other physiological sensations. Your new physical body is now *remembering* the past that was stored in your Soul's genome.

Anyone who has had this kind of experience, returning to a site they visited in the ancient past, can attest to the profound and mysterious sensations that can arise. In our modern world, we have few educational resources that provide context for this kind of experience, so throughout these books I will be providing insights for practical integration of these powerful metaphysical and physical experiences of past-life memory recall.

For those avid adventurers ready to embark on the journey of recovering their lost hard-drives, and restore the memories, skills, wisdom, relationships, and emotions of their extensive journey through time, there are a few ways to enhance and amplify your reconnection with the past.

First, if we are resistant to any memory because it is painful or scary, we will create actual *resistance* in the information flow we can receive from something we have entangled with in our past. This is like constricting the flow of a hose, and while the flow is decreased, the pressure also increases as energy builds up wherever we are rejecting the energy of the memory. With enough time and continued re-entanglement, it is nearly inevitable that eventually our resistance will be broken and the energy of the memory will flood into us like a tidal wave. While this is a common path Souls take to obliterate patterns of thought and ideas that have been limiting to us, it can also be exceedingly difficult to process and integrate. I strongly recommend practicing receptivity in every area of your life, learning to accept feelings, ideas, people, and even scary and horrible things with equal measure. If we do this, we can quickly integrate the painful moments in our past and unlock the skills, ideas, and blissful memories all around them.

Second, we can recreate conditions of our experience in the past and accelerate memory restoration by recalling language, singing specific sounds or songs, doing physical movements, using similar objects or tools, allowing ourselves to experience similar emotions (which will probably happen naturally in certain environments and sites), or surrounding ourselves with one or more people who we feel like may have been with us. If you have always felt some familiar fascination with a particular object, tool, or instrument, try to find a version of it that is close to what you would have used in the past.

Third, it's important to have a starting point. How can you even begin to know when and where you lived in past lifetimes? What if you haven't had an experience at a powerful megalithic stone site like Stonehenge, the Pyramids in Egypt or Mexico, or other ancient sites around the world? If you ever took history classes in school, you may feel like there were certain periods or cultures you studied where you felt excited and energized. You felt like every picture was familiar somehow, and some of the stories too. Maybe you had a particular resonance with a certain God or Goddess, or with some other specific aspects of the people or culture. Then, your history class moves on, and for some other time periods and cultures you feel like you could fall asleep in an instant. The information feels boring, not interesting, and you find yourself thinking about other things... What time periods and cultures are fascinating to you? There is a reason for this, as we discussed how mental entanglement can create physiological and emotional responses, and this can happen through ideas and concepts just as easily as through physical contact with the Protons in ancient sites.

Someone in our lives may also be the starting point, as we feel a deep sense of familiarity, "as if we've known them forever," with often profound levels of emotional and mental connection. Sometimes simply the way we relate with people can be a trigger of memory, whether that engagement happens through intimacy, conflict, or anything in-between. Our connection can be rich with trust, or barren and anxious. Regardless of the nature or content of the connection, the link itself contains an energetic and holographic glimpse into part of us in the past.

If you lived in another town when you were very little, you might not remember much about that town. It's a blur of a few places where you have strong memories, and it would be hard for you to provide too many details about the location. What you remember is more likely to be feelings, thoughts or ideas you had, or meaningful relationships. You know you were there, but not much is "there" in your mind, just some mysterious parts of you. Now, if you find a toy or piece of clothing from that time, reconnect with a friend from there, or visit the location, and a huge wellspring of additional memory and information will be restored. In addition, reconnecting with painful moments that stand out in our memory, and focusing on them with our acceptance, forgiveness, love, and acknowledgement can also restore many other memories.

Just like some people are thrust into dealing with their past by going to a high-school reunion, others are thrust into past-life memories by returning to places they've been, receiving gifts connected to that time in their memory, or meeting people who they had significant relationships with in another time. For me personally, it was encountering people who had not only shared experiences with me in one lifetime, but across a vast array of them, which provided the existential pressure to light up a complex array of my quantum wormhole networks entangling me to past moments. Yet each experience was unique, encoded with a very specific moment and visceral sensory pattern that was infinitely individuated, and at times also containing a general sense of culture and archetype from the time period involved.

# INTRODUCTION - PART 4
# EXPERIENCING TOTAL RECALL

Orellana, Wu and I were in the Founders Hall Dormitory at the University of North Carolina in Asheville. I was still in High-School, living in Cullowhee about an hour further into the Blue Ridge Mountains. It was Orellana's dorm room, on the fourth floor, just across the hall from where I would eventually have that fateful cup of coffee in Rastara's room a couple years later.

We played chess, and as usual the conversation began to open into spaces of logical inquiry, with lucid waves of insight and satori leveling up our co-creative session. I woke up with these brothers at 15 years old, in 1996, and have only shared glimpses of our many adventures in my talks, and will share more of our story later in this series.

The topic at hand shifted to manifestation. Our observations of the process of conscious awakening, along with our innate occult understanding of the Planes of Existence, led us to exploring how the force of creation and manifestation can come through an individual.

We talked about how the mind and Astral Body constructs geometries, containers which hold the Astral essence of a new creation. The emotions and Etheric Body can fill those containers with juice, charging the Astral idea forms until they begin to emanate. When we have a strong or inspiring idea, our feelings about it can be strong, passionate, forging it with our creative desire.

Then, a physical action must happen; the Gross World of matter and mass responds to the worlds of energy and the structure of intent. As the Tai Chi Master Chen Kung would say, "When control of the mind is achieved, the Ch'i will follow," and "The mind-intent is the commander, the

Ch'i (etheric energy) the troops, and the blood like the camps." Mind is driven by the mind-intent, and this commanding force moves Ch'i like an engine. This engine can mobilize our blood, breath, and other vital essences within us, but it can also create change in the world around us.

"As above, so below; as within, so without." This ancient Hermetic philosophy based on teaching attributed to Hermes Trismegistus points directly to this phenomenon. When we move energy and act within our bodies, we can mirror that energetic change and action in the world around us. The worlds inside and outside of us are holographically interconnected because of the quantum wormhole networks which make up the living light structure of spacetime itself.

This is why many ancient wisdom traditions would use a "focus," an outer object they could act upon such as an Athame (Dagger/Sword), Chalice (Cauldron/Cup), Wand (Staff/Spear), or Crystal (Stone/Diamond/Pentacle) sourced from the Tuatha De Danann lineage as a tool to enact the ritual of changemaking. When the mind-intent makes a cup represent the land, and the emotions of the practitioner feel the joy and gratitude of experiencing rain, then the physical act of pouring water into that cup has the power to bring rain upon the land. At heart, all creation is that simple.

I summarized these realizations, saying simply, "When the mind, emotions, and physical world are all in alignment, creation must happen." And in that moment, we were no longer in the dorm room.

::: ⧗ :::

The three of us stood wearing long beautiful robes of different colors around a solid clear crystal pillar.

Protruding waist high out of a shimmering while crystal floor, the pillar extended down into the darkness of the earth, yet the top glowed gently from light deep down at its base optically traveling up to the top. The pillar was often used for scrying, linking, or as a creation altar…yet in this moment, it served a very different purpose.

We were inside a massive temple with thick white crystal pillars soaring up to an arched ceiling. Between the rafters, dark blue tiles glittered behind shining stars in mother of pearl decorated the curving expanses of stone. Gold and silver touches shone on stone statues along the temple walls, and wove in threads up wall inlays.

The three of us were speaking powerful statements of Truth, the most complete phrases of Wisdom we had regained in this life, and channeling the energy and structure of those realizations into the crystal pillar, and down into the heart of the Earth. We were storing data, backing up the massive archives of Galactic and Gaian knowledge we had attained, and imprinting the planet for recovery in later lifetimes.

We all knew what was coming… The massive tidal waves had been foreseen, and while some fled our white city on a peninsula, others had determined to greet the rising oceans standing open-armed on the beach, watching as the water was eventually pulled out beyond the reef. We spent our final hours in the temple, building our time-capsule for future incarnations. The Akashic-Library we were creating was also encrypted with a few specific insights, one for each of the three of us.

Then, in a flash, we were back in the dorm room. The air felt thick like liquid, the palpable and tactile feel of energy vibrating so strongly that the entire room was electrified.

"Wow… I feel like we've said this all before," said Wu, eyes wide behind his thin rimmed glasses, shaking his head of curly brown hair.

The smile on Orellana's face was contagious, "Damn." He laughed, and I had to laugh as well, my body shaking as I processed all that I just felt.

"Yeah." Was all I had to say at first.

Wu looked pensive for a moment. "Guys, I think we were just in Atlantis." A sense of relief poured over me, as I knew he had seen exactly what I saw. Orellana nodded emphatically, affirming that he had seen it as well.

"That was definitely Atlantis," I said, "I could feel the waves coming in and the flood happening… That crystal temple was amazing." Both guys agreed with me.

That night, we all had dreams about Atlantis.

In my dream, I could see familiar people, places, and the structure of the white city, climbing level after level up to huge buildings with domes, towers, and temples. At the top, our Crystal Temple overlooked the city, with pavilions and gardens extending out on top of the peninsula from its entrance. The domes were gold and purple, but almost the entire city was brilliant white with silver and gold decorations. It was stunningly beautiful, and had a warm feeling of home that seemed to wrestle with another feeling, a longing to be with the Stars.

When the waves finally came in, the sound that came before the crash was unimaginable. Only in the age of airplane jet engines and roaring trains can one begin to describe the continuous thunder that grew as the leading wave approached. Dwarfing the city, the wave swept up everything in its path, crushing every sea-wall and building along the ocean, then consumed level after level of the city and anyone remaining in it. I opened my eyes in the dream, and was standing in the temple with my two wizard brothers around the crystal pillar, and then the walls collapsed inward with a thunderclap rush, and all went silent. My Soul was able to still feel through my Astral and Etheric Bodies, aware of being within a swirling ocean, and rising from the surface towards the light of the sun. Emerging from the waters in my Spirit Body, I had one glimpse at the endless churning whitewater and rainbow mists filling the sky, before the radiant light of the Sun consumed me and I let go of my first lifetime on Gaia.

This was the first time I recognized that a dream might be much more, a memory of another time in another incarnation. I became deeply curious about the concept of reincarnation, exploring its gifts and looking for limitations in the spiritual philosophy around it. The more I considered it, the more I found it made complete sense. Why would we go through all the trouble of individuating, entering the physical world, learning growing and experiencing, storing information for the future and leaving legacies, only to die and "go to Heaven forever?"

# Introduction - Part 5
# Of Heaven & Hell, and the Story of Good & Evil

I was always troubled by the construct that if we failed in some way to meet the "standards of God" that we would be punished with eternal damnation in "hell." My experiences of God showed me that every action and event has an innate perfection, and that Divine Love is the essential force permeating All that Is. If God is infinite and eternal Love, how could there ever exist a place where one is punished and suffers for eternity? The idea seems ludicrous.

I eventually discovered a lot about this construct, and how it was essentially used as a marketing and recruitment campaign strategy for the Roman Catholic Church and Empire as it rolled across Europe. It was a well known Roman strategy to turn the symbols and cherished beliefs of their enemies against them. Pan, the Greek god of nature, fertility, and sexuality, was transformed from the playful inspiring Satyr to the fearful horned devil of Satan.

As the Roman armies expanded across mainland Europe, the symbol of Satan grew to encompass similar deities of local indigenous traditions, including Cernunnos of the Celtic peoples, Puck of the Anglo Saxons, and the Green Man or fertile nature spirit of many European traditions. All of these gods were connected to fertility, and the Romans knew that they could decimate these peoples through depopulation, rape, and out-breeding them.

About a year after my experience with Orellana and Wu, I also realized the Pentagram was the key to the physical world, the elements, and physical manifestation, due to my work on the Unified Harmonic Matrix. It couldn't be a coincidence that the specific geometry related to gravity, the creation of mass, physical beauty and proportion, as well as fertility and physical creation, would also happen to be the main symbol of Satan. It didn't take long after I woke up at fifteen years old that I stopped believing in coincidences. Everything contains meaning, and is synchronistic whether we can perceive its interconnections or not.

Furthering my work on the Unified Harmonic Matrix as a senior in high-school through my project, "The Unification of Science and Spirituality Through Unified Field Theoretics," led me to another startling discovery. The vibrational geometry of the Third-Eye Chakra should be 18, as the vibrational progression from Sacral Chakra (6) to Heart Chakra (12) should naturally increase in frequency to Third-Eye (18). The "two-petal lotus" is then 9 and 9, visually mirroring the shape of the yin-yang ☯ as the balance between masculine and feminine forces. However, it is also $6 + 6 + 6 = 18$... If the Third-Eye is key to our capacity to discern the Truth, have empathy and compassion, and unlocks our psychic abilities, why would its vibrational geometry be considered the number of Satan, 666?

In our modern era, we are finally quite familiar with the way disinformation campaigns, fake news, and media propaganda can manipulate people. If techniques of psychological manipulation were used in religious wars and strategies in the past, what would they look like? Perhaps the threat of an all-powerful evil deity that could claim your Soul, torturing you and punishing you forever in a realm of fire and brimstone if you step out of line or go against the "rule of the Church" precisely illustrates the nature of such an ancient propaganda campaign.

The effects of this "curse" on sacred symbols is more vast than you can imagine. The result of believing that the fundamental archetypal force of nature is evil led to Puritans burning forests, the Inquisition burning hundreds of thousands of female herbalists accused of Witchcraft, and sexuality being demonized. The wave of Christianity spreading across the planet brought with it an intense fear and need to control nature, *tame the wild,* and is partially responsible for our industrial disconnection from the natural world that has laid waste to countless areas of our planet.

Even Rene Descartes, one of the founders of modern philosophy and physics, reinforced this disconnected belief system by defining the entire physical world as a dead and unfeeling machine, an "automata." The physical world in his belief is dead, and only the Soul's expression of mind in a human body is special. This has permeated Western philosophy and psychology so deeply that even today in "New Age" communities, people have reinterpreted the Eastern and Hindu concept of "Maya" as the "illusion," the "fake world" we are working to escape to experience "reality."

However, the name Maya has only one of its roots in the Sanskrit word "māyā" which can mean illusion, but also means magic or creativity. The Maya were also an ancient civilization in Mesoamerica, where its meaning is "the few people" or "chosen people" as "ma'ya'ab." In Buddhism, the word maya can refer to a psychic power, often associated with emptiness and non-duality. In Spanish it refers to a type of woven textile, while in the Yoruba religion of West Africa it means "she who has made something out of nothing" and is associated with the orisha Oya of change, transformation, and the power of creation.

Though many spiritual teachers would have us believe that the physical world and time is just an illusion we're trying to liberate ourselves from, what if this is only part of the story? What if the common interpretation of this teaching is entirely wrong? As we've explored throughout this introduction, the process of creation and magic is only partially about learning to transcend our apparent physical limitations, but once we realize we are physical, energetic, mental, and spiritual beings, the process reverses itself. Once we've achieved some sense of holistic self-awareness, we can begin integrating our higher-states of awareness back into the world of the physical. This is the pathway to miracles, transmutation, manifestation, creation, and is the Art of the Avatars across Time. However, many attempt to continue going "up and out" into "higher frequency," so focused on "Ascension" that they begin to lose touch with the beauties and pleasures of the physical world they've chosen to experience through their current lifetime.

If you have ever held the belief that the Pentagram, the symbols of the horned beast often referred to as the devil or Satan, or the symbol of 666, or countless other *mudras* (hand-positions) or symbols are fundamentally *evil*, then you have been influenced by these long standing programs of behavior. Whether we like it or not, it is historically verifiable that these are ancient *hate campaigns* designed to disenfranchise, disempower, and essentially destroy European indigenous traditions and mystical traditions around the world. It's not your fault; everyone gets programmed from birth with ideas and concepts passed down across generations through our language, culture, and traditional "holy days" or holidays.

As people practice new rituals and ceremonies, we often forget where they came from. The Christian holiday of Easter comes from the Pagan celebration of Ostara and the Goddess Eostre. The playful mockery of Halloween arose from the Celtic ritual of Samhain. Many of the symbols used at Christmas, from the lights on the tree to stockings over the fireplace and the giving of gifts all come from Nordic traditions and Yule celebrations.

The karmic backlash inside Christianity itself has been severe. In the last few decades, the number of stories that have revealed deep sexual psychosis in countless ministers and pastors is sickening. Sexual abuse has been documented in orphanages, Christian schools, Sunday schools, special Camps, and many Christian communities. I've personally worked with and supported hundreds of people who have shared stories with me about their abusive childhoods in "perfectly pious" Christian families.

Yet these issues have gone far beyond their religious roots. Sexual repression is so rampant that instead of teaching actual sex education in public schools, we teach kids abstinence and force them to memorize images and names for sexually transmitted diseases. Sexuality has become synonymous with shame, so most young people exploring their sexuality end up ashamed of their experiences, whether they were supportive to their development or traumatizing and harmful.

While all of these topics truly deserve their own entire book, we cover them at high-level here because they are also essential to understanding our longer journey through time as a human species. As I share my experiences across lifetimes with you, there may be many places where you have a hard time accepting what I'm sharing without casting judgement upon me. While I understand this well, having had to face my own processes of healing around self-judgement, and diligently work to disarm my own trauma patterns and shame, I can offer you one insight here that may serve your personal journey of self-discovery:

Every judgement we apply to the world is based on a belief, and these beliefs are often deeply entangled in our perspectives and emotions. Some judgements are valuable, supporting us in discerning whether or not we should step off a cliff. Other judgements are ignorant, based on a limited perspective of someone or something, though we are not aware that our perspective is limited. Racism, hate crimes, prejudice, psychotic controlling behavior, borderline personality disorder, religious persecution, and other forms of psychological warfare are all forms of ignorant judgement. They are all *semi-unconscious* expressions of judgement, and they are usually accompanied by emotional defenses, self-righteous armor, and hypocrisy.

Take a moment and consider how many judgements you make each day that are consciously supportive of your life, and which ones may be causing you suffering due to ignorance. How many times have you reacted to someone's post on social media in a way that created conflict and pain, lashed out at a friend for their political perspective (or confusion thereof), were shocked and terrified by the "revelation" of someone else's beliefs and immediately rejected them (and their beliefs), or struggled with acceptance of someone's personal choices including sexual orientation, vocation, practices, or religion?

These are not simple dances to contemplate and reflect upon. However, when we begin to look at ourselves, and begin to unpack our own pain and trauma, softening our armor and opening our hearts, we may begin to discover that many of the things we judged are not simple black and white determinations. Many modern movies and stories now reveal to us that what we think is good or evil may not be what we assume… Sometimes the character you think is good is actually deeply traumatized and manipulative, while the characters in the shadows is actually the one humbly facing their darkest experiences to bring forth beauty, grace, and honor.

On this journey together, I invite you to open your heart and reserve your judgements. While some of what I share in this series may feel extraordinarily familiar and resonant with you, other parts may trigger places inside of you and bring up emotions, fears, or judgements. Pause, breathe, recognize that there may be more to the story you have not yet come to understand, and proceed with curiosity and gentle inquiry. With care and compassion, turn your awareness inward, and consider that part of you may be resonating with my story in a different way, perhaps as a participant in similar experiences or traumatic events in the past.

In our journey through time, we often will play out both sides of a karmic lesson, experiencing cultures from both the perspective of the colonizer, and that of the colonized. Through these opportunities to experience all sides of a situation, we can alchemize the pain of our past and forge the glory of self-realization, compassion, and love.

# INTRODUCTION - PART 6
# SOUL CONTRACTS & SOUL FAMILIES

The past-life and between-life recall experiences in this Prologue are a detailed example of the source material for this book. The writings here are not "channeled" as communications from other Spirits or Souls, but rather the direct visceral memories that have arisen from countless experiences with my Soul Family in this lifetime which surfaced our past adventures together.

As we enter the main timeline of my Soul's journey through this book, I will dive directly into the interconnected moments of memories I have assembled, and the personal transformations and realizations that arose for me during each lifetime. After sharing the bulk of each lifetime's journey and the most significant memories I have to share, I'll provide some post-lifetime notes and commentary, along with lists of my Soul Family from that lifetime who have given me permission to include them in this book. They may choose to keep their names obscured or remain anonymous, and for any of those who I have not been able to reach, I will obscure their identity by default, while still referencing the general time period along with events and the region in which my memories with them occurred.

My ongoing series of past-life recall experiences with other people helped me to understand that as Souls, we do not make the journey through time alone. We are part of Soul Families or groups of beings who share memories, resonance, and lessons with us. Just as my memories with Rastara were not isolated to one lifetime, I also discovered other lives with Jon, and a cascade began in my life of encountering many other Souls with whom I had deep connections across many other lifetimes.

For over seven years, all of my clear and visceral past-life memories were on Earth. However, eventually I would learn that Rastara and I forged a Soul Contract as brother and sister in the Sirian Star System, and that we bonded with each other at a deep genetic and energetic level before incarnating on Earth. That Soul Contract, forged on another world over 13,000 years ago (before I incarnated in Atlantis) and released in the middle of the desert that night of destiny at Burning Man, would enable us to locate each other wherever we incarnated, and in finding each other, we would trigger the release of our memories and come to know who we are across time.

While we were not always able to remember everything in each life, we did our best to keep a strong anchor to the reality that we were not from this planet. Yet in the cycles of karmas and Sanskaras we faced as humans, we eventually lost that awareness in the countless tangles of memories across our lifetimes on Earth. The last twelve millennia on this planet have been very primitive compared to these Galactic Civilizations, so the cultural contexts of society were even more unprepared for the truth that we're part of a greater family of worlds.

In this life, I was finally able to restore that memory, thanks to the rise of more advanced technologies and transportation methods, which helped to remind me of some of the ways we lived on other planets. Yet more importantly, I was able to access this period in my Soul's journey through a massive healing journey, and resolved many of my blocks since the time of Atlantis, mostly in one night in the desert. In addition, it revealed the true nature of this Soul Contract.

When my memory of the Soul Contract was fully restored, I knew it was finally time to let it go. Clearing the contract with Rastara enabled each of us to access more of ourselves, as well as many codes from each other's experiences along our journey. This restoration of myself catapulted me into a higher state of awareness that enabled me to make physical contact with an extraterrestrial being that night, and enter a great Galactic Council chamber in the Astral where I met 73 ambassadors from different star systems across the galaxy. Much of what I experienced from this powerful Galactic Reunion event, stepping back into my long-held role as a Galactic Ambassador, was the trigger for the cascade of experiences and memories which comprise this first book.

Therein lies the critical lesson: while Soul Contracts can have great benefits, releasing them can often have even greater rewards. We take our journey though time with many beings, and whether by oaths taken, promises given, or magic words spoken, we create contracts and bindings. These may serve us deeply for a time, but like all attachments, they eventually must shift. We can not always force this change, but in the great Sacred Journey of our purposeful path these bonds will naturally arise to teach us, awaken us, reconnect us, and then free us even more deeply as we release them at last.

# Introduction - Part 7
# Archetypal Memory
# vs Individual Memory

Students often approach me with the following question in one variation or another: "How do I know if my memory is really my past experience, and not just my imagination stimulated by films or books or other archetypal stories?"

There are Collective Energy Streams that bear Archetypal information between sets of Souls. These Archetypal energy flows best inform each individual of their personal potential, but they also carry on the resonance of the Sacred Service of others that has been able to change lives, transform places, and clear and transmute the most challenging of collective traumas. This is why we love heroic films; we identify with the energetic resonance of certain leaders and "Superheroes," because we aspire to their qualities, abilities, breakthroughs and exaltation in our own Soul's journey.

In doing countless healing sessions and past-life integrations, I've found that people often have layers in their field in which these Archetypal memories are resonant, where knowledge of a specific famous character in the past or a "fictional" character triggers an emotional or energetic memory stream within an individual, but these Etheric and Astral constructs are quite different and distinct from the Physical visceral memories of being embodied in specific bodies at certain specific times. The Archetypal field can inform an individual of what their Soul is seeking, and can help describe their broader Astrological path of Purpose in life. Yet the Archetypal field does not directly enable one to identify their individual incarnation; rather it often will cause projections of identity, as we attempt to support our own sense of self-worth by identifying with the most important characters of a specific time in history or particular story.

Think of it this way: historical narratives, mythologies, and Archetypal stories give us a broad sense of potential cultures, time periods, roles and experiences we may have a resonance with from a past-life. Then we must look inward and to our relationships to actually begin to access our personal experiences and Physical memories, which will then clarify our Emotional memory, and finally allow us to cartographically map our lifetimes with Mental precision, reincorporating each layer of our individuated Energy Bodies into our Present Incarnation.

I encourage individuals to get to know who they actually were in different lives as an individual Soul Stream so that they may know their own personal path more deeply and fully, and give their precious and distinctive gifts more fully. As we integrate our Energy Bodies from past-lives, we regain the skills, abilities, emotional bandwidth, and knowledge from lifetimes of experience.

To this end, I invite you to embark on your seeking with rigorous questioning. As you look into your past, make note of the Archetypal energies that come forth, but do not assume individuality or identity from them. Look deeper, peel through the layers asking more specific questions about your birth, life, and death. Ask about your most challenging experiences, and be careful not to seek for something you already know about, or that is historical.
I've found that even in my most resonant lifetimes that I'll remember the specific feel, smell, and emotion of a battle or powerful event. If you notice others in that memory that you recognize, or it is the recognition of another person that triggers the memory, explore further with them. Ask them about it, and if they are open to it or resonate with it, ask them if they remember how it felt. See if you can remember what you did before and after

that, and what your relationship was. These are keys to the individual Soul Stream.

I personally chose to ignore any similarities between my memories and historical events in order to get as much detail about my personal journey as possible, without distorting or filling it with false information. Only after I had full confidence in my memory stream, experiences, and many confirmations with others who were there with me, was I willing to look for the actual time periods and events. Even then, as I have come to know personally, where our actions happen to be recorded in history, direct memory turns out to be far more accurate and clear than historical records. There are many time periods in which only certain individuals of specific religious backgrounds, often with agendas and political alliances, recorded what happened in detail.

When we dive deeply into a personal memory, we access the Physical, Emotional, and Mental state of that moment of being. If we allow ourselves to feel this fully, a whole world of sensations will bloom within us. The first step is embracing all of this feeling, all the sensation, and all the memory it represents. Emotions may flood our being, and these may carry a combination of frequencies across the spectrum of passion, elation, intention, creation, relation, and ascension... From anger to bliss, fear to gratitude, sadness to awareness.

Our lives are full of experience. Those experiences are a stream of energy flowing into us. We can either accept all of it, or we can deny and resist its current. Yet when we go with the current, we gain the currency of the wisdom, skills, power and love across lifetimes.

Start with however you feel in the moment, and begin to explore the many ways you felt across that lifetime's journey. These ripples of feeling will often carry visions of places, of Archetypal expressions we've seen in movies, of deep moments of questioning ourselves...are we like... this?

Who are we really? The answer is where we start, and where we end to begin again. We are everything we remember, everything we have experienced, and we are the memory of Spacetime itself. We are made of Stars.

The journey of healing lifetimes is not just a path to acceptance of the Self, but also a Spiritual Journey to the Origin of Being. Perhaps you have lost your faith in Creation itself at times throughout your journey, but it is the Returning to the experience of the Infinite Within that Restores this Faith, for it is only in falling in love with our own Divinity that we truly discover what Faith means.

You are perfect, in all the ways you have ever been. Accept them, one by one. Face each relationship with a curiosity about it's depth and origins. Discover each other through engaging the questions that come alive in your hearts, and be Courageous. Ask the questions, and embark upon the Quest of knowing the Souls in your Family.

These are friends that will not ever fade, no matter how long it is between times when you see them. You have shared such powerful experiences together that those experiences have shaped WHO YOU ARE. And so, the myriad Songs you weave in your life will inevitably lead you back together... After all you're playing the same Symphony.

# Introduction - Part 8
# Notes on my Translations
## of this Journey

It is important to understand that in each of these lifetimes I used different languages, and different methods of communicating. However, the only way I can transcribe these experiences is through English as my native language in this incarnation. At times I will introduce specific words from these lifetimes in other languages that carry great significance, but will always clearly define them for you in my usage. I may also incorporate specific words from certain "fictional" sources, when those words closely match words in the original language and thought forms of past-lifetimes covered here. Some of the ways of speaking may also seem modernized with characteristics of current communication flairs on Earth, but these are intentionally added as there were similar cultural flourishes and various linguistic stylization in the original languages.

You may also notice parallels between some popular fictional stories and a few of the story arcs contained within this book series, just as I did. In many cases, perhaps by grace, I had pieced together my direct visceral memories and experiences with others into a timeline of events long before I realized correlations with these fictional stories. This brought up a deep and profound inquiry for me, many years ago.

Where do our fictional stories come from? When an author sits down to write a book full of stories that "never happened," where does he source his material? In my studies of J.R.R. Tolkien in high-school, I found it extraordinarily fascinating that he was not originally an author, but a linguist with fluency in many languages. He had set forth to create a "new language," and as he began to bring it into form, he had dreams and visions of the people who spoke this language. In his own words, he described the stories as having come from somewhere else, another world in another time. Eventually his stories evolved to become "The Lord of the Rings." Yet the original language he translated is the Elven language, Sindarin, and it is a complete and working dialect, as I would eventually come to discover that it mirrors the language of an actual Galactic Civilization: the Sirians.

George Lucas similarly starts his Star Wars films with "A long time ago, in a galaxy far far away..." There are many stories of the wild process of creating Star Wars, where many of those working on the story had visions, and the whole production team had to go through many iterative processes to reveal the final storyline. It is now my belief that these films are a rough echo of the Orion Wars, as I discovered many people (some of whom had never seen the Star Wars films in their lives) who remembered detailed accounts of events that had connections to this film storyline.

Perhaps there is a tapestry of Truth underlying some of the most powerful visionary fiction on Earth, and there is a reason why so many people resonate with these stories at such a deep level. If they contain hidden keys to our lost past, then we will experience the resonance of the memories being triggered, and we will experience a profound sense of belonging and connection with the story.

Of course, we must also recognize that the story is coming through a filter: a person or people who are *translating* those deep subconscious (or sometimes conscious) memories into their fictional art. The more conscious the memory, the more accurate the art matches reality. In addition, the more people who access the memory together, the more clearly it renders the prior relationships and events that were experienced by those people.

In forging this series, I have attempted to gather as many data points from as many people as possible, both through memories we shared together, and memories they had which I could not yet access. I tested their memories against the stories of others, as well as my own. I tested my memories against those held by others. As I mentioned before, in the final published version at the end of each lifetime, I will include the list of people who I had past-life recall experiences with, as transparently as their permission allows.

Over the last 23 years, some of my earlier understandings were corrected with more comprehensive integration across lifetimes. Remembering who we are is a lifelong journey, and I'm still on this one, so I fully acknowledge that I may come to remember more than I have so far, and that these newly access memories may change the way I look at those which I have published here. If these additions and changes become significant enough, I will provide new editions of these books. It is my goal to give you as accurate a picture of my experiences across time as I possibly can, so that you may find resonance with your own personal journey through your lifetimes.

For the first time in my life, I have determined to unveil my own journey in comprehensive detail and make it available to anyone who reads these books. While this feels extraordinarily vulnerable, I now know that these memories can help many others in better understanding their own Soul's journey and their own spontaneous past-life recall experiences. It is also clear that sharing these stories often triggers memories in others for the first time, and so with all my love and deep dedication to the service of All Life and the Awakening of Consciousness in All

Beings, I offer myself upon the Altar of your own Self-Realization.

Aloha Ke Akua *(God is Love - Hawaiian)*
Blessed Be *(may you be Blessed, and are Blessed - Celtic)*
In Lak'ech *(I am another You - Mayan)*
Wopila *(with Infinite Gratitude for the Divine in You - Lakota)*

Love All Ways
Always Love,

Adam Apollo

# Book I

## In The Beginning

# CELESTIAL - CHAPTER ☉
# BEFORE INCARNATION

The shifting weave of spectral threads spun through space, a tumbling knot of ribbons shimmering with light, forming geometric knot-work as they gracefully tightened into a form. Arches began to form a ring, merging a rainbow of streams into a scintillating torus of brilliant waves, reverberating outward into an egg-shaped field. Within this field, new threads of light spindled into curling vortices from growing stars emerging at the poles of the egg, and began dancing into the architecture of a vehicle.

My being, a hovering consciousness aflame with the creativity of a Soul discovering creation, focused lines of imaginal energy, emergent from a spring of ideas, guiding the shape of the weave of spectral light ribbons. From the depths of my heart, I could feel the way the ring of all colors was bending the void, moving space itself, harmonically resonating with the lattice of the quantum plenum. There it was, the key to commanding the flow of spacetime, a secret inherent to the patterns of Stellar and Galactic generation which were spilling out across the Universe.

The vehicle in the heart of the field was becoming more and more dense, its shape serpentine, extending into a long neck and tail, with a four-legged body expanding from its center. The large vibrating ring and field surrounding the body interacted with it, as arched ribbons of light began to shimmer into the form of wings between the ring and body.

What was this strange body, borne of intuition, imagination, and inquiry? So many structures had issued forth from these creative sessions, but there was something different here. I had made physical form templates connected to the layered torus ring geometry which could adjust spacetime, and thus gravitational fields. Yet this was not just a vehicle, but a Species.

The field and forms slowed in their vibration, growing brighter and more substantial. The ribbon-like weaves of light flowered into trillions of mini-vortices, shaping spacetime into protons, atoms, molecules, and the coiling flow of acids forming the codex of life itself, DNA... A language code in letters of fire-light blazed across the body surface, becoming a chromosomal formation guiding the DNA. The ring pulsed and all the flame letters were encapsulated in a sphere of light, which went through a swift fractal division, further populating the shape of the body of the emergent being. These cell-nuclei bloomed into cells, tissues, organs, systems, and then...

The head slowly turned to look at me, a face both ancient and young, gentle and fierce, metallic skeletal points framing glistening smooth cheeks, a crown of gleaming sword-like bones stretching back from the forehead, and eyes enflamed by the hearts of Galaxies bore into me. I could only take in the glimmering rainbow scales that decorated its body, the gleaming gems embedded in energy centers like its heart, the ripping waves of light moving across its web-like wings stretched between long staves of silver and gold, before I was drawn into its gaze completely.

I felt a jolt of panic, a feeling both unfamiliar and exhilarating... Was this fear? Had I made some mistake by creating, or facilitating the emergence of this being? The stability of my confidence as a creator shattered, and the deep stillness of the void all around me collapsed into a cloudy lightning storm. The being before me became more fearsome, its eyes red-hot ruby embers drilling into me, exposing a whole realm of self-doubt, fear, concern, and a deep dissatisfaction that I had not known was there. This being was...powerful...beyond me somehow, and something much more than my creation...

Was this emerging being making me feel this way? Was it to blame for these unusual feelings? Why was this happening to me? Had I done something deeply wrong?

I felt as though everything in creation was pressing in on me, and as painful and terrifying as it felt, there was something familiar about it... A flicker of memory, a wink about some secret, a question I had held, and the desire for an answer beyond all that I knew... I felt this deep sense of Omniscience coming directly into contact with the Mystery, the sense of knowing everything and knowing nothing, and in this moment, I was in touch with the infinite alchemical dynamic that could arise between the two.

Suddenly the being's eyes changed, red blooming into white petals in a wave of rainbow colors, and in the heart of these eyes a sharp slice as dark as the void opened like a slit. A symphony of feelings expanded out of the spaces of anxiety in my being, songs of exquisite beauty blooming from places of contraction and doubt. I could feel a swell of Love radiating from my CoreStar in direct rhythm and resonance with the light pouring from the black pupils in the eyes of this Great Master. I felt awe, wonder, gratitude, shock, relief, trust, surrender, excitement, and so much more in a single instance.

The field all around me exploded outward like the pyre of a supernova, and I could see the unexplainable beauty that would emerge from the gift of this Species in the Universe. This being was an embodiment of the dance between the Ray of Creation and the Mystery, incarnated with the unlimited power of the template of existence, while able to navigate and traverse the veils of the unknown, and bring an entirely new evolution to Consciousness and Being itself.

My Soul instantly called me to this being, and I knew I had to experience this form, become one of these beings, and experience the Universe through this perspective.

And so, I fell in Love, cascading into the layers of Matter, following an inner beacon of intuitive knowing into a pool of many star systems, to a large planet around a brilliant white star. I could feel the threads of creation itself again, now shaping themselves around me as I shot through space faster than a beam of light. I slowed above the planet, and felt the specific frequencies of the local Sun encoding the layers of my energy bodies with light language. The weaves of light surrounded me like an egg, creating a tapestry of every color brilliantly individualized in red, orange, yellow, green, blue, purple, edged in violet flame and golden glows, decorated with white star-points.

A sequenced formula of choices flowed from my CoreStar effortlessly, configuring the field around me, until the whole structure pulsed with total coherence...and all went dark.

...

# Dragon
# Andromeda Galaxy
## Khashakhanantian'oea

# DRAGON - CHAPTER 1
## BIRTH

The pulses rhythmically woke me up, a feeling of deep and profound warmth surrounding me, with waves shaking my whole body from the pounding of a brilliant luminous heart in my chest. Huddled in a ball, wrapped in my limbs and wings, I raised my head slowly and began to see. Riversheds of pulsing veins and arteries stretched around me in a cocoon, and I could feel the liquid around my body vibrating with each beat of my heart. I could feel something else, something just beyond my reach, but gently fluttering through the edge of my senses as it moved across my little world bubble. I began to sense its light, the fine frequencies carrying emotional current into my being, and the feeling surrounded and penetrated me deeply.

Love, care, protection, presence... I felt relaxed and comforted by these waves of light, my heart beating slower and yet more full, vibrating my whole being. Deep rumbles resonated in overtones of my heartbeat, and I felt as though I was ringing.

I slept and woke, always finding this presence around me, comforted by its love, at at times I would feel as though I was riding on waves of sound that would ripple through my world with a feeling of anticipation and gratitude, coming from this other world I couldn't see, but could feel stronger and stronger with each awakening.

Then it happened... This brilliant star of light emerged above me, beckoning my head upward again, and I felt a strange sensation as my eyelids parted and my world came into crisp view. Where I had seen rivers and currents of energy, now I saw deep red and blue blood vessels subtly glowing and resonating purple light, and see the slightly sparkling sheen of my body reflecting this light, and the nearly blinding starlight above. The star was more than a star... I could see a geometry pulsing into form, three points of light forming smaller trines of light forming yet smaller and smaller triangles of light, a fractal weaving into my blood pulsing from my heart through the network of vessel trees around me. It got brighter, and the field around me began to become translucent.

Brighter and brighter, this triangular star structure seemed to be opening, lightning tongues stretching out from its heart, piercing my eyes with such luminosity that I felt my head pull back in reaction and my eyelids tighten together. For a moment my heart raced, and an uncertainty caused my whole body to contract. Yet as a blinked in the blinding light, I felt a familiar rumble of sound soften my body, and a waterfall of emotions cascaded into me through the light above.

My eyes widened, and I could see two forms emerging from the edges of the light, their colors and shapes more beautiful than any of my dreams. One white and gold, the other silver and black. The two shapes came closer and I saw that they were beings looking at me, elongated snouts with large nostrils sniffing, while large eyes embraced me with gushes of feeling in my heart.

With a jolt of excitement, I pushed outward, reaching towards those faces, the warm cocoon cracking and giving way to my efforts. The light poured in from every direction, but all I wanted was to be closer to the shimmering white and black faces that were both familiar and mysterious. My heart vibrated with long rhythmic strums, causing my whole body to shake and fluids to fall from my wings, stretching out for their first time. My legs stretched downward and my arms upward, and they looked like they were made of light, reflecting all the colors and shapes around me.

The two heads came swiftly down into contact with my face, pressing against me with a tender embrace that stabilized my little body attempting to hold itself up, and their glints of gold and silver were reflecting on my own face. The rumble inside my heart burst forth up my spine and my throat and suddenly a sound creaked forth from my own body, a squeal that was both surprising and joyful.

I looked into those deep eyes as the heads of my Mother and Father pulled back from me a bit, though staying close. I fell forward and caught myself on my front claws, which were just nubs of shimmering chrome. I moved my torso and felt the weight of my wings almost pull me over, and I stretched them out to balance. I could feel the song of the ground beneath my feet, the music of the space around me in the breeze caressing me, the warmth of the star which was still above me. I craned my head back to look up, and between my parents was the same brilliant light, though now far far above me in a field of light blue with puffs of white that matched the belly of my Mother.

*I am alive. I am Dragon. I am here.*

# DRAGON - CHAPTER 2
## THE CONCLAVE

"If everything is made from Elementals, and we are part of those Elementals, then are they part of us inside too? Do we have other beings inside of us?" The small female blue dragon's eyes peered into mine inquisitively, the clarity of the questions shining within them.

"Yes," I responded to all the initiate dragon students gathered before me under the soaring peaks of the white stretched tent, "but the part they play within us does not compose our minds or emotions, only our Physical forms." I clenched my large muscular clawed fist in the air, "Each of our bodies are connected to the Elementals that form us, and so we are in relationship with them. As harmonic expressions of the Source, they move with us in a synchronized dance with our wills, evolving their own essence through participating in our experience, just as a muscle in your body gets stronger every time you use it. And like your muscles, the Elementals inside of you move with your intention and are guided by your feelings. They cannot, and will not ever, be able to control you, as it is not in their nature to control."

The little blue dragon stared out across the valley below, blinking with comprehension. "Elementals are like fields then, right? They permeate everything and respond to everything, but are raw forces rather than thinking and feeling beings?"

I smiled at my student, admiring her astute conclusion. "Indeed, Elementals are just like Harmonics, coherent fields of vibratory information at specific frequencies, and each serves specific purposes in their interactions with the rest of the Lattice of the Universal Field."

Teaching was one of my favorite ways to express myself. Since I was first scrambling around on the ground as a baby dragon, everything just seemed to reveal itself to me. The information was everywhere, moving and flowing in currents, showing me their geometric and vibrational secrets. While often irritating to my elders, I found great joy in expressing my knowledge about existence, and took great pleasure in seeing their old eyes widen in new realizations on occasion.

After class I headed to the top of the massive peak that tore into the sky above one end of the valley, soaring on the swift lifts of the evening winds hitting the jagged ridge extending down one of its arms. I found this mountain to be a refuge for my own contemplation, and a growing gnawing inside my heart was telling me this might be my last opportunity for some stillness.

Landing on the wide jutting rock protruding out the side of the peak facing where the sun would set, I tucked myself in by folding my wings around me and laid on my belly, enjoying the sensation of the warm rock against my cool silver scales. As the wind whipped in short gusts, I let it lull me into deep meditation. The mountain was moving underneath me, a living organism of rock and minerals, sprouting other forms of life all over its surface. Deep below the countless layers of hard stone, I knew there was also fire. I could feel it like I felt the power of the elements within my own body. I had Fire within my roaring heart. I had Water surging through me like geysers gushing from a volcano, my Sacred Blood. My whole body rose and fell in waves as I took in Air with each breath, fragrances wafting from wildflower fields mixing with the many mineral smells in the mountain's stone. The weight of my body feeling as heavy as if it was made of pure silver, yet the force of Earth mixed with the other elements to decorate me with a balance of hard steel and soft flesh, iron bones and flexible tissues, sharp nails and sensitive fingertips.

The core of my heart began to vibrate, and I closed my eyes, relaxing into the hum.

*It is time.*

My eyes shot open as the voice boomed inside me. My head lifted with long neck, craning around to see where the voice had come from, though I had a feeling it was not sound that I had heard.

A ruby wingspan gleaming in the golden light of the low sun came into view over the ridge, as a large red dragon glided gracefully onto the rocks closer to the peak, and began to climb towards me on the outcropping.

Gusts of wind issued from a quick flap were louder than the soft touchdown of the Red Dragon's claws touching down on the rocks. With blazing eyes, lit with an intensity I had not seen in a long time, he boomed, "A Conclave is Called. Che-karak Vale, in three Arcs of the Stars. You are Summoned."

:::

I had never seen so many Families in one place, the massive valley decorated with splashes of glimmering color and shimmering metals from thousands of Dragons assembled in the greatest Conclave of the Age. The energy was a bit tense and restless as the Great Star reached its peak, and the light was focused by gathering clouds along the valley sides to form a spotlight on the wide flat valley floor, like a great amphitheater.

The Eldest of an Ancient Red Dragon Family came forth, his gargantuan body crushing the ground beneath his feet as he stomped on all fours into the center stage of the valley floor. The sun's light caught fire on his scales, setting off the illusion of flames rolling over his smooth and glossy dark red and golden tipped scales.

Thundering forth, he roared with rage, and he declared:

"My brothers, my sisters, we have been wronged! My very blood has been taken from this world. It has been carried across the great seas of the Aether between stars, and it is now in another sea of stars far away. I can feel my Grandchildren being born in another world. I can feel their spirits crying out, 'Where is my family, where is my home?' Our life blood, our flow, our Ancestral Gift has been stolen! And we must go reclaim it. We cannot travel this great distance between Galaxies in these bodies, so we must drop them and go. And I know of these beings who took our blood, who have taken our life code, and they are little, and they are dishonoring, and they have taken from us that which is most Sacred to our Families.

"These fleshy beings of five fingers and toes are soft, and they crush easily between our claws. I will go, and I will CRUSH them. I will DESTROY them. I will make them pay, Teach their Spirits the way of Honor, that you cannot take our lives, our Families!"

There was a great roar among all the Dragons present, cries of anger and rage and grief all at once. The pain was tangible, the rumble of fear and electrical crackle of nervous systems lighting up, the pure power in the valley swelling to dangerous proportions. And this was the opening statement...

In a flurry of brilliant sapphire refractions of light, an Elder Blue Dragon came forth, roaring "Our bloods have been stolen too! We have Family that has also been taken from us. This is the Truth!"

The roar through the valley began to resonate the mountains themselves. These were not the only Families who had lost their kin, many others came forth confirming this Truth, crying out for justice and retribution.

The Great Elder Red Dragon who led the conclave had heard enough, and with a roar so strong he ejected a fountain of liquid fire from his guts like in a vertical pillar of death, his claws began to tear into his own body, ripping forth his heart of hearts in seconds of all consuming terrifying rage. He became a pillar of black smoke, a smoldering body extending into a towering Spirit of darkness that blocked out the light of the Great Star, spreading a pool of shadow from the center of the valley out to the edges.

The smell was awful, but the horrors had only just begun. Elder Dragon lords from many different lands and worlds followed, tearing apart their bodies in rage, filling the valley with gore and fountains of Elemental explosions. My Soul felt ripped open by this display of passion, and stabbed by the painful revenge that drove these actions.

By the time the valley was thick with smoke and ash, a hellish landscape of violent self-destruction, many remaining members of the Dragon Families were leaving, dismayed and concerned. Would all of these family members be lost forever to another galaxy?

My Mother had bolted from our Family's roost in the valley, and I had seen glimpses of her addressing other Dragons around the Valley. As I flew across the landscapes, heading back to our homelands, I began to see groups of other Dragons across various other Families heading in the same direction. Some of those Dragons were sired by the very Elders who had just torn themselves to pieces, and left to travel as Souls to this other Galaxy.

# DRAGON - CHAPTER 3
# A COALITION OF CARE

Far from the scale of the Great Conclave we had all just witnessed, it was still profound how many Dragons arrived to the huge white stone amphitheater on the side of our home mountain range. My Mother stepped into the sonic nexus of the theater and her voice was soft but thunderous as she spoke to the gathered Families.

"Many Souls in our Families now migrate to this other sea of stars, some by their Souls bound to blood, following their incarnation path, and others by their anger, hate and desire for revenge. This is True, yet we must ask ourselves in honesty why this has happened. We do not know the ways of these other beings who have taken our blood. We do not know why they failed to consult with us, yet we can be certain that they do not know our Ways. As little as we know of them, it is almost certain that they know far less of us.

"We are guardians and stewards to the life in our worlds, and if these beings from another sea of stars had lived here, we would not be so hasty to wipe them out based on their ignorance. We all feel the vast and terrible pain of the loss of our Elders, and those Great Elders who had already passed, traveling along the lay-lines of their blood to these other worlds, rather than incarnating into the next nests of our Families' eggs. Yet we must look upon this moment for its Wisdom, and discover the Great Purpose of this juncture in our Paths as Souls."

Her long shimmering tail whipped around her white, gold and silver body as she moved to speak to all those present, speaking with immense authority and gentle grace at once.

"I propose that we learn about these beings and their relatives, spending time traveling the Astral to explore their ways of life and the Purpose that drives them. Let us not hastily destroy ourselves in anger, but open up ourselves to the elation that may come with greater realizations. There will be time to make our decisions, to determine whether we will join our Elders in their fight for revenge, or to stand with our Principles as stewards and offer our lives to stop this passion-driven war, or to wait and observe what comes of all of this for our Families in the cycles ahead.

"My Heart shall not wait idly, but I will also not condemn thousands of unknown worlds to potential destruction without clear cause. I implore you all to join me in this action of inquiry, and travel together right now to see what these worlds are hiding. Let us begin with understanding, before we move to choose our actions."

She came to a halt, sitting back on her haunches and opening her hands before her to focus her consciousness and energy. Her wings began to wrap around her body, forming a shield wall of shimmering pearlescent skin.

I quickly moved to follow, stepping closer to her from the audience and sitting back on my tail as I wrapped my body inside the silver glittering foil of my wings, closing my eyes and tucking my head down to focus on my inner awareness and energies. I reached out my inner senses and could feel her breathing, vibrating, humming in an entrancing rhythm. I felt her attention move to me for a moment, and it was a warm summer dance among flowers and a rolling laughter full of joy and love. She always knew how to ease my heart, and I relaxed further into awareness of my Astral body.

As I did this, I began to see more clearly all around me through my inner vision, watching as Dragons made of light appeared in my awareness in every direction. My Mother's form grew, and I felt her extending an energy ring, spreading her wings around the entire circle of Dragons. I sent that ring my own surrendered support, adding to its field density and clarity, and I felt others begin to do the same. Soon we were all wrapped in an Astral lattice, a great vehicle of light that seemed to grow more solid and uniform, and yet more transparent at the same time. Our senses were now extending from this shared vehicle out to the Physical world around us, orienting in spacetime.

In an instant we began moving, rising together off the surface of our planet and quickly gaining speed as the blue sky fell away, the warm glow of the setting sun shifting colors across the rainbow as it passed through layers of atmosphere. Finally the black beauty of the glittering star filled expanses surrounded us, and the distance of our Great Star became more visibly perceptible as its light cascaded across the sphere of our homeworld below us.

Awareness reached out from us, listening for the energetic frequency of our Elders who had traveled to this other galaxy, and moments later we were shooting between other star systems, accelerating into a blurring field of passing starlights zipping by in every direction, and then suddenly they were all gone.

I expanded my attention and moved my awareness to be able to witness our entire collective Astral field together as a group, and it looked like a mushroom headed rainbow serpent made of light in the vast expanse of the void, tracing a series of lines of dark and violently vibrating threads left behind by our Elders in their passage between galaxies.

Then I began to feel them… Billions of stars with trillions of worlds, every one of them a rare and special spectral crystal of light, in a Great Sea of Stars that felt both similar and vastly different from my own home galaxy. The beauty and magnificence of the endless variations immediately ignited my curiosity and excitement, and I could feel many of the other Dragons traveling with us also beginning to brighten with interest, hope, and excitement.

The trail of our Elders led to a remote citrine colored star system with one sun and two habitable planets. There were only a few other stars nearby, one of which was a massive primarily red star with a deep orange glow, and other which was a sharp white with an aura of amethyst and magenta ruby. I felt something around that white star even in my momentary passage of attention, something that felt...different than anything I had felt before.

Our collective intergalactic Astral starship slowed as we approached the planet in the star system where our Elders' trail ended. The feeling of this world was one of confusion, domination, anger and pain. I had images of battling beings that looked a bit like Dragons, but they had various distorted bodies that stood more upright, with longer arms and legs and...short or non-existent tails! I only saw wings on a few of those fighting, and the battles were ruthless and ended with either submission or death. These beings used objects to slice and pierce and blast apart each others' bodies, and many wore metals and other materials like a second set of scales over their scaled bodies to protect them from such assaults. These must be the softer and more delicate bodies the Elder Red Dragon had spoken of, needing protection.

The scenes were repulsive, and while we could feel our Elders' Souls among the frays, they were obscured by such thick clouds of intense hatred for themselves and others that it was difficult to discern anything with clarity. It felt impossible to reach their consciousnesses, and I could feel my Mother accept this with a seasoned sigh; somehow she had known this would be the result of their suicides and reincarnation impulses. Where would it lead? If they got off this planet, how many worlds would they destroy, campaigning in unconscious revenge against the humanoids? Briefly, I saw images of interstellar war and endless destruction, before I shook it off and cleared my mind, wanting nothing more than to be away from this place.

With a huge sense of relief washing over us all, we moved away from this conflict ravaged planet and out into the empty space between local stars in the region. Coming to apparent stillness, we could begin to feel and see stars in every direction throughout the waves of this Great Spiraling Sea.

As our collective awareness relaxed, releasing the emotional grief that had crashed over us all, we began to expand our attention in all directions to these other star systems across this new galaxy. Suddenly I felt them, worlds upon worlds ringing out with rainbows of light and life. These worlds and their stars were each like a different Dragon family, with different colors, energies, and geometries forging the shapes of life and lands upon them.

A very specific inquiry arose within our field, coming from my Mother's warm heart: "Who are those responsible for our blood coming to this Sea?"

Instantly I felt a warm and bright red star, along with a mountainous rocky planet. The planet felt ruddy dry and barren, but with this warm wet and brilliant glow of many colors inside. I felt the layers of resonant memory inside countless gems and massive crystals geometrically gridded throughout the planets surface, and the luminous metal lattices forming tunnels, millions of chambers, flying crafts, and patterns upon the great geometric crystal stone structures in pyramid shapes across the world.

Yet the true marvel was the luminous Astral geometries that surrounded the people of this world. They were small, but their weaves of energy bodies seemed to dance in glorious integration with the crystals and structures all around them. They moved and created and spoke with an elegance that could be felt, like a soft pulse of love that resonated among the caverns and architecture.

Then there was the brilliant central pillars, their vertical energy alignment, which revealed their genetics. These beings had integrated their genome with many other types of species and life. They had found a way to weave the exquisite architecture of the Spiritual Spectral Field of the genetics within bloodlines, adapting new gifts and evolutions by their own experimentation and apparent Mastery.

I was not the only Dragon in our Family that noticed this particular gift in the Astral fields of this planet as we soared through its Atmosphere in our Astral Bodies, projecting and remote viewing from our home world in Andromeda. I felt a dawning of understanding in me; these people had taken our blood to attempt to integrate it into other forms...perhaps like theirs. My thought passed among our Dragon Tribe and I felt it link with similar arising thoughts in the other Dragons, and all of our hearts began to relax and open, feeling the deep and profound seeking that this desire embodied.

Then we noticed that the Astral Geometry of this idea was not ours alone, but linked to us and radiating from a specific cavern within the planet. We moved as one towards this link, connecting our intention to the location, building energetic tension between us and the place of origin. As we passed down into a deep canyon, we came to the entrance of a pyramid, nestled between the cliff walls of the base of the ravine. The entrance was a glorious series of huge decorative rectangular alcoves with massive statues guarding the entrance. The statues reflected the form of the people of this planet, regal and gracious with deep focus, and they wore metal lattices that covered their bodies in areas, decorated with symbols.

Our collective attention as we entered the massive doors in the base of the pyramid went immediately to one being who was standing with their arms wide open, beaming a feeling of love and gratitude directly into our Astral Hearts as our wave of Dragons swirled into the space. Others stood in a circle around her, cloth flowing elegantly over their bodies glittering with metallic symbols and soft weaves. Our Dragon Family quickly filled all the space between stone, and expanded out, dancing in and among the solid rock structures and labyrinths of tunnels throughout the pyramid. The few of us that moved directly in front of this powerful being condensed our Astral fields to make our light-bodies smaller, and came to stand before her.

She was definitely the female form of this species, and her eyes pierced the veil between worlds as she looked in a relaxed and considering way at each of us. When her eyes met mine, I felt a tingle ripple through my scales and I heard her speak into my mind…all our minds, as we were all linked with each other, and now with her.

"You have come far, and you grace us with your presence, Great Dragons of Andromeda. Once we knew you, as your Elders visited our worlds long ago. Cycles nearly beyond remembering have passed since then, but We are Keepers of Memory, and our Stones never lie. I Antara also know that I was once one of you, and I chose to journey here as a Soul many incarnations ago. Forgive me for leaving you, dear Family. It is with our love and our fervor that we seek to reconnect with you, and have brought your blood to worlds within this galaxy to call upon your presence once again."

Her words rang within all of us, a cascade of bells resonating deep wells of feeling, memory, grief, love, and gratitude. They had *called* upon us? Part of my being growled in anger, knowing the pain this *calling* had caused. Another part of me was confused, curious, and desperately wanted to understand these beings. This *Antara* was *one of us*? So it was possible for Dragons to incarnate into these peoples...

But then why had they done this? She should have known that our blood would draw our Souls as we followed the trails of our genome to our next incarnations, and that this must offend some of the Dragons whose family members were drawn away from our home? She must have known how much pain this would cause!

The thoughts were not mine alone, and Antara's eyes widened as she felt the intensity of our inquiry and the fires of anger flaring up among our Family. She took a shuddering breath, and spoke clearly with her high and resonant voice along with her mental projections.

"My dear friends, it was not I who started this project to bring the blood of the Dragons to our worlds. When the Mission began, I was not yet born. As it progressed in the years after my birth, I had not yet accessed my Dragon memories, and I did not know all the details of the Mission. It was only as I came of Age to be an Oracle, and went through a sequence of initiations that I began to remember my Dragon heritage, and I learned about this Mission in detail. When I found out, I did my own investigations on the project, and discovered the intensity and violence on the world of hybrids created by my people's scientists.

"I know now for certain, as I feel your grief and pain, that we have wronged you. I can see in your visions the Conclave of Dragons, I can feel in your *Eldunari*, your Heart of Hearts the precious care for those among the Dragons that lost so much as a result of my people's actions. We have taken your blood...without permission. We have broken your covenant of Honor, though I plead with you to understand that my people do not understand your ways. They had no harmful intent.

"I knew you would come, and I am here because I have awaited your arrival. My purpose in this lifetime is to pass to you this message, and to show you the codex of my own process in incarnating into this species. My visions have shown me that many of you would come to this Galaxy and stay here, becoming part of our Star Families, a vast spectral rainbow of beings from different stars and worlds, many of which are now interconnected in a beautiful culture of exchange and wisdom sharing.

"It is my great honor to welcome you to this Galaxy, and to help you find a way to support your Family members that migrated here due to our experiments in unifying Dragon and Humanoid genetics. I know that this task will not be easy, and many stubborn leaders in our planetary community are arguing over whether to somehow eradicate this entire living world of their own experimentation, or wait and allow these new beings to develop on their own to whatever results it may bring. I believe their hearts are good, and I know they will not choose to hurt these children of their science.

"Yet it is not my people's goodwill that concerns me, regardless of their mistakes... It is the great danger I can feel swelling within me, a force arising from this planet we seeded with lost Dragon Lords and volunteer beings of various worlds, caught in an experiment gone wrong. We have seen where this may lead, in our Council of Oracles, and it is terrifying. We need your help."

Antara's words rang within our hearts as Truth, and we could feel her anguish at the mistakes of her people. We could feel the grief, and knew her care was genuine. We could also feel her fear, which stoked this emotion within all of us who had gathered. There was indeed a terrible danger coming, and these beings were not prepared for the eruption brewing in their own planetary experiment.

With a grace of lifelong practice, she relaxed her body into a seated position with her legs crossed and hands laid open on her knees, and effortlessly stepped out of her body in a single breath. Her Astral form was luminous and beautiful, billows of light like thin fabrics swirling into the field behind her, giving the impression of wings. Her eyes twinkled and burned with an inner fire of commitment and dedication, and she beckoned us to follow her with a wave of love.

# Dragon - Chapter 4
# Exploring Worlds

It was in this way that we came to explore the key Humanoid worlds which had some of the same fundamental genetic codices as she had. These were also the same worlds that had seeded the experiment merging Dragon genetics with Humanoid forms. The Arcturian scientists had figured out how to link and weave aspects of several Humanoid species with several Dragon species, and in doing so had also inadvertently uncovered some of the keys to allowing Dragon incarnations.

Antara had furthered that work in her lifetime, and discovered that there was a pattern of stellar frequencies, specific rainbow spectra of light, which allowed an energy matching between certain species and colors of Dragons with certain Humanoid species. Incarnating into this vastly different species was simply a matter of finding our already existing harmony with specific stars bearing planetary systems where they incarnated.

In my inner eye, I saw each star system's central sun as a gateway, a locked door which only certain Soul frequencies could pass. I saw each of our Dragon colors as keys that could unlock specific doors, and the basics were so obvious. The Ruby Dragons could unlock access to into the cooler red star systems, Sapphire Dragons to the young hot blue star systems, while the golden and neutral white star systems could be accessed by many Dragons from Gold to Silver, Pearl and Emerald. The stronger the specificity of the stars color, the more limited the frequency of Souls which could incarnate there. In a star's life cycle, this naturally limits early and late incarnations as the star's spectrum moves further to the red or blue end of the spectrum in temperature, and invites wider incarnations into the peak periods of the star's life.

On the Astral, we visited:

## YAHONIA - YAHONIAN STAR SYSTEM
## BETWEEN ATHEBYNE & θ DRACONIS
## DRACO CONSTELLATION

A world almost entirely covered by lush jungle, with a heavy fog-filled atmosphere trapping sunlight in a wide tropical band extending almost to the polar regions. The cloud-cover near equatorial regions is thickest, so it's temperature is more protected from the solar heat, while sun bakes through the lighter coverage towards the poles, warming the planet everywhere. Green as an Emerald Dragon, the Yahonian planet is a biodiverse world beyond imagining, where life finds its way into every tree and nook and crevice. The humanoid species there live inside of the bases of massive trees, building structures over countless pools and swamps, and their villages glow in spindling golden networks like mycelial fungi woven throughout remote regions of the planet. Most of this humanoid species have skins as dark as night, absorbing all the light they can soak in, and perhaps telling of earlier eras on this planet. Their love for life and plants is visible, as their lives seem to interconnect entire aspects of the biosystem into more evolved circuits and cycles.

As we explored, we noticed some of these beings sitting inside of trees, who turned their full awareness to us as we passed over the landscapes. Suddenly we found them moving with us on the Astral, dancing among us with joyful abandon, and the sheer glee of the man was contagious. We found ourselves bobbing and diving and playing with his Astral form, before we headed further out of the planet's atmosphere until the highest blues became deep black space. The Man with the Astral Tree Starship body followed us there, then waved his arms around and sent us all more joy and gratitude. Many of our kind lingered for a moment, in awe and curiosity over this wise little creature, sending him gratitude in return. Then in a concerted shift, following Antara's leadership and guidance, we angled ourselves in the stars towards a dual-sun system.

## XANTHIA - SIRIAN STAR SYSTEM
## SIRIUS A & B
## CANIS MAJOR CONSTELLATION

Nestled between a bright golden star and a smaller white star, there is a diverse planet of snow capped mountains and endless deep forests woven with rivers and bounded by snow white beaches and large seas. In the joy of sunlight flickering between leaves, dancing with a rustle in the gentle breeze, held in the embrace of the ancient trees, the Sirian cities weave from the purple mountains to turquoise seas. They stand steadfast in the elder boughs, high above the shadowed ground, where the golden light plays among bridges and arches, courtyards and temples. Some rise from the ground, fingers of white stone pointing to the sky, glittering crystalline walls carved with reflections of the simple beauty of nature, whose graces consume the cities inside and out. Some cling to cliffs between cascades, where water gushes down endless indigo rock surfaces that turn violet in the sunshine, flowing from melting glaciers on snowy peaks. From villages in forests deep to waters edge, cities on mountain cliffs to the silver Starports on the icy tundra of the polar caps, Sirians accentuate their natural surroundings, magnifying the inherent beauty with honor and grace.

The various humanoid species populating this world have distinctive long pointed ears, almond shaped eyes of various elemental hues, deep penetrating gazes, and embody various heights and skin tones. Agile and lithe, they find joy and strength in running, swimming, and dancing. Their clothing and jewelry is often decorated with fine lattices that resemble the patterns in leaves, vines, and other natural life. Those that live in the forests often have light skin tone. Those in the forests edge, hills and coasts often have much darker bronze skin, hardy from the endless light of two suns. The lightest skin is that of those who live at the massive stations made of illuminated metal arcs in the icy polar regions of their homeworld, and board the gargantuan star-bodies shaped like sleek chrome birds. Star-Ships, as Antara clarified to our awareness, shared vehicles they could use to travel to other star systems.

The beings in the Star-Ship-Base as well as many others around the planet noticed us as we moved through their atmosphere on the Astral plane. We should have been invisible to these Sirian beings, just as much as the Yahonians, but they seemed all too capable of noticing any significant movement on the Astral plane overlaid within the Physical world. The Star-Base teams immediately reached out to connect with us as we came over the horizon towards their citadel in the heart of ice, one of the darkest places on the planet up here at the pole, and suddenly we found ourselves with a sort of energetic dashboard of options being shown to us.

They provided illuminated energy patterns like pathways, showing us where we could approach and land at the Base, revealing many other Starships in outer orbit and on approach or departure. They also sent us curious inquires as to our origin Planet and System, perhaps not realizing we might be from another Galaxy altogether. Our collective Dragon smirks sent the answer, with a lightning quick mental rendering of exiting this Galaxy, approaching Andromeda, then diving between two nebulas into our beautiful home system. The response was unexpected. There was a huge swell of excitement we felt emanate from the Star-Base, and it got stronger as we approached and felt many beings within it's metal and glass spires suddenly focusing their attention on us, tentative but full of curiosity, awe, and honor. We did not follow any of their landing paths, but instead showed them our trajectory, back down across another continent of sky-scraping mountains with stone citadels and cities woven into the forests, then onward into the stars.

We felt their longing and their gratitude pour into us as we traveled on, and it was though a ripple of light went through the planet, a transmission to beings all over their world. As we sped up and emerged from the icy landscapes and snow covered peaks back to lush green forested valleys and riverbeds, we found something even more prolific than their Starships. They had Gates all around the planet, Portals that seemed to link spaces so any of these beings could take a few steps and be on the other side of the world... Perhaps even to other star systems? They had found a simple and elegant way to live locally to their own homelands, while traveling and connecting with each other all over their world, and other worlds, practically at will.

## MAYANA - PLEIADIAN SYSTEM
## STAR MAYA
## PLEIADES STAR CLUSTER

Entering the deep blue pools of the Pleiadian cluster and surrounding nebula, we immediately felt a drastic shift in our energies. In the heart of this bright stellar nest, there was a feeling of timelessness, and it grew stronger as we approached a single blazing blue star, receiving its harmonics as we passed towards a luminous blue planet. A rainbow aura surrounded the ocean covered world, as the full light of the blue star behind us caught the wet yet sparsely clouded atmosphere, setting off a sunset-like ring around the whole world from our view as we approached.

The endless oceans were dotted with scattered island chains and atolls that seemed to have only primitive villages, huts, and small caves carved into temples. Yet the simple way of life here seemed oblivious to the massive underwater cities, countless floating structures just over their horizons, and the nearly continent sized Starships just floating in stillness just outside their atmosphere.

Almost like two distinct species or cultures on a single planet, the Pleiadians had found a way to preserve the most simple primitive way of life of their ancestors, and yet build advanced cities and technologies that were the most complex and fascinating structures we had ever seen... How they managed to have so many beings living this anachronistic way on the same world as their interstellar culture was a curiosity that drew immense interest among all of us Dragons.

The rhythmic resonance of the ocean waves, soft walls and flexible pathways bending and flowing with the wind and water, living structures woven with water, their Pleiadian island cities bloomed from tropical atolls and bubbled deep within the seas. They were woven into the landscape, artfully crafted to disappear into the biosphere. Underwater tunnels, domes and spheres decorated the ocean floor, covered in coral and spilling into trenches and caves. The few cities and villages populating the sparse island chains were only a tiny fragment of the population spread throughout the deep seas, and orbiting in the outer atmosphere. From gargantuan transports to moon-sized Motherships and more personal Starships than stars in the sky, the Pleiadians seemed to enjoy being more spread throughout the Galaxy than floating around home.

Generally taller than the average human, the Pleiadian humanoids' skin tone ranged from an icy white to deep blue. Their large, often deep blue eyes seemed to engulf everything in an ocean of acceptance. They sing to their lands, to the water, and they seemed to have learned how to control the structure, shape, and density of water and other objects through sound vibration. They can communicate readily with Dolphins, Whales, and other Cetaceans, and treat them as they would treat any family of their own species.

Pleiadians seemed to exhibit an extreme level of empathy, feeling our group and sensing into connecting with us long before we could see them. They apparently could feel emotions of another individual, a group, or even an entire species, as easily as they felt their own currents of energy. Groups would often gather to meet us before we flew over, openly gifting us with singing abilities, musical talents, sound healing energetics, and visions of sciences or technologies involving water.

There was a subtle sensuality to it all, in their deep intimate regard for us felt in our awareness, and through to their movements and closeness with each other. They would look upon us, touch foreheads together in communion, and send us the feeling of love and connection they felt. It was all quite stunning and beautiful, and the feeling of appreciation I had for all these Humanoid beings continued to grow within me.

## SHIHAELEIO - SHIHAELEI SYSTEM
## NEAR STAR BETELGEUSE
## ORION CONSTELLATION

We moved on to a brilliant white star with tinges of indigo, violet and magenta in its light, and swooped in towards a pair of planets that happened to be fairly close in orbit and position around the star at this point in their elliptical journey.

One of them was wet and lush, with massive oceans and cloud-covered rainy continents. Areas of deep verdant forests and open plains, interrupted by jagged black stone cliffs, mountain ridges, and coastlines. Beautiful towers and warmly lit structures made of white stone and black stone presented themselves like great temples at the edges of cliffs on the ocean, rising from high-ridges, and boldly reaching forth from the highest hills of endless grasslands. The humanoid species here seemed to be in some constant form of ritual, whether in dynamic movements shaping the air with metal blades and rods, or draped in robes standing in circles in halls full of firelight. Their focus and discipline was both inspiring and exhausting to witness, and they all seemed to be guiding each other through initiations of one form or another as a way of life.

We shifted back away from this beautiful dark and rich landscape to arc back through space and towards the other planet with life, a little closer to their primary star. The difference could not have been more drastic.

The second planet in this system was bone white, entirely covered in deserts and lacy white crystalline mountain ridges. Unlike a sandy beach or the thick dirt of deserts on our home worlds in Andromeda, this desert moved like plasma, a powdery dust rippling in serpentine formations and whirling funnels across endless flat expanses with spidery cracks in hardened clay, and smooth exposed white crystal faces of rock. Here the cities were all built as massive white assemblies of crystal stone, and carvings cut directly out of the glittering mountains. The dust covered everything, but the occasional glimmering refractions like sparkling snow, and energy of the stone itself did little to hide the majesty of these cities, and the extraordinary magic hidden just beneath them.

We could feel beings not just on the surface, but down inside the planet's mountains in huge caverns. We brought our Astral forms down inside the ground, and found ourselves winging through huge crystal caverns lit with bioluminescence, with endless streams and pools of water surrounded by lush vegetation. We could feel creatures much deeper, beings hiding in the darkest depths of the water channels into the planet that held an expansive intelligence we acknowledged as potentially being as Ancient as our own. We could feel their curiosity towards us, and the immense respectful regard they held for the Shihaelei people.

On this planet, the Shihaelei were more similar to the other species we had witnessed on our journey, and they seemed to involve themselves with every kind of art form and work imaginable. It appeared that those who had mastered the initiations on the other planet were leaders, guardians, guides, and oracles here. That was when we noticed that the oracles on this planet had been tracking us all along our exploration of both planets; they had been watching us without any of us even being able to sense their awareness upon us. I was stunned by this realization, and I was not alone in our Dragon Family having that reaction.

An Oracle's consciousness then reached directly towards us, and said into our mental field, "We are Watchers. We are Guardians. What is your purpose here?"

Antara intervened on our behalf, expressing that we were travelers from a distant Galaxy exploring new worlds, and that she was from another planet in this Galaxy.

We could feel a distinct electrical *shiver* come from the Oracle, and immediately her mind (and voice within the great stone hall she stood within, surrounded by hundreds of other Shihaelei) boomed forth: "A time of great terror comes on the tail of your arrival! Worlds will die, and our people will lose nearly everything. Yet we will rise with Purpose, and gather a thousand worlds under our wings.

We will be enslaved in servitude, and lead countless lives to liberation. We will become you, but only to become ourselves. We will know you, only to know ourselves. The time of the Great Forge has come!"

There was a swell of energy that rang through the planet itself, and we felt city after city light up with the same energy. It was as if someone lightly touched a huge leaning stone and knocked it loose, its massive weight crashing against another precarious stone, and another, and another, all falling in sequence. Yet while the energy was electrifying, the peaceful and methodical motion of the beings of this world taking actions in response to this oracular revelation was so precise, so composed, so artful, that it immediately soothed our own troubled Dragon hearts.

This revelation was clearly connected to the planet where our Dragon Tribes were incarnating into hybrids. This world was not far from the star system of that planet... perhaps it was the closest inhabited system. Antara's consciousness confirmed this, and expressed that this is why she had brought us here. That she had felt our resonance with these very special beings, even though they had not yet joined the other species who were part of an extensive Galactic Community of interstellar travelers. The Shihaelei had developed the ability to travel between their two planets in orbit around their star, but they had not advanced their technology enough to travel to other star systems, yet. She felt that they were culturally the most capable of handling any potential attacks from another world, but that they may not have the technological capacity to stand a chance in an interstellar war. Her energy dipped into grief, as she added that *none* of their worlds were prepared for something like that.

It was true. All the worlds we had witnessed were ill prepared to face any kind of onslaught, and certainly not one by raging Dragon Lords, regardless of the weaknesses of bodies they now inhabited. The only world that might stand a chance would be this one, where the species embodied such poise in the face of danger, preparation in the face of mystery, and levels of physical skill in movement and action that were far beyond anything we had seen in other worlds. They may not have the most advanced technologies, but they moved *like Dragons*, they anticipated and listened and struck like lightning.

I felt my Soul begin to vibrate right through my Astral form and into my physical body back on our home-world like a massive bell, a resonance of deep knowing that I would be Shihaelei. Dragon would become Shihaelei, and the Shihaelei would protect life on other worlds just like Dragons in Andromeda. Even with this powerful vibrational sensation nearly pulling my entire awareness back into my physical form, I managed to stay focused in my Astral awareness and linked with my Dragon Family here in the Shihaelei Star System.

Others could feel my resonance, and my resolution. I could feel some of them building in their own resonance, many harmonizing with this world, and many with some of the other worlds we had witnessed. Suddenly, it all seemed very clear for all of us; we would come to this Galaxy and protect these beings, serving life on these worlds, and stop the onslaught of those in our great Tribes who had been lost to pain and trauma.

Feeling the massive shift in our energies, Antara quickly led us back to her own star system.

## ALCHAMETH - ARCTURIAN SYSTEM
## STAR ARCTURUS
## BOOTES CONSTELLATION

Back where we started, approaching the crystal gridded red planet under the light of the large red-giant star, we now determined to study this planet and species in more depth as well. Resonating deep in the hearts of mountains, the songs of the Arcturians boomed through ancient stone halls and passages deep within the surface of their home planet. From secret pools illuminated with fluorescence to high-speed transit tunnels, Arcturian cities burrowed into the red stone of their world, leveraging expert technological craftsmanship of stone along with the delicate shaping of metal hulls and crystal windows. Pyramids dotted the surface cities, and giant gates opened in the walls of canyons accessing gargantuan halls and atria under the ground.

While the surface of the planet was mostly dry and dusty, like Shihaeleio, there were hidden oceans of ice and liquid water following passages through the deep places of the world. Some of the tunneling canyons underground were so large that Starships fly through them, docking at various villages blooming from the rocky cavern walls. Starports sprouted from cavern openings, and the magic of Arcturian stone work was everywhere.

Antara shared with us that over the millennia, Arcturians intermingled with other species, and adjusted their own genetics in vastly diverse ways. For this reason, there was no fixed archetypal appearance for the Arcturian humanoid, though they all appeared very similar to the other humanoids in general shapes and sizes. Showing us their their root genetic form, Antara gave us the visions of how they evolved themselves from a tall, strong humanoid race with reddish bronze skin and dark eyes.

The energy of their harsh homeworld and giant red star were apparent in the sense of "solidity" and strength they emanated, and they still always chose to keep parts of their root lineage, often bearing darker hair and darker eyes in their incarnation lines. These beings took their initiations in the darkness of caverns and temples, and were taught to see the light in all shadows.

Antara continued to elaborate about her people, as we observed their many qualities. Arcturians were determined and many of them strongly mission oriented, traveling the galaxy on secret or overt missions to enhance consciousness and heal ancient traumas. While most species tend to get caught up in worrying about unsolved problems and overwhelmed by shadows and challenges, Arcturians tended to thrive on solving problems and finding the silver lining in issues. Their hearts were as strong as the stone mountains and canyons of their homeworld, and instead of retreating when times get rough, they would often advance quickly in a new direction. Yet with all these gifts, they also tended towards hubris, taking risks and advancing things without full knowledge of the potential results of their actions. She shared with us that it was a well known practice for Arcturians to purposefully block out specific knowledge of certain situations in order to face them with fresh, "untainted" minds.

They had clearly taken risks in taking our Dragon genetics and creating a new species, and indeed, their hubris had kept them from seeing the massive pain this would cause. Yet within our Dragon Family of Astral visitors to this world, we all felt a greater understanding and compassion for these beings after learning about their humanoid kin on other worlds. Their particular gifts made more sense; they were a piece of the puzzle of the consciousness evolution for this galaxy, just like each of the others. And for some of our Dragon Family, this particular piece of the puzzle was most resonant for them, and they would become Arcturian.

It was time to return to our physical bodies and home-world our distant Andromeda galaxy. It was time to bid farewell to our Dragon ways and our Dragon lives. We were a family with a mission, much like these Arcturians. And our Mission was leading us into new bodies, new ways of life, and hopefully a swift end to the inevitable conflict we felt brewing within our brethren.

Antara had completed her Sacred Task, and expressed more gracious energies towards us as we prepared to depart. My attention was already back home, considering what needed to be wrapped up in my world, in my life, before my last death as a Dragon.

:::

It wasn't long after we had returned to our bodies, that many of us were ready for the Great Transition. Our beautiful little home planet in the Andromeda Galaxy now seemed more stark and plain after experiencing so many diverse worlds during our Astral Travels to this other Milky Galaxy of humanoid worlds. I was afraid I would have to let go of so many beloveds here in my life as a Dragon. Sweet dances with the serene Pearlescent Dragon, silky sensual play with the Amethyst Dragon, and so many amazing Souls I had spent Ages around… But nearly all of them were coming with us. We would all consciously drop our Dragon forms and migrate as a fleet to incarnate across these other worlds in another Galaxy.

Where our brethren had left these worlds in rage, we would leave these worlds like a luminous comet of light and compassion, offering ourselves to the mystery and discovery that we must inevitably face in standing for All Life on these other planets. It seemed that time was in a slipstream, days cascading like a waterfall as everything I had ever known was seen and celebrated. And perhaps, for the last time. And then, it was time.

:::

A vast tapestry of rainbow colored Soul Fields billowed across the endless empty fields of spacetime between Galaxies, the wave of Dragon Souls curling around each other in spiral dances the way smoke rings spin in still air. The luminosity of Souls was stunningly brilliant, and traveling in my complete Spiritual Bodies after dropping the physical form of my Dragon revealed so much more to the energetic Tapestry of the structural lattice of spacetime.

That is to say, we didn't really travel in a traditional sense, but rather slowly and gently reoriented ourselves together into proximity of the worlds of the new whirlpool of stars in this new and foreign Galaxy. It was like a rippling swirl of feeling our connections with each other and our growing connection to the new worlds we had chosen, our Souls gathering in fractal self-symmetry with similar Dragon Soul colors around shared vortices of purpose and presence.

Each fractal whirlpool of specific harmonic vibrations began to spread out to different Star Systems, matching energies like musical notes played in beautiful harmonies, and each star began braiding our Soul genomes with its own energies. It was like a Sacred Song being imparted into our Hearts, the Song of the Star.

The Song of my chosen Star seemed so sad at first, a symphonic tragedy that wrenched my lower spiritual bodies in cries of anguish, but within that grief was something far more... A light so brilliant that it bloomed up into every part of my Soul, a beacon of Divine Purpose that swelled from the darkest notes of the Song, bringing every layer into a higher order of beauty and harmony. I felt my *Eldunari* explode with love, gratitude, and a profound acceptance woven into me just like my old

Dragon scales, a sort of Sacred Armor I would carry into this incarnation. This next lifetime would require sacrifice from me on a level I could barely comprehend, but it would also plant seeds that would grow into a precious Sacred Garden in my Soul's near future.

The symphony reached an ecstatic crescendo, and my Soul was propelled from the Shihaelei Star like a beam of light straight to one of its two populated planets, and everything faded into a dark and comfortably warm dream...

:::

# EPILOGUE: DRAGONS

For a long time, I didn't know why Dragons were so important to me. Growing up, they held the same allure as swords; whenever I saw one I felt a surge of energy, interest, and excitement. I ached to wield real swords in my childhood, but instead I danced around and battled with sticks. Similarly, while they were seemingly completely absent from my physical reality, I would often draw and paint Dragons, as they decorated my dreams.

As a young child, I saw a film called "Excalibur." The entire movie had a very strange affect on me I would not begin to understand for a decade. I felt every emotion and pain deeply, yet some parts felt confusing and irritating, as if they were wrong. While there were no visible Dragons in this film, at one point Merlin calls the Dragon with magic to enable Uthar to bed Egraine, and later the Dragon is key to the initiations of Arthur. The spell which Merlin used to call the Dragon forth felt very real to me, as if it was calling me, inside my Soul.

My first acrylic painting in middle-school: a Dragon with fire-like scales among the stars and a crescent moon. My first stencil cut for spray-painting as a freshman in high-school: a Silver Dragon wielding all the elements in swirling magical patterns, all contained within a circle that would be imprinted on the back of the first clothing I ever made, a set of violet velvet robes. I wore those robes the first Halloween after I woke up and realized I had an energy body, and that magic was indeed very very real.

After reading "The Hobbit" and "The Lord of the Rings," the first fantasy novels I ever explored in middle-school, I found myself drawn to a series of books called the "Dragonlance" series. Years later, I was in an airport and picked out a random fantasy book before boarding a flight called "The Eye of the World" by Robert Jordan, the first book in "The Wheel of Time" series. It turned out the main character of the book was known as *The Dragon Reborn*.

As I began to have past-life memories surface, symbols of the Dragon seemed to always be there, following me through time as Sigils on my armor, signets on rings, tokens of protection in my homes, and more importantly, in direct experiences with Spirit Guides across lives. I thought of Dragons as some kind of Astral or Spiritual Archetype, something that was part of me for some reason, but purely mythological or spiritual in nature.

In 2006, the year after I had my first Galactic Contact experience and began accessing my Galactic lifetimes, I was working in Santa Rosa with Denise G. and the late John Orava doing design work for his nano-ceramic building material company. They felt that the household was under psychic attack, computers failing and Denise's kids getting sick daily. That really upset me, and the first night in the house I could feel it, like a strange energetic invasion. An ancient power arose within me, and I decided that any outside entity attacking this home would have to go through me first. I called on all my Guides, Angels, and Ascended Masters, called upon the Four Watchtowers of the Four Directions, and commanded through my Higher Self that protective Wards surround the house. Basically, "none shall pass."

I went to sleep easily after that, and immediately found myself in one very very long dream: the early part of my lifetime as a Shihaelei. The next day, everything was different. The energy was good, kids felt better, computers were working. Everyone asked me how I had done it, but I felt that the answer had more to do with my dream than just my prayerful Commands. That night I had the same exact dream. And the third night as well. The lifetime's memory was emblazoned into my consciousness as if I had just lived through it all again, three times in a row. In the next chapter, I will share this lifetime in its full depth, as I wrote it all down in detail after I had integrated the experience. Relevant to our current explorations however, it was in this lifetime that I temporarily transformed into a Dragon using advanced technology (along with others) in order to try to stop a Galactic War. Even with these memories, I only knew for sure that these Dragon forms we inhabited were seen as some sort of Gods by those who sought to destroy us. I thought I finally understood: I had once transformed into a Dragon to end a brutal planetary battle, that's why I loved them.

Then in 2014, I experienced a profound healing through my friend Caitlin. As she tuned into the depths of my vibrational field, she brought my awareness to an ancient memory within me. It was hidden behind symbols, sigils of light and patterns that I did not yet understand. Encouraging me to speak it all aloud, I found myself describing a wave of light traveling between Galaxies that felt like countless Souls in migration. She urged me to go back before that with subtle cues and energetic support, and I found myself looking at a pulsing triforce geometry that seemed alive and electric, branches of something glowing and fluid swelling in perfect rhythms around me. The shape began transforming into pure shards of light, breaking open, and I found myself looking up from inside of an egg, seeing my Dragon parents for the first time.

It is profound to remember your moment of birth, and seeing your parents as you emerge into the world. This is something most of us never get access to, as it is extraordinarily difficult in a humanoid body. Yet I remembered every detail of my Dragon birth, and all my ideas that Dragons were simply an archetype were shattered like fragments of my egg. I *was* a Dragon, and I knew it so deeply and profoundly that there was no question in my mind anymore. Now I *knew* why Dragons had been woven throughout my lives. How could I ever *not* be myself?

# Dragon Shared Memories

✦ Silver Dragon - Apollo
✦ White & Gold Dragon Mother - Kaia R.
✦ Black & Silver Dragon Father - Justice
✦ Red Dragon - Hart Wood
✦ Blue Dragon - Jack Senechal
✦ White Rainbow Dragon - K.J.R.
✦ White Dragon - Greg
✦ White Dragon - Shaina
✦ Red Dragon - Dakini
✦ Purple Dragon - Leila
✦ Black Dragon - Knowa

✦ Dragon - Shaina
✦ Dragon - Ehren
✦ Dragon - Renee
✦ Dragon - Finch
✦ Dragon - Shiloh
✦ Dragon - Daniel
✦ Dragon - Agustina
✦ Dragon - Leandro
✦ Dragon - Anna B.
✦ Dragon - Carrie
✦ Dragon - Rael
✦ Dragon - Caitlin

✦ Dragon - Ashaweh
✦ Dragon - Phoenix
✦ Dragon - Karen
✦ Dragon - Layna
✦ Dragon - Juniper
✦ Dragon - Karen
✦ Dragon - Sasha Starseed
✦ Dragon - Michaela
✦ Dragon - Alexis
✦ Dragon - Anna N.
✦ Dragon - Stephinity
✦ Dragon - Verdarluz

…and more discovered all the time…

Are you a Dragon?
Let us know at TheDragonKey.com

# SHIHAELEI
# BETELGEUSE REGION
# ORION SYSTEM

# SHIHAELEI - CHAPTER 1
# A SUDDEN DEPARTURE 熏

The air was cold inside the long terminal, sticking to the steel arches that framed the tunnel every few paces, and penetrating skin like a sharp blade.   Even with a swift pace, our bodies could not overcome the chill after leaving the dry heat of the Desert sun.   I winced as my father's hand clamped down on mine, his long strides almost dragging me along as we rushed toward the entry of our Pod.  Most of the other gates were closed already, and only a few people were left in the halls, boarding at the last-minute.

Reaching the large pressurized door that sealed the gate to our Pod, my father quickly swiped a small token in front of the security panel. A hydraulic burst hissed as the outer doors quickly retracted into the walls on either side of the entry, and a smaller door smoothly opened inward to our little spherical room.

Climbing inside, I looked around at the disheveled bed, sets of open books, and dirty platters scattered about the Pod. My stomach tightened reflexively, and I glanced at my father wearily.   He seemed not to notice, as he activated the interior control-panel and the small door moved back into place, seamlessly sealing with a gentle hiss.  The room was always perfect when we traveled, with everything precisely in position, organized with efficiency and ease in mind.   For even the slightest mess to persist, my father would have to be very distracted.  In this case, I thought nervously, this was either someone else's mess, or something was very wrong.

The subtle sinking feeling that I had been having all day was quickly becoming a free-fall, as my father almost frantically moved from sealing the door to rustling through books and pulling out maps. He constantly got up to look at the screen above the control-panel, which showed the status of the other Pods during the boarding process, and the expected time of departure.

"Faherin?" I tentatively asked, using the most formal and polite fatherly title I knew. "What is it?"

"Quiet." He said without so much as a glance in my direction. "Now is not the time." He continued shuffling through the pile on the floor until he found a book he was looking for, and quickly flipped through to a certain page with strange markings. He pulled over an old map he had set aside, and began looking at the page and map next to each other. His face darkened, his slightly reddish skin becoming saturated, and his eyes narrowed even further, brows knotted together.

Suddenly there was a jerk, and a quick beeping sound, indicating that our Pod was engaged with the Transport Ship's docking system. The usual loud mechanical hum died away quickly as our little sphere was secured in position. The whole room rocked slightly, as if floating on water, and old steel joints could be heard creaking as we were pulled away from the gate and into the air. A low whirring tone began and quickly rose to a piercing pitch, sending a wave of tingles through my body just before it fell silent, indicating the gravity field settling into place. At least on the outside, there would be absolute stillness and perfect silence for the rest of the journey.

It was not as cold in the Pod as it was in the terminal, but I wrapped myself in the heavy blanket on the bed anyway. The warmth settled in to my skin, but could not melt the icy lump in my belly. I tried to ignore my father's stress, already a thick fog in the small space, and focus instead on the display monitor.

The bright screen had a diagram of the Transport ship on the right side, showing a long rectangular craft with several hundred spherical Pods like the one we were in lining its sides. The pods were arranged in layers, and undulated slightly with the subtle curves of the ship. The left side showed a graphic rendering of the Planet's surface, with a few layers of atmosphere. A small moving circle left an illuminated trail from the surface to the outermost border of the atmospheric layers, indicating we were already entering the vacuum of space. There were also some basic digital gauges, the largest of which showed that we were gaining speed to enter orbit.

I stared at the screen, letting it wash away everything else, and watched the display change to show the entire Planet, and our orbital path. My father was now making elaborate notes and sketches, and rolling them up to slide them into mirrored cylinders, which he placed into a delivery rack embedded in the inner wall. After a while, he seemed to become exhausted, which made it easier for me to ignore his anxiousness.

It seemed like we hadn't stopped moving in days, and I found myself sinking deeper into the blankets. My feet hurt from all the walking, and the lump of ice in my stomach made me both hungry and nauseas at the same time. It was difficult to relax, but I began to realize that sleep didn't care about tension if you were tired enough.

A meter on the bottom of the display monitor slowly filled up with colored cells, and our path showed that we were already close to completing an orbit of the Planet. I wanted to stay awake for the jump, though my eyes seemed to be growing very heavy.

The meter was almost full, the charging of the superluminal systems almost complete. Things started to blur, and I struggled to stay conscious... Leaping in four degrees...three degrees... ...my eyes jolted open. I suddenly realized I had momentarily slipped into sleep. One degree left. The screen showed the ship's marker meeting the point where it entered orbit, and in that instant it flashed, brilliantly displaying hundreds of star patterns and constellations in rapid fire.

A moment later it returned to normal, showing the orbital rings of another Solar System, then zooming in on two Planets. Our ship marker was now entering orbit of one of these, discharging its residual energy.

Smiling to myself, a warm sense of satisfaction finally settled my stomach. I knew it would still be many hours before we reached the other Planet, our final destination. Thinking of all the wonderful people there, it seemed as if I simply slipped forward in time, and had already arrived...

:::  :::

An orange sun lit the terminal with a golden light, and other kids, my friends, were running around laughing. I ran with them, playing tag, dancing, and everything was perfect. There was an old man playing an instrument with many strings, his smile almost as warm as the large sun that was slipping out of the big bay windows in the ceiling. It seemed all the secrets of the Universe were contained in his voice, the words of his songs creating the very air around me, the melody setting the pace for every event in existence.

I was watching everything move with his music when my father appeared before me, grey and haggard. His eyes were dark and full of sadness, his face twisted in pain, and the color in the room began to fade as if it was being sucked out an airlock.     Everything suddenly began shaking, and I tried to grab something to steady myself, but all the things I reached for slipped through my fingers like mist.  I wanted to shout, and I opened my mouth, but the sound that came out sounded like metal rending and twisting in a horrible mechanical scream.

::: ⧗ :::

I sprang upward in the Pod bed, my father's terrified face in front of me, flickering in and out of existence with the lights of the Pod.  The metal rending sound continued, and the room lurched violently.   Looking up at the control panel, I saw that we were just entering an atmosphere before the screen flashed and went dark.

The room lurched again, and suddenly everything was shaking with bone-breaking force.  "What's happening!?" I heard myself shout, as I gripped the blankets and tried to steady myself on my hands and knees.

"We must be on another ship!"  My father shouted from somewhere across the room.  Another ship?  Meaning that we were not attached to the Transport ship any longer, and no longer in the peace and quiet of its Gravity field...   A smaller ship then, one without a Gravity drive...but what kind of ship?

Before I could even begin to conceive what was happening, the noises outside the Pod overtook my thoughts and drowned out the sounds of objects flying about the room. Explosions, blasts, roaring wind, and the piercing screams of engine machinery all flooded my ears at once.  It was madness, and all I could do was try to hold on and not get hit by flying books, canisters, and cups.

Eventually, what seemed like an eternity in chaos came to a slamming halt. The lights flickered once more before the room went completely dark. My heart pounded in my chest; I could feel the pressure of my blood behind my eyes, and through every muscle in my body. Several frantic breaths in silence gave way to the loud hiss of decompression, coming from the Pod door. It sounded distant, almost as if it was underwater, beneath a steady ringing sound that filled my head.

With a loud crack, blinding lights poured into the room. I thought I heard my father's voice screaming and saw him silhouetted against the lights for an instant, but then the light was on top of me. Pain gushed from my shoulders as strong claws clamped down on my arms, and I gasped for one last breath before a piercing pain bloomed in the side of my head, and I knew nothing more.

# $S$HIHAELEI - $C$HAPTER 2
# $C$APTIVITY 火

They were beautiful and endless. Without their constant companionship, flashing and dancing in the cloak of black velvet that seemed to be just out of reach, it would have been easy to be consumed in the vast seas of crust and lava. Sometimes they danced in my vision, moving with the thick pulse of my heartbeat as it pounded the blood into my arms and legs. Though I should have been slick with sweat, the many layers of sleeves that wrapped my body simply molded to my flesh like a second skin, absorbing my fluids and heat and returning just enough to keep my muscles warm. Connected to sensors and resistance cables that detected even the slightest motion, there was an incredible fluidity in moving such a massive vehicle.

Almost three-stories down, massive feet of steel crushed the young crust of shiny rock to a graphite powder. Canisters built into the sides of the powerful and complex hydraulics of the lower legs occasionally released jets of super-cooled gasses into the ground as sensors detected the depth and integrity of the solid crust. Kneeling down for a moment, supported by one of the massive titanium shields that served as kneecaps, I drove a massive hand into a semi-molten soft spot of the ground.

My display cascaded with geometric and physical data projected from a spherical chunk of crystallized steel I could "see" under the ground. Noting some of the rough knobs on one side of its form, illuminated in my virtual screen as chaotic three-dimensional grids of light, I slammed my other arm under the surface of the dried lava and used both hands to begin pulling out the meteorite.

Leaning back in my body-suit in the cockpit, the exoskeleton's anatomy reacted instantly, shifting its weight backward over the kneeling leg, and I jerked my outstretched hands back toward my chest. The resistance my robotic arms felt was echoed in the cables holding my fleshy arms in place, but the quick movement was enough to crack a surface plate that was covering over part of the metallic sphere in the ground.

Rocking forward for a moment, I leaned back again, pulling hard with my hands and pushing down with my left foot that was flat on the surface. The lava plate burst off, floating upward swiftly, then gradually slowing in the low gravity, as I rolled all the way back into standing position. The meteorite in my mechanical hands was almost ten feet thick, yet I hefted it easily.

Thousands of spectral highlights of all colors danced across its surface, as complicated crystalline patterns were revealed in the shifting light of the distant sun. With no atmosphere, the great central star of this planetary system could not overpower the brilliant light of thousands of other stars in the dark sky, so they danced together in reflected glory.

Forcibly pulling my eyes away, I sent the meteorite soaring and bounding across the dried lava-field with an easy toss. It was caught in a large wire net, where other, smaller mech-suits were being used to gather the crystals and load them into large mobile containers.

A few times during the day, large transport ships would arrive and pick up the containers, gathering several from different stations spread far apart on this side of the moon. Then, they would carry these containers to the massive black Mothership, always hovering over the same area many leagues away, visible above the horizon.

Thousands upon thousands of amber lights covered its surface, curving downward like the crescent of a black moon. The lights flickered and wavered in the ripples of rising heat so that they looked like the campfires of a distant army in another Age. They were indeed the fires of an army, for behind those lights an entire civilization of cruelty and malice dwelt.

This place was their forge, and I was an anvil.

I glanced over at the guards in their smaller mechs. They moved like birds, riding in small bubbles of glass and steel, gracefully running on legs that bent backwards. Clearly built for mobility and speed, they had no problem guarding the miners with the massive missile and laser batteries mounted on the sides of their cockpits. A moment longer, and they would have been turning toward me if I didn't start scanning the surface again for meteorite impacts.

This is how it went, every single day. This was life, lived through a giant, humanoid mechanical vehicle that at times felt more like my body than my own flesh, blood and bone. Being out in the fields of endless fire, and the vast emptiness of the stars above, was comforting at times, at least compared to the alternatives. I let my mind drift away for a moment, staring at one of my favorite constellations. Those stars often served as a perfect escape route from the dark roads of thought that crisscrossed the back of my awareness. A few twinkles and time stretched out to a thin whisper; everything retreating into the velvet of the void.

A streak of light shot forth from the heart of that emptiness, as a small reminder that time was indeed flowing along, and massive chunks of metal were still plummeting to the surface of this nightmarish place. Another one followed it, from the same spot in my constellation; then another, and another...that seemed to curve upward at the last moment. Wait. They were all curving the same way. In an instant, it was as if a fleet of thirty shooting stars cascaded out of that constellation, turned, and vanished into another.

As if they had transported themselves straight into my bloodstream, I felt as though sparks of light were coursing through my entire body. My hair stood on end, and my skin felt like it was on fire. I closed my eyes for a moment, and symbols flooded my vision. Fractal geometries blurred into vibrant memories and back again.

My mother, in white robes, speaking before a massive hall of people... My father, leading me down a long hall with windows overlooking a white planet from a very high orbit... Sitting next to an old man playing songs and telling stories about the universe... People looking at me strangely, almost fearfully, and me winking at them... Giant caves opening out into endless white desert... Armored men standing around my mother, guarding her... Riding in the transport pod with my father...

Jolted back into awareness of my body, I suddenly realized where I was, and how I had gotten here. There were huge gaps of darkness, but I remembered hearing my father's shouts and everything going wrong...what must have been almost 20 Solar Cycles ago on my home planet... My home planet...

Almost as if on cue, a high-pitched ringing sound pierced my ears. Cringing as a shiver ran down my spine, I instinctively turned back towards the barracks and headed "home." I watched myself go through the motions, considering just how normal this whole process had become. It was not the first time I noticed "the program," but this time was very different. With a glance toward the Mothership, I could see that the Planet this moon orbited was just beginning to rise on the horizon. We were herded like gears in some angry clock, sharply snapping out the measure of each moment.

After a decent march, I reached the barracks with the rest of the mining group. Each of us walked our mechs up to our specific loading docks, and stepped onto the plates that would magnetically seal our steel bodies to the dock housing. A few guard-birds bounded by, scanning for damage to our vehicles as airlocks hissed and pressure was released from our mechs' hydraulic systems.

I held my breath. If they noticed any damage, I would not eat until I had finished the repairs myself in one of the big hangar bays. Sometimes this was an opportunity to make some "extra" modifications, and install a few "specialty" items to the cockpit or mech systems, but today I felt like I could have eaten that last meteorite, and was eager to get into the mess hall. It would also be my only chance to share what I had seen. Pointless and futile as telling my slave brothers might be, my heart still pounded with the intensity of the vision, my blood flooding with the energy of each moment of the memory.

A quick buzzer sound signaled the airlock was in place, and the cockpit of my mech opened in sync with several layers of retracting doors in the barracks. The restrainments of my interior suit released simultaneously, and I wiggled my arms and legs out from the rubbery sleeves and unbuckled the straps and support pads wrapped around my waist. Climbing out of the cockpit, I stepped onto legs that were wobbly for a moment adjusting to my "slightly" different body, and felt as though I just lost a few thousand pounds. Some of the mining work involved very heavy lifting, and even walking around in the mech required a great deal more strength than my flesh needed.

As I regained my balance, I attempted to keep my body from breaking into a run, moderating each footstep and keeping my expressions under control. A few Guards lined the halls, watching the mining groups heading back to their cells. Narrow, angry eyes with a yellow glow and black slits quickly scanned each of us for signs of "damage." Leaning back against the wall in their black and red lacquered armor, it was obvious that most of them disdained having to complete this duty, and not just from impatient feet or the occasional tail slap. Nostrils on many of their scaly lizard muzzles flared every time we passed, as if we could possibly have a worse stench than their stinking hides.

I used a few brief glances to memorize, for the ten-thousandth time, some of the possible vulnerable spots in their armor. Always polished, the scattered interlocking plates on their bodies were like insect exoskeletons, hard as crystallized steel, but not without chinks and a few visible buckles and straps. There were definitely a few weak points in the ribbed support webbing, where it stretched around areas of ribs, arms, and legs to hold the plates tightly in position. They wore it larger than needed, as occasionally some of them seemed to go through some kind of strange growth spurts. I only took note because it meant that some of us might fit in that armor, though almost all of us non-lizards had near to a foot or more of height over our common slave drivers...though their leaders could be much bigger.

Turning down the next hallway, I came to my "living quarters," a few cells down. Everything in each area of the barracks was as close as possible to everything else that area needed. Short walks meant longer work hours, and more work for us meant more of whatever the lizards wanted. There were few lights, just a couple dim white bars in the corners of the hallway ceiling. The only thing they illuminated was dirty graphite walls, greasy grated floors, and metal bar grids on cell doors. Darkness would have been preferable.

I quickly stripped out of my tight and stretchy bodysuit, designed for working in the Mech, hit a button on the wall that blasted me with steam, and then put on a fairly clean pair of my loose "living clothes," which were barely more than cloth folded and cut into smocks and loose pants. That's about as complicated as things got. Living, and working. If we were lucky, eating decently might be added to that equation.

When I eventually stepped into the dining area, it was almost a relief to be in the brightness of the sterile white space. Everything was white, and the lighting had an almost bluish tint that seemed to make the room all the more vivid. I walked in silence at the back of a line of miners, but noticed when my few friends came out of the serving area and made their way to our usual table.

I wasn't sure what friends meant, in our situation, and we certainly didn't see each other or communicate often. Yet we ate together, and sometimes we talked when there were only a few Guards around, or those that remained dozed on duty. They were all I had, and it felt good to think of them as friends. I was honored to think of them as friends.

Haggan, as we called him, was almost the last of our group to make his way over to the table. I watched his hulking body movements from the line, gracefully stepping between two other tables to come around to one of the far side seats. His fluidity of movement always struck me, though it was not much different than the grace that I experienced inside the gigantic Mech suit. He spoke no language we could understand, and spoke very little at all, yet there was an awareness about him that seemed to say everything we needed to know.

His skin was a reddish brown, thick and muscular, with a mane of dark red hair around his neck and shoulders, hanging low down his chest, along with a thick beard. His deep-set eyes gleamed like dark pools within the squared structure of his lighter skinned face and jaw, with two larger bottom incisors which subtly emerged over his upper lip. There was a catlike quality to his features, but not enough to overwhelm his manhood.

I received several servings of food onto a white square tray, and went to sit. Everyone seemed to feign intent focus on eating, though the chunky mush was neither tasty nor colorful. It was filling, however, and our bodies desperately needed the nutrients after another long day of intense physical labor.

By the time we each had put down a few servings, there was only one guard left, his body slumped back against the wall, and his scaled snout hung limply on his chest, nostrils flaring in his dozing snorts. I looked over at Kritos, a Shihaeleian brother of the same planet I came from, and spoke very quietly. "I saw something today..." He looked up at me quickly, eyes intense and hopeful. "From a constellation-"

"Ships!" he whispered fiercely. " I saw them too; we're not supposed to be here!"

"Shh..." I said, "I know...I know. I remembered..."

Haggan looked at us both with wide eyes, and a sharp pain bloomed above my left temple. The memories of my childhood had opened some new space in my head, but the old mental constructs still seemed to be resisting my new awareness. In the empty places in my mind, I was dimly aware of the dark memories and intense torturous physical programming that had attempted to wipe out all traces of my real life and true origins.

One of the rare blue-skinned beings in the barracks, Jassan often joined our table, and now he was staring off into space intently. He often did that also, and said he could hear things, when he said anything at all. Though Jassan was also a different species, with his bluish skin and large deep eyes that could swallow planets, he spoke our native tongue perfectly. It was rare for him to say more than a few words, however, as he communicated much more quickly with a glance and slight expressions, which somehow seemed to carry whole monologues of information.

"I remembered too..." said Kritos, the fire still blazing in his eyes. "We gotta get out of here."
I nodded, and looked over at Haggan. He seemed to take in my thoughts, then frowned, brow furrowing. After a moment, he seemed to resolve something in himself, and nodded with intensity.

Smiling slightly, with a nod in return, my gaze shifted to Jassan. He looked up at me instantly, his eyes piercing my Soul. He seemed to look through me, through time itself, and was deeply inspecting everything he saw there. I maintained my gaze, and let the images I had seen in my flashes of memory flow through my mind again. My smile returned at thoughts of my parents, and this brought warmth to Jassan's face as well. He nodded once with solid affirmation, then looked away in thought.

I wasn't sure how he did it exactly, but beyond viewing my memories, I knew he was reviewing all the possibilities for how we might escape, and that was exactly where my thoughts went next. Kritos seemed to be lost in strategic calculations as well, while Haggan got up to get more food.

Though I knew very little of these "friends," I trusted them completely. They were there, every day, and we supported each other in what small ways were possible. Whether it was hiding bits of extra food when someone's Mech got damaged and they were locked away for days repairing it, or distracting a guard just long enough for one of us to take a breather, we were constantly watching each others backs.

We often passed each other info about new technology shipment arrivals that we aided in unloading or storing, so we could identify crates in the repair docks to install "custom additions" to our suits when we had the opportunity. It was dangerous, but these subtle modifications provided the marginal comfort that made our daily grind bearable, and also afforded additional protection to enable us to stretch beyond the rules when necessary without getting ourselves killed. From systems for cockpit temperature regulation to high-performance hydraulic additions, audio insulation to retractable thrusters, we made many special adjustments to our exoskeletons over the long solar cycles of our captivity.

To apply these adjustments to an outright offensive strategy was far more complicated and difficult, and it was many days before we began to formulate an effective plan of action. It emerged from dreams and scattered inspiration, noticed only through the contrast of such thoughts from the drab, hopeless thought patterns of living as a slave.

The strategy was a feeling, a space where energy and life seemed to pour forth from an ancient crevice within. It quickly and suddenly illuminated spaces and times of shared confusion, while forming new pipelines of translation in our unspoken communication with each other. It was as if solving the riddle of our freedom was a process of engaging the feedback patterns of ease, agreement, and complete understanding amidst the persistent waves of doubt and terror that threatened to consume our minds.

# $\text{S}$HIHAELEI - $\text{C}$HAPTER 3
# $\text{H}$ACKERS 水

The communications outpost was a small structure about twice the height of our Mech suits, located not far from the barracks. It had a series of circular rings with spherical pods suspended in the centers angled in different directions around the upper areas of the tower. The lower section was simply a black steel box covered in cable lines and conduits, about 20 feet cubed. There was a small access station in the front for maintenance, like a protected porch for smaller Guard vehicles to stand on, or for larger engineering crews to disembark.

It was not heavily guarded, considering it was not much more than a relay station. The only reptilian Mechs about were Guarding the mining detail, which was not much more than the four of us today. Knowing the simple patterns that their lizard brains worked with, it didn't take a Gravitation Engineer to figure that Kritos's plan could actually work. The trick was not getting ourselves killed in the process.

He was already making his way over to the far side of the lava field, looking for meteorites just over a low crater wall. Having not fully scoured that area previously, the Guard watching him seemed to be fine with him going that far, but followed not far behind anyway. Jassan and I, on either side of the com outpost, tried to keep from glancing too often in his direction, and focused instead on finding a few smaller balls of crystallized metal.

It wasn't long before we heard a loud warning horn and looked to see Kritos's Guard bird tumbling backwards on the lava field, bouncing long distances in the low gravity. A large chunk of meteorite was spinning off into space, having slammed into the small Mech after what must have been a truly epic throw by my Shihaeleian brother. The other Guards were now bounding across the lava field, shooting plasma blasts at Kritos's Mech as he began to run hard in the other direction.

Quickly glancing about to make sure there were no other Guards or Patrol Ships in range, Jassan and I ran toward the com outpost. He got there first, ducking into the low porch, and pulling open the access panel door. Extending his Mech's wrist, a small panel flipped open and a network key telescoped out. Plugging perfectly into the rotary port, it began to spin, and Jassan looked over at me with what I could only imagine was a thick grin inside his cockpit.

Cringing at each blast that tore into Kritos's Mech, I made a motion for Jassan to hurry, and he opened his other robotic hand with a helpless gesture. Then Kritos went down, knocked to the ground by a Guard's missile blast, and I found myself leaping in his direction. Halfway to the low crater wall, I glanced back to find Jassan closing the access panel door, and hurrying after me.

Even at a full run, the Mechs were not that fast. It was the only frustrating movement, since the tension cables constantly kept you from trying to move the vehicle any faster than it was capable of going. I almost tested the rockets I had secretly built into part of the back ventilation paneling during my last repair session, but I didn't dare waste the opportunity to use them in the future, and likely sentence myself to death at the same time.

By the time I reached my brother, his suit was heavily damaged, and the Guards were practically on top of him, shooting him at the slightest movement. "WAIT! STOP!" I shouted through the communications system, "I'll take care of this! I'll get him out of here! No more trouble, I promise!" I carefully stepped between the small Mechs, and shielded Kritos's Mech with my own. "I'll get him out of here… No more trouble…"

I knelt down, rolling his Mech over onto its back, then worked to get him standing upright again, while supporting him from under one blackened arm. By the time I had him limping forward, Jassan showed up, and got underneath his other arm. The snarling Guards bounded after us, keeping their guns aimed at our backs all the way to the barracks.

Yet as we walked, Jassan transmitted all the data he had downloaded from the com system into our suits' backup storage. Though it would be a hard couple of days for Kristos, repairing his Mech and starving, we knew his sacrifice was worth it. He knew, we had won today. For the first time, we had beaten them.

# SHIHAELEI - CHAPTER 4
## ESCAPE 隘

The distant sun sparkled across the sphere, illuminating dancing rainbows in overlapping circles that bubbled on the surface. Fitting, that this beautiful fallen star should be my last harvest. If those wishes my Mother once spoke of were true, this meteorite would never reach the freighters.

I almost felt her warmth around me for a moment, wrapping me in brilliant bliss as if it were a blanket, her shimmering eyes smiling down at me. Those eyes were stars now, watchful and steady, counting down the moments as they imperceptibly drifted across the sky.

We each worked within a tight area today, our four Mechs positioned within an exact arc curving across the dark lava field. Hanging like a dark cloud, the mothership felt closer today, its orange lights seeming to glare menacingly down at the forsaken moon. The Guards seemed occupied with pouncing around and snarling at each other, headless steel birds determined to threaten each other to death. In slow motion, the small fleet of Patrol ships came over the distant horizon, preparing to do a final sweep over our positions before heading back to the mothership. Four of them…perfect.

Watching them from the corner of my eye, my mind instinctively went over the plan again. I still didn't understand how Jassan was able to create a program using the Draconian code language, but I trusted him. His description of the "realm of Blue Crystal Fire" seemed to push away the knots in my stomach, and I found myself drifting into a space of endless blue cascades of perfect geometries and rippling storms of light. "Here", he said, "all language emerges…all translations are the same."

In that moment, as his words finished drifting through my memory, I felt that strange gap between logic and the feeling of Truth. I hoped he was right, but more than hope, something in me Trusted in his Truth. It was like a light piercing through the darkness. All I had right then, was this feeling, a feeling which seemed to peel back everything around me and reveal one powerful rising sensation: the Patrol ship was approaching right behind me.

Almost without thought, mostly quelling my spiky nerves, I squatted slowly, reached over to my right sidewall controls and slid open a small panel. The ground began to rumble through my suit and into my body in resonance to the electromagnetic vibrations pulsing from the bottom of the approaching ship. The scanning lights swept over me as the front passed about 50 feet overhead, shaped like the head of a massive beetle. I waited one more breath, glanced at that constellation which sparked my memories of another time, another life…then drove my legs against the ground as hard as I could.

The moment my Mech's feet leapt from the cracked surface, I slammed my hand against a small knob in the panel I opened, and was jolted by the immediate g-force of the rockets kicking in on my back. Fighting the gravity pulling me down inside the cockpit as my Mech was driven upward with immense force, I held my arms up and aimed for the docking rails that straddled the main fuselage of the Patrol ship above me.

A split second later they slammed into my steel palms, my hand reflexively closing like a vice grip as the sensation transmitted to my gloves. At 300 feet long, I hit the bottom of the big beetle ship slightly off center to the rear, and it tilted forward violently from my momentum. As soon as my rockets gave out in another second, the Patrol ship's thrusters would be propelling it toward the surface of the moon...not good.

Releasing one hand while I still had the vertical support of my thrust, I ripped off the central paneling on the fuselage of the ship just above my head. Exactly where Kritos said it would be, there was an access port just like the one on the Com outpost.

Rockets sputtering out behind me, I started to drift down and swing backwards as the direction of acceleration shifted, and I prayed the ship would autocorrect it's course as we began swiftly descending. I tightened my grip with my left hand and flexed my augmented muscle, bringing my Mech body close enough to open my right wrist and slide my rotary key into the port.

It clicked in just as the Patrol ship started to automatically reorient its pitch to the horizon line after diving briefly, and I initiated the virus upload.

My heart pounded and I felt soaked with my own sweat, though this was no workout. Alternate plans flashed through my head in a blur, spinning out scenarios, options, and actions to take if this failed to work. A single second seemed to stretch out through Eternity, leaving me anxiously waiting at the crossroads of life and death, good and evil, freedom and slavery.

With a gentle hiss, the tension cables securing my arms disengaged. My display flickered and shifted to show navigation systems and autopilot route settings. Sounds crackled through my communications relay, resolving into muffled voices shouting. Leaning forward, I frantically looked out my cockpit to the right. The shouting became laughter, just as I saw the other Patrol ships. Each of them had what looked like a big armored beast hanging off the bottom, and they were all on course towards the mothership.

I slid my arms out from the tension sleeves as I realized my Mech was locked in position, holding on to the Patrol ship. I tested a few commands in the navigation system on my display. All of the ship's functions were under my control, and it appeared that the only system that was disabled by the viral program was communications. Yet through some backdoor function Jassan had enabled, he, Haggan, Kritos and I could all hear each other, and we began coordinating our approach.

:::

The putrid amber glow of the orange lights spread further apart, and the gargantuan black surface transformed from an impenetrable wall into a maze of conduits, weapons batteries, and docking bays. Even from a thousand paces, the curvature of the dome-shaped Mothership had all but vanished, and its darkness seemed to consume everything in sight.

Still set to navigate on autopilot, continuing its original course, the Patrol ship my Mech hung from headed straight toward one of the gaping docking bays. I took a deep breath, letting the tension in my stomach release slightly, but could not help a subtle shaking that took over my body. Was it fear? Anticipation? Excitement? I wasn't sure, but there was nothing to do but let it flow through me.

I closed my eyes for a moment and let myself go into the feeling, and the shaking immediately became more intense, each wave become stronger and larger, jerking my body about until I felt like sparks of light flooded my veins. At that moment, my shaking stopped.

My eyes popped open, and the black surface exploded into flashing light. Blinding strobes surrounded the outside of the docking bay, which lit up with a pale white flood of light. It was immediately crawling with black armored lizards forming ranks and firing plasma blasts in my direction. In a moment, I would either be pulverized, or thanking the stars I was facing unseasoned guards. With the flash of alarm strobes, I couldn't tell which was more likely.

Either way, the bay was approaching very quickly, and without thought I shut down the autopilot and opened up to full thrust. At the same time as the thrusters kicked in and launched the Patrol ship forward, swinging my Mech hanging off the bottom backwards. I directed the nose of the Patrol ship downward and to the right, rolling it onto its left side slightly to form a shield. Letting momentum carry the motion forward, I disengaged from the ship controls and slid my arms back into my Mech's tension sleeves.

They responded, and I was jerked back into the position of hanging on to the ship's bottom guide-rails that were quickly tilting sideways. I swung my Mech body back forward again to brace my feet on the approaching edge of the docking port. An instant later the front of the ship slammed into the floor of the bay as it entered, continuing to accelerate. Piercing the atmospheric field, I could suddenly hear the screaming sound of the metal sliding and the blast of alarm horns, even from inside my sealed cockpit. The scraping scream shifted quickly to a torrential crunching roar as the ship slid sideways and slammed into other objects in the bay, crushing everything in its path.

Letting the ship drag me inside, I hooked my Mech's foot on one of the bay floor's catchment cables, and gave a last twisting shove with both arms on the rails of the big Patrol ship, and let it go. Tumbling down on one of my kneeguards, my Mech slid a few feet further in. The ship continued careening across the huge area like a huge black wave of metal, sliding on its side until it slammed with a deafening crash into the back wall.

Using the shock of the guards that managed to avoid being smeared across the floor to my advantage, I got up and lumbered towards them as quickly as I could. Grabbing one of the large toolboxes to the side of the bay, I threw it like a meteorite, plastering three of the lizards to the far wall.

Another close-by assailant had begun to shoot my Mech frantically, so I reached down my huge Mech arm and crushed him with my free hand. The stillness that had somehow consumed me like candlelight was being ignited into a raging fire storm, as all my anger and hatred began to surface. I threw the gore in my hand at some of the other guards, who were beginning to recover and fire their weapons.

I ripped a railing section off a raised work area, and used it like a sword. The twenty-foot long metal pipes crushed their armored bodies like bugs, as I charged through their blasts swinging viciously in my giant death machine. Gritting my teeth and roaring, I slammed fists as large as their bodies into floors and walls, leaving behind insect shells and pools of dark blood.

Everything faded into blistering destruction, as I delivered carnage to wave after wave of lizards. Plasma shots tore into my robotic arms and legs, and many of my shielding plates fell to the bay floor in ruins. Even these battered pieces of my suit became weapons, thrown across the space to sever bodies, and slammed down like a tray to the crunch of beetles.

I screamed as anger ripped through me, and killed as if I could kill the pain inside me.  They were the darkness taking my father away from me; they were the fear in my mother's eyes.  They were the sadness in Jassan's gaze, the coldness in Kritos, and the anger in Haggan.  They had eaten away my life like parasites, and now they faced their exterminator.  Now, at last, they faced Judgment.

One of them had run around behind me in my charge to the back of the bay, and before his blasts could tear open my hydraulics, I turned and swatted, sending his body flying through the magnetic atmosphere field of the bay entry.  The glow of the red moon below caught and held my eyes, and my Mission suddenly pierced through the fire of my rage.  It came like a firm hand on my shoulder, and a cooling wind on my face.  I became aware of my breath again, and everything came back into focus.

Turning back to the area at the back of the bay that wasn't filled with flaming wreckage from the Patrol ship, I saw an access panel next to one of the entry portals that had swarmed with guards only moments before.  Now only corpses littered the walkway, though it wouldn't remain that way for long with the alarm horns still blaring.  Ignoring the carnage, I walked to the panel and ripped open the door.  Seeing the rotary port, I opened my wrist and slid in my network key.

As it began to spin, I noticed that I could hear nothing from my brothers over our Com system.  My heart began to pound as the system display appeared in my vision.  With a deep breath, I focused on the data structure and tried to remember what Jassan had told me.  *"Move backwards,"* he seemed to say into my mind.  *"Everything they do moves forward in a simple pattern, a simple chain… follow this chain back, and you will find its origin."*

Somehow, even as his words touched my head, I was already speeding through layers and layers of data, following what appeared to be a tree of commands that systematically broke apart and came together in repeating forms. What almost distracted me from this process was the clear awareness that Jassan had never actually said those words to me at all. It didn't matter. I heard him now.

In moments, I began to see a different pattern, a directory tree that expanded in two primary directions, like a pillar extending through the center of millions of spiderwebs. *"There,"* Jassan said, clearly speaking to me inside my own head somehow, *"upload it now, into the Core."*

Initiating the command, I watched as the viral program packets began to populate this central directory, and ripple through the data structure. An instant later, the alarm horns fell silent, and I knew the program had taken hold. It worked!

The virus would be rolling through the whole Mothership's networks, disabling communications and shutting off alarms and automated security lockdowns.

Manually disengaging my suit's tension cables, I depressurized the cockpit. Pulling out of my Mech's restraining straps and rubbery sleeves for the last time, I jumped from the cockpit to the entry walkway. I grabbed the nearest plasma gun and stepped between the sickening piles of gore toward the portal.

A sudden hissing sound made me instinctively leap over and press myself against the wall. Sure enough, a snarl of shock and anger proceeded a lone guard running in to see what had happened. Before he could grasp what he saw, the side of his head was torn apart by a torrent of plasma from my blaster, and the portal door hissed shut behind him.

I was suddenly reminded of the existence of my own heart pounding, and my bound up muscles relaxed as gratitude flushed through me. Here was an unexpected gift. Quickly moving to the corpse, I removed his armor as quickly as possible. My habitual inspections had paid off, and I managed to strap into the slick black and red plate armor in minutes. It fit perfectly, and I almost laughed.

Taking the swords and other nasty blades, I fitted them around my form in a way I had seen the more seasoned guards use, giving me easy access to any of them. The one longer curving blade went on my hip, tilted almost horizontally and slid around on my waist belt toward my lower back to stay clear of my arms and legs while running. The shorter blades were strapped in a curved V down my upper back, their hilts sticking up above my shoulders. A smaller three-pronged blade was sheathed on my opposite hip, and a throwing dagger was strapped to the outside of each calf plate.

One of the open-faced helms lay on the ground nearby, and I considered putting it on. Without the long lizard snout, there was no mistaking my true form. Still, it might add to the confusion or work to my advantage if approached from behind, so I slid it on and buckled the strap under my chin. It fit tightly around my forehead, then flared out a bit to cover my jaw and the back of my neck. A bit awkward, and the smell was almost unbearable, but it would have to do.

I jumped up and headed toward the door, when I suddenly heard the voices of my brothers. Stopping for a moment, about to glance around, I realized they were coming through the helmet's Com system. "Ki'Shen, in!" I responded with excitement.

*"Stop there, that channel Jassan!"* I heard Kritos's voice chime in quickly across the coms. He must have been scanning across their channels for communication from the rest of us.

"Haggan?" I asked.

*"Not yet,"* Kritos replied.

Jassan's voice came through, tight, fast, and precise, *"Enter the main corridor, and keep heading left and down. We'll meet at the docked freighter."*

"On it," I responded, and ran through the entry portal.

As it closed behind me, I scanned both directions for sounds and signs of guards.  I heard some distant jabbering down the hall to the right, and nearly breathed a sigh of relief.  Instead, I didn't breathe at all, and headed to the left as quietly as possible.

Once I could see around the next bend ahead, I sprinted forward at full speed, rolling my feet to keep the sound of my steps as soft as possible.  The hallways were only slightly different here than in the prison mining barracks down on the moon.  Snakes of black piping and cables ran along the ceiling, splitting off at regular intervals to enter the sidewalls.  The floor was hard steel grating with a small space underneath to catch refuse falling through, which all looked like it was slick with black oil, and encrusted with yellow sulfur in places.  Pale light from two ceiling panels running along the tops of the walls provided the same old cold light, but here the walls were supposed to be white.

Approaching a T-junction in the hall, I slowed quickly on the balls of my feet.  My head kept impulsively turning to glance back the way I came, as I crept up with my back against the right side wall and shuffled my way to the corner. The left turn of the hall across from me opened up only a few paces and then turned down a stairwell.

I held my breath again, and concentrated on relaxing my heartbeat. There was silence. Leaning my head very slowly toward the corner, I let one eye slip around the edge. There were two guards, standing about ten paces down the hall, guarding another hall entry, but they were not facing my direction.

Hearing the crackle of a Com suddenly bursting with loud commands, my head jerked back, and I immediately walked swiftly and quietly across the hall, keeping my back to the guards as I entered their line of sight. Turning quickly the moment I reached the stairs, I nearly ran down them, and held my Plasma blaster ready.

On my way down, I could hear booted footsteps running closer, and then receding down the hallway I had come from. I almost grinned, but couldn't help thinking about the guards' Com unit. Apparently some of their communications were still functioning even with the virus engaged, but perhaps only the short-range local networks. If their communications and security systems were fully online, these halls would already be swarming with hundreds of lizards.

At that moment two guards came around the corner at the bottom of the stairs, heading straight towards me as fast as their springy legs could carry them. At first they saw another guard in armor coming down, but then plasma blasts from my rifle tore into their faces, and the hard truth seemed to dawn in their gaping eyes.

So much for the quiet way...

In a few bounds I was at the bottom of the stairwell, dodging twitching arms and legs, as a snarling shout boomed down the hall toward me. It was accompanied by a few blinding blasts from a plasma rifle, so I leaped into an alcove on the right, in front of a door the two brain-dead carcasses had come from. Through square window I could see a room running parallel to the hall, where it looked like a few unarmored lizards were scrambling to get suited up.

*No need for that*, I thought, and punched the door button. By the time the door slid open from a hydraulic burst, one of the half-dressed lizards received a large melted hole in his chest, and I almost lost my own head to a blast that took out some of the conduit behind me. I dove into the room toward a large storage container, tucking into a somersault as I hit the ground. Rolling back to a kneeling position, I caught sight of the guard blasting at me coming in at the end of the room. Firing a few quick shots, I heard a squeal of pain.

The other dressing lizard had his pants on and was now leaping toward me with fangs and claws bared in a nasty display of deadly force. I rolled back to kick upward, slamming my boot against his chest and sending him flying against the wall behind me. En-route, his frantic slashing of claws drew blood on the exposed flesh of the top inside of my left elbow, and knocked my gun from my hands.

Without thought, I clenched my teeth, rolled upright, and pulled one of the shorter curved blades from my back. He had come down the wall to land on his head on the floor, and very quickly rolled his feed back to the ground and was swiping a clawed foot at my face in a snarling reverse roundhouse. My blade swept up and to the right, meeting his foot as it came down toward my face, and I sliced straight through it. Turning my face quickly as the blood spattered on my helmet, I leapt forward and drove the blade straight into his neck in his moment of shock, and he fell backwards against the wall again.

In disgust at his gurgles of pain, I tore the blade free and grabbed the plasma gun from the ground where I had dropped it, and scanned the room again. Still hearing moans further down the room, I crept low along bunks on the left side, watching for any movement.

Sure enough, a moment later the wounded guard was rising warily, eyes flickering around my side of the room. I aimed carefully from my hiding place behind another of the storage boxes, and shot him in the muzzle.

Jumping up, I ran the rest of the way through the room and took the door at the other side to get back into the hallway. With a quick glance in both directions, I ran on to the right, soon coming to another T-junction just like the one on the level above.

Creeping to the corner, I checked the hall to the right again, but this time there were no guards present. Crossing the hall, I nearly jumped down the stairwell, leaping two to three steps at a time. The next hall below being empty, I ran full speed, and almost ran right into a guard coming out of a door further down the hall.

Without slowing, I drew the larger sword at my waist as I ran past him. As he jolted around in surprise, I skidded to a stop in a sideways squat, and leapt back towards him with an angled slash that slit into his neck under the jaw. It nearly took his head off, but I barely noticed as I landed, turned, and continued running to the next T-junction.

As my body surged with energy and renewed excitement that I was "winning," I didn't even slow down to check the hall, but instead bolted to the left and headed down the next flight of stairs. Everything seemed to fly by in a blur, hallway after hallway, always the same design, same pattern, same program.

Then suddenly I came to a different junction, where there was no stairwell. Instead, there were a series of large hexagonal pressure gates in the left wall, with large windows in between that looked out at the conduit lines on the side of a large freighter ship. I made it.

The ship was docked, and I ran over to one of the data panels next to the nearest pressure gate. It showed the ship's energy storage and payload information, and had access buttons for entry. As I tapped the screen, each of the pressure gates hissed and opened to give access to the interior of the freighter.

Sudden movement further down the hall caught my eye, so I spun, raising my plasma gun to end the confrontation quickly. Something made me pause, however, and in a second I realized the guard was way too large for his armor, and his orange furred body was not lizard-like at all. Haggan pulled off the helmet shading his face in the cold light of the docking hall, and I laughed in relief. I quickly pulled off my own helm to make sure he saw me clearly.

His big beastly smile never looked so charming.

Then a door at the end of the hall opened, and Jassan stepped into the hall. In the same moment, a side-access door opened, and Kritos sauntered in. They both looked at me and at Haggan in surprise, then grinned and shouted with joy. "Ha! We showed those stinky greaseballs where we come from!" Kritos roared with excitement on the edge of rage, and I felt exactly the same way.

"Let's get out of here," I said, becoming serious in my focus again, knowing that we were still far from victory. I jogged into the freighter and headed toward where I thought the command deck would be. "Kritos," I yelled back, "get us disengaged. Jassan, check the energy core levels, and Haggan, check on the food and other supplies." They were already on it before I closed my mouth. We were in sync.

Locating the command deck and the manual flight control seat, I sat down and looked over the system. It was exactly like the navigation controls for the patrol ship, and the supplemental Mech controls for running loading cranes and the small freight transports.

The command deck had huge windows with triangular crossbands reinforcing them, where you could clearly see a few angles out each of the sides of the ship, and most of the forward view. From where they wrapped around the edge of the floor in the front, you could see the waves of heat rippling over the surface of the black lava fields below. One of the volcanic mountains in the distance was erupting, ejecting brilliant orange chunks of molten metal into space. It glittered like sparks of sunlight as it seemed to hover, then it would darken, and slowly drift back down onto the surface many thousands of paces away.

It would have been beautiful, if it wasn't such a place of pain and terror.

The main engines suddenly rumbled to life, as Jassan activated them. Kritos ran onto the command deck saying, "We're clear." Without waiting another moment, I grabbed the thrust lever and slid it upward gently.

Jerking with the sudden burst, the ship began to drift forward, and I lightly shifted the guidance control pads to the right to activate the side thrusters, moving us away from docking port of the mothership.

# SHIHAELEI - CHAPTER 5
## RESCUE 濟

Far ahead on the moon below, the dim amber lights of the barracks were barely visible. Using the trajectory monitor, I lined up the ship's angle and pushed the thrusters as far as I dared. A freighter leaving the mothership at this moment of chaos would hardly be noticed, as long as it wasn't blasting away at full speed. Thankfully some part of me was surfacing bits of flight training from childhood, and the controls here were similar to others I had seen my captors operate, and other mining vehicles I'd used over the years.

Kritos and Haggan went to the rarely used weapons batteries on either side of the ship, just in case we encountered any trouble. Jassan went on calculating energy supplies to determine if we could make a jump.

Within a few minutes we were on approach to the barracks, so I initiated some of the reverse engines and cut the forward thrusters. I used the guidance pads to shift the ship into position as if we were going to land in the loading area, and held that trajectory right until the last moment.

Then, instead of hitting full reverse and stopping the ship to lower it to the ground, I slammed the thrust lever forward for a split second to give us a violent burst forward. Pulling it back again, I shifted the ship to the left to bring us over to the main-entry side of the barracks.

I heard Kritos running over to the secondary battery on the right side of the ship, and as I began to lower the ship into docking position with the entry, I heard the chugging cry of the freighter's massive blasters and saw a couple of the guard towers on the barracks exploding into molten stumps.

"They didn't see that coming..." I said to myself, and pulled up the docking screen to line up the hydraulic seals. The ship shuddered from a few impacts on left side, away from the barracks, and again Kritos went running across the ship. A second later I saw most of a bird-like guard Mech cart-wheeling across the lava field and bouncing into the distance from a few high-powered blasts from the turrets on the other side of the freighter.

Lining up the docking seals, the familiar mechanical screech and *ka-chunk* signified the airlocks connecting with the barrack entry. As the hiss of compressed air engaged the seal, I jumped up and ran out of the command deck and toward the portal. I found my three brothers immediately appearing at my sides, two with blasters raised, and Jassan quickly using the docking interface to start loading in the virus, just before the airlock door opened.

Entering the barracks, the hall revealed a wall of reptilian flesh, immediately shattered by our preemptive firing. Fearless and full of dedication, we charged forward behind a constant array of searing plasma, and shortly found ourselves dancing through fallen bodies in an empty cathedral of broken conduits and raining showers of sparks from exploding lights.

Chaos seemed to be echoing down the halls by the sounds of shouting, crashes, and blaster sounds. The virus must already be working, and deeper inside the complex someone had noticed...

Coming to the first juncture, we turned toward the miner's cells, taking out a couple more guards in the halls en route. Hefting the main locking lever, each of the cell doors slammed open in sequence, as the men within shouted and ran towards us in joy and surprise.

"Quickly," I said, "to the women and children."

Now a mob of intense and focused force backed with rage and anger, we streamed toward the mess hall. The miners picked up weapons and armor where they could from the fallen bodies, and several of the men split off to load the larger Mech's onto the sides of our docked freighter.

Upon approach of the stale white space that had poorly nourished our ravaged slave bodies for so many years, the sounds of blaster fire, metal bounding off walls, and small explosions were now very loud. Slowing to cautiously approach the entry, I peeked inside.

Children were ripping weapons and armor off of fallen guards while punching their twisted dead faces and kicking them with rage. The security systems going down had awakened their attention immediately; they heard us coming, and had taken their chance to overcome the guards themselves. And they had won.

"Xīnghuì[4] young brothers!" I shouted, to let them know we were there without startling them into firing at us. They turned as one, a terrifying fire in their eyes, and suddenly broke into cheers of joy and smiles of hope.

As a group, we came into the room fully, but the children did not run to embrace us. Their eyes were still glazed steel underneath the relief, and they worked to straighten and fit their armor and weapons to their small bodies. Those fathers who knew their sons clasped their shoulders and held back their own tears. Perhaps there was hope for

---

[4] Xīnghuì - From the Ancient Chinese "Star Gathering Fortune," meaning "it is fortunate to meet with you under these Stars" in Shihaelei form.

these kids, waking up from their programming so much earlier than I had…

"It's time. We must hurry…" I said.

One of the youth, a gangly tall boy with fierce eyes looked up at me and said, "Some of us are already on the way to the mothers." I couldn't help but gape at him, but was not so surprised at this display of courage, now that I had seen what they had already overcome.

"We must go now then!" I replied, and ran back into the simple maze of corridors that lead to where they kept all the females. I trusted my brothers were behind me, and charged forward at full speed, finding only dead lizards in my path.

Hearing more blaster fire ahead, I tried to run even faster, and found myself suddenly bounding into a room full of explosions and blinding plasma streaks. Diving into a roll to keep my body low while taking in the situation, I saw reptilians falling left and right, with both women and children armed and systematically taking out the waves of guards who were entering this large juncture room used for storage and research.

"Xīnghuì family!" I shouted, before hasty plasma blasts could tear me apart.

"Xīnghuì!" was the response, more a challenge then a cheer. A young leader came forward, sending a few of the other youth and women down the side corridor to check for any more incoming guards, while sending the rest to run past me. Bringing his attention to me at last, his focused eyes seemed to pierce my soul.

"They are all released. We are clear for departure." Spoken like a true warrior, simple, clear, and to the point.

The intelligence that radiated from him was stunning, matched only by his fierce gaze and set jaw, but I sensed that he wasn't entirely sure of himself. It was time to get off this cursed rock, but we were not leaving *anyone* behind.

"What of the birthing mothers?" I asked, noticing only younger women and daughters running past.

"Where?" the young warrior said, his face flushing slightly with either anger or embarrassment.

"Below," I said, immediately springing up to run down the side corridor, and heard one of the young women already shouting for aid somewhere ahead. Coming around a corner, I saw her blasting down a stairwell. Another beautiful girl was on the ground beside her, lifeless face torn open by the liquid fire of a blaster, with two young daughters crying next to her.

Rage bubbled into my belly again like a storm, and I almost dove into the stairwell. Instead, I dropped my body to the floor at the top of the stairs and with tightly held focus, shot each guard at the bottom in the head.

In the next blurring moments I was at the bottom of the stairs, leaping between plasma rays and littering the floor with lizard bodies. As the madness and noxious smoke cleared, I made my way through sparking cables and flaming terminals to a space where there were many rows of pregnant women laying on operating tables. Fluid cables ran from ceiling pods to injection points in many areas of their bodies, and the biofeedback monitors showed that many of them had been killed either before or during the firefight.

Swallowing tears that welled up, and trying to calmly breathe out the choking sensation that suddenly left me suffocating, I grabbed a pile of large white cloths from a shelving system. Other mining brothers came down the stairs, and I handed them sheets quickly to keep their attention on the task at hand. We went to the mothers who were still alive, and carefully removed the cables from their bodies, then tenderly wrapped them in the white cloth and carried them from the room.

It took several trips to make sure everyone was loaded onto the freighter, and there were few other encounters with reptilian guards who had evaded our initial assault. Jassan assured me that the virus would keep any communications alerts or alarms from triggering armed response from the Mothership.

We also loaded on all of the food and energy supplies that were available, which Jassan coordinated and began to calculate as we began to disengage from the docking platform. As Kritos and Haggan took positions with me on the command bridge, we glanced at each other anxiously, awaiting word from Jassan on our energy capacity.

His eyes were a cold blue when he entered, making the flutters in my belly suddenly freeze over and fall like a lump of ice. "No... We don't have enough energy to make a jump."

I tried not to let them see my teeth grinding as I focused on the navigation panel. After a long silence, Kritos spoke as he hunched over the mapping system, "What about this other Moon? It's on this side of the planet also, and we could reach it quickly from our current position. It looks like they have an outpost in orbit there..."

No one was going to argue, as it was clearly the only option. Attempting another assault on the Mothership now was simply suicide. Not to mention the almost unbelievable fact that we had somehow slipped away and rescued everyone from the barracks without attracting notice. At least, with their communications down, even if they had noticed, they couldn't coordinate anything well enough to do anything about it.

Gently drifting clear of the barracks by popping a few light bursts from the side engines, I tilted the nose up and eased the main thrusters into action. The gravitational stabilizers began to engage and counteract our tilt and acceleration, smoothing the ride and easing the pressure of the g-force. With a deep breath, I pulled up the other Moon's outpost from the navigation database, and set the autopilot.

# SHIHAELEI - CHAPTER 6
# INTO THE DEEP 堕

*"zz-Krackti chanka ke arankata chati kranka.-zz"*

Everyone looked at Jassan, eyes wide and hopeful, as the coms buzzed at us, a security check on our approach. His eyes were closed, and he seemed to be repeating the words in his head. A moment later, his eyes popped open, and he leaned forward. "Che chanka aran sithara ka chita," he responded in a gutteral and choppy dialect. Kritos and I looked at each other, a grin splitting our faces.

*"zz-Krakti nochaka. Akansa kara.-zz"* The reptilian voice on the other end of the com seemed to take the bait, and Jassan began to transmit a series of codes from his communications terminal on the freighter ship bridge to the outpost command. He then had one of the freighter's onboard droid bots plug into the access port under the terminal, and upload the virus he had transferred to its databanks during flight.

Jassan nodded to me as the readout finished issuing a docking command, and told me the location to enter into the autopilot system as we made our final approach to the Outpost.

It was a massive, dark grey vertical structure with a large disk at the top, extending about ten-times the width of the freighter, which itself was at least 50 paces from side to side. The disk gently expanded to about five-stories high in the center, and the long vertical stem of chambers and docking platforms running out its bottom was ten-times that height.

As our craft slowed, coming to dock at one of the lower platforms, our ship was a flurry of motion. Groups of miners and youth tightened their armor, reset their weapons, and readied themselves for the moment the pressurized entry doors would open. Our mission was simple: knock out their communications, secure energy cells, and recover any supplies essential to survival.

The first step was accomplished as soon as the ship engaged the dock, as conduit cables attached themselves to the main information arteries of the ship and the virus began uploading into the outpost's mainframe system.

Securing the energy cells was a matter of finding them, and disabling all hostile forces keeping us from them. As the outpost was built for loading and unloading freight cargo, there were few guards and fewer trained warriors onboard. As our hot-blooded miners flooded into the main vertical corridor, they swept away any resistance like a boiling torrent of red and black acid, with frothing waves of violent plasma explosions.

Within what seemed like only moments, all the available energy cells and supplies were loaded onto our freighter ship, sweat-soaked warriors returned, and commands were initiated to disengage from the outpost.

As the ship began to drift freely, I added thrust to bring us out of range of any last minute strike attempts by reptilian survivors. Those of us on the command deck were silent, each of us nodding to ourselves, knowing that there must be enough energy cells now. I steered the ship up and around in orbit above the grey dusty moon where the outpost was located to bring the constellation into view.

The constellation that awakened my memories. The constellation that held the secrets to my past and future. The constellation that led home.

Just as the curvature of the moon slid low enough in the main bay windows to reveal the beautiful set of stars that changed my life, Jassan returned from loading the new energy cells. My head refused to turn and see the answer on his face. My mind was focused on one thing... He would say yes, and we would begin calculations and preparations to make a hyperspace jump.

We were not sure of the exact star-system, but there was a catalog of at least a few inhabited planetary systems referenced by that constellation in the databanks. It didn't matter, as we would find somewhere safe, and work our way home no matter what the odds.

When Jassan did not speak, I allowed myself to release my tension for a moment, and took a deep breath and simply feel. It was cold again, my stomach slowly tightening into a knot. Kritos cursed and punched the wall. Haggan growled, and I looked disbelievingly at Jassan. "There is not enough?"

His cool blue eyes spoke clearly, and I let my head slide into my hands, pressing my fingertips over my scalp as if to clear the dark thoughts that tried to infiltrate my mind. "There is another planet." I said flatly, staring out the bay windows toward the distant and familiar stars. "It is nearby, relatively speaking. I saw it in the databanks on this solar system, its orbit is adjacent to this one and it is within a quarter of its solar year from us now."

I could feel the eyes of my brothers on me, and sense their frustration. Again, they were left without argument, and without another suggestion. I roughly tapped the navigation screen to bring up the planet from the database, only to find that there was a complete absence of data other than its position and location. I brought the ship around, and we could all see the dim yellow glow of the planet in the distance. It was only slightly larger than the other stars in our view, and would require almost all of our existing energy cells to reach.

It was a painful choice. If the planet was terrestrial, we could likely find the material resources we needed to fill our energy cells. However likely, this was still a hard option that would require long searching, mining, and refining work. If there was a Draconian outpost, we could raid it, although that option was very unlikely considering there was no information about it in the database. As to other options, and other locations, there were none within our range. It was not much of a choice at all.

I looked at each of my brothers in turn, and there was confirmation and hope in their eyes. Locking in the navigation coordinates and the autopilot, I set the ship for its top sub-luminal speed, and slid out of the pilot chair.

"We should all get some rest," said Kritos. "I'm not sure we ever have."

The wind pressed into my face, and violently rippled my loose sleeves. I sank lower into my seat, straddled between curving bone ridges, two smaller bone plates rising to my hands from the backs of shoulder blades, but somehow sitting with ease and comfort with my thighs pressed against a massive breathing body beneath me. The world spun, and gravity vanished as we hurled downward through the clouds.

Massive silver wings cut through the mists to each side of me, stretchy membranes of skin vibrating with a deep bass tone as air pressure folded over and under them. As the ground suddenly became visible again, I twisted, tilted and pushed hard on the right shoulder bone plate, and the being responded with a smooth rising curve that compressed my intestines and seemed to pull my eyes lower within their sockets.

The trees blurring by below gave way to jagged stone foothills that rose into snow-capped peaks that pierced the cloudline ahead of us. Nestled in a shadowed valley, I could see the fortress, laced with fire from above and below, and surrounded by glittering tendrils of color that danced with each other in the sky.

The long neck stretching out before me undulated like a serpent, and I could feel the creature's whole body wiggling with anticipation as we streaked towards our freedom, or perhaps towards our doom. The sun broke through the clouds, and everything was ignited in blinding light as thousands of mirrored scales all over their body caught the reflection.

We were a comet of light, at One with each other in breath, movement, and blood. I was riding this creature of liquid metal, soaring through the sky. Then I could see through the eyes of the beautiful beast... I was...the...*Lóngshén*...or *ancient skyborne winged serpent spirit* roughly translated.

Together as One, no fear could stain us, no fire could burn us, no pain could harm us. Our voices cried out as one, a spectrum stretching from the roar of an earthquake to the piercing song of the Stars, and battle became Us.

Opening my eyes, I found myself sitting upright in my bunk, my skin hot and tingling, and everything seemed full of light. I looked around at the familiar space, with the same old black conduits snaking over walls and sickly glowing panels that barely illuminated anything.

Shaking my head to clear it from the strange dreamspace, I started to get up as Kritos appeared at the entry. "We're here," he said, his voice callous and disturbing.

Walking onto the command deck after these many long days of travel, I still had a sense of excitement, even though I had already started to feel the old knots begin to tighten in my belly after hearing the tone in my Shihaeleian brother's voice.

The planet loomed before us, almost filling the bay windows, with yellow and white clouds streaking across its surface and curling here and there where massive storms where raging. We were entering orbit, and the planet was very slowly drifting to the right in our view.

It didn't take a glance at our sensor readouts to know that this was not a terrestrial planet. It had screamed "gas giant" at us for days now, but we had to be sure. There were no outposts here, no material resources to gather, and no place to find solace but in the darkness and cold depths of space.

Our resources had dwindled, from food to water to energy, though we reused and renewed everything we could. This was clearly the end of the adventure. We had gained our freedom; the freedom to die by our own choices, by our own mistakes, by our own fates.

I sat down in the pilot chair, letting myself relax and sink into thought. Soon, I would have to share this news with everyone on board. *Congratulations everyone, we've made it, we're free. Now, we're going to die.* I could hear the sardonic tone in my own mind, just thinking about it.

Sighing deeply, I looked around at each of my brothers. Kritos simply stared out at the planet, arms crossed and eyes narrow. His face was set firmly in resolve, and disappointment.     Haggan's bushy eyebrows were wrinkled in worry, and his huge beastly form seemed hunched over and defeated. As I looked at Jassan, his eyes closed, and I watched as his face became peaceful.  He had entered the "Blue Crystal Fire," as he called it, the place where he was able to understand other languages, decode and recode information, and somehow, where he found a deep sense of peace within.

In those moments, I wanted to be there with him, to see those endless halls of beautiful blue light cascading around me.  I wanted to see the rain of symbols passing by like falling stars, and feel the gentle cooling and warmth flowing through my body.  It was there, in me, somehow, but it kept burning up in a smoldering fire of anger and failure.

After a long time passed, barely containing the rising explosion of rage within me under each breath, I slammed my fists against the arms of the pilot seat. I wanted to scream and roar with pain, but I held on to my voice, and my sanity, by a thread. I finally managed to forge it into steel and stillness inside of me, and rose from the seat to bear the death toll to our family of freed slaves. My tight shoulders shook and slumped as I started to turn towards the passageway that led deeper into the freighter ship.

Then, something strange happened.     Blue light was suddenly cascading around me, illuminating everything inside the command deck.  I looked down at my body, stunned, then glanced swifly over at Jassan. His eyes were still closed, but a smile was creeping into his features.  I looked at Kritos, and found him staring wide eyed and slack-jawed out the bay windows.

Coming down into view ahead of us, pulsing with liquid flows of radiant blue light, dancing with flashing points in every color of the spectrum, rotating slowly like a gargantuan blue crystal disk, was a Mothership.

It was unlike anything I had ever seen before; its bottom was finely lined with brilliant turquoise channels, like a perfectly arranged labyrinth of conduits on a circuit board. From the center of its base extended fine filaments, towers of light blue with cascades of white light spiraling up and down their lengths.

Small craft with blinding white and colored lights emerged from the ship, silently dancing passed the bay window, flying behind and around our whole freighter ship faster and more deftly than I had ever seen anything move. They did not seem hostile, and if they were I would not have been able to move to do anything about it, as the beauty of the Mothership was hypnotizing.

As it came closer, it began to fill our entire view, as the forsaken gas planet vanished in the radiance of its surface. We began to realize just how large the ship was, as the towers of light at its center extended far below and above us, and the labyrinth of turquoise channels became canyons in an endless ocean of deep blue.

Soon, we were being drawn up into one of these canyons, which was a busy corridor for many other small lightships. Some were lazily drifting by, and others passed in a streak of light. Rows of lights which I assumed indicated levels of the ship extended endlessly above and below us and we drifted further into the gently curving channel. It looked as though we were surrounded by two undulating planes of stars that were reflected on softly glowing water.

As our ascent slowed, and we neared the left sidewall, the smooth gloss of its surface revealed crystalline structures that extended to form a dock that would interface with the freighter. It took only a moment longer for the ship to reach perfect stillness. No loud crunching, squealing, or whistling pressure releases signaled our arrival, so I found myself having to work my way out of my dazed state of complete relaxation on my own. I had slipped back down into the pilot seat at some point, and was stunned by my state of calm and peace.

Logic returned, along with the realization that I had no idea what this ship was, what kind of species created this kind of technology, and how in the Universe we had made it all the way into the ship and been docked before any of us even reacted with more than gaping awe. Uncertainty came with this logic, and a jolting return to my state of protective guardianship over my people.

"Get your weapons and armor, quickly!" Instinctively, I was already strapping on my insect-plate armor and situating blades around my body, taking up my plasma blaster last. Kritos was staring at me with an eyebrow raised, and still looked dazed. "Come on! We don't know who these beings are, and we must be prepared." I found Jassan looking at me with calm amusement, clearly not going to gather any weapons or armor of his own, and Haggan already armed to the teeth with a blaster in each hand.

As I moved back into the main halls of the freighter, I found a small group had already suited up, as someone had picked up that we were docking in a strange and unfamiliar place. This group of around twenty armed miners, my brothers and I stepped up to the docking entry, and found that the pressure had already been equalized. The door opened easily with a slight hiss, and we found ourselves looking down a long, gently curving hallway that was completely empty.

The white hallway had a glistening shine to its surface, and felt almost soft beneath our feet, like the very slight flex of cartilage. It had five sides, which as we walked forward began to slowly transform into six, and then seven. With each permutation, there were subtle rings of multicolored light that circled the hall like illuminated arches.

Surrounded by this inspiring beauty, I had a moment of reflection on my own appearance and that of our group. We were dirty, skin stained with grease and ash, wearing armor that was encrusted with blood. We bore tools of death, instruments of pain, and carried them like honored treasures. We emerged from a realm of endless suffering, displaying the scars of demons and the fires of destruction openly on our faces. We were an army from Hell, and we had entered Heaven.

As the walls continued to morph, gaining more surfaces and gently becoming more and more rounded, my steps became more certain and my breathing more full and relaxed. I didn't feel dazed this time, but simply clear, and composed.

Then, the hallway opened. I led the group into a large atrium, where the floors were made of glossy blue tile that was finely laced with spiraling curves and geometries. White pillars lined with curling webs of gold and silver extended upward on all sides of the egg-shaped room, supporting two balconies that surrounded the room.

The first had three beings standing on it, looking down at us as we entered. One of them had green skin, and large oval eyes like dark purple glass. His forehead extended back at an angle and split into two lobes that formed the two sides of his elongated cranium, and he wore white robes with golden lacings. Next to him, some paces apart, was a woman with blue skin in blue robes that reminded me of the surface of the Mothership. She was ageless and enchanting, her face partially obscured by a veil that hung from a crowning head-dress. Further to the right was another being in white, whose head-dress extended to a point, and veiled his entire face except for two dark slits. This being's broad shouldered robes were also laced with golden symbols and cords, elegant yet simple.

As I came to stand in the center of the atrium, I noticed the ceiling looked like a sapphire blue flower with swooping and pointed petals. They spiraled out from a large red crystal woven with a golden grid, and further balanced and illuminated the light in the space. Every color in the room was rich and brilliant, perfectly in harmony with every other color, shape and form.

Yet, everything vanished when she entered. Her movement was silent, and she glided into the room as if nothing touched the floor beneath her elaborate dress. It seemed made of everything in the room, and yet all soft cloth in precise layers. Her hair was the same, braided and woven into a head-dress that made her seem much taller. As she approached, I saw that her piercing and breathtaking blue eyes were only as high as my heart, and this is where her gaze focused.

When she stopped just out of my reach, she looked into my eyes, and penetrated through to my Soul in an instant. I felt naked, as though nothing stood between us, and nothing I could say, do, or think could conceal my Self, and how I had come to be here. The hardened steel of my forged spirit was also present, bare as I was to her, and I could see compassionate sympathy soften the intensity of her eyes.

It melted me, and her voice sung gently, clearly, and in my own tongue, "Be disarmed..." Her lips almost curved into a smile, as I felt every muscle in my body relax, "You are welcome here."

All my armor could have fallen to the ground in that instant. Perhaps it did, for all of us who stood before her in that moment. For all of us who suddenly realized that we were safe. We were free. We had made it. We were welcome.

My heart melted, my eyes filled with blue stars, and I knelt down in the heart of the egg. In that moment, I was born again.

# SHIHAELEI - CHAPTER 7
# REBIRTH & DEATH 死

The first real and full experience of any newborn is Love. If we are not feeling love, we are dying, and each time we receive the gift of this experience, it is a kind of birth. Yet in the emergence from darkness, as the wet layers of the known world are peeled away to reveal pure beauty, it is the ambassador of that freedom that calls forth a symphony in the depths of our hearts. This being was far more than that, and the tides that surged through me carried as much charge as any memory of my Mother's love. Yet now, I had much more body for that charge to surge through.

She was stunningly beautiful. Her physical form was similar to a Shihaelei woman, but with pale skin that had a tinge of sapphire blue. She was short, but her energy felt like a giant. Her eyes though... Like the depth of the ancient seas on our wetland world, Mizu'no waku'sei[5] where I had spent time as a young child learning and training before I was taken by the Draconians. Then those eyes were gone, as she swept away to somewhere else on the ship, leaving attendants and healers to surround us and guide us to places where we could rest and recover.

I felt like all I needed was more time with this being, as even this one brief moment with her was enough to ease so much of the pain I had been carrying.

Still, in an echo of some old wounds I began to remember from my childhood, she was as distant and illusive as my Mother was; an Ambassador not only to my rebirth, and my awakening heart, but to an entire civilization of beings.

---

[5] Related to the Japanese translation of "
"

They called her Ama'dali'shkala. The Mothership was vast, and she seemed to be everywhere at once, and always where she could not be reached.

Our arrival had seemed to set off a chain of *protocol initiations*, in which we were gently but insistently herded to different areas of the starship city to cleanse ourselves, nourish our bodies with long lost foods, and select more *appropriate* attire for this peaceful existence.

Our guides varied, but generally said little and answered very few questions. Jassan, being a Pleiadian himself, stayed with our group of ragged refugees, and helped us to understand certain things, yet even he would simply offer a knowing smile when some unspoken message was whispered into his mind from other blue-skinned guides.

We were fed excellent foods that were immediately familiar and stimulating, and I began to have memories triggered simply by eating them. I soon realized that they somehow knew how to recreate the traditional Shihaeleian meals I ate with my parents as a child, though to my frustration, they would not answer how they knew these meals or attained the food. Still, the rich sauces with a complex weave of spicy, sweet and sour, and the alternating crunchy, soft, and fibered roots saturated with flavor satiated my hunger and my appetite for information. The strange green strands with a nutty oil and small seeds woven through them tickled my memories, visions by the ocean on a stormy day, dark clouds menacing above sharp black stone cliffs where the lush green plant life seemed to glow in its brilliant verdant splendor.

My own mind was revealing many stories, and I began to understand pieces of my species' history and the nature of our current situation. I remembered my father most often, like a pillar within his long brown cloak, seeming to command spaces with his silence and his simple words. He was often an agent of Justice, and I remembered certain people shrinking in his presence, their faces contorted with guilt that seemed to effuse from their pores. It seemed that in facing his gaze, no accusations ever needed to be made.

Waves of anxiety would wash over me in the middle of a meal, remembering my own mistakes, and feeling the overwhelming urge to reveal them to my father and beg for forgiveness. Yet I only remember him smiling, his heart opening and pouring forth love. Gratitude would well up inside me, along with oaths and promises to never make those mistakes again! It was in my father's eyes that I discovered forgiveness, but underlying that gift he revealed to me an ever-present space of peace… With stillness, silence, and a quiet mind like the surface of a pond, he was forever undisturbed by the waves of existence.

My mother was something altogether different, and my feelings about her were much more present than visual memory of our times together. She was a mystery, endlessly revealing the unknown, and always maintaining a deeper enigma.

I remembered large meetings, where my mother sat on one of several large chairs on a raised dais, overlooking a crowd that was in a smorgasbord of states from concerned to angry. I felt the tension in my father as we stood to the back (or sometimes the side) of the room, and underneath that, a tender sadness as he watched my mother fielding questions as skillfully as any D'jedai danced with sword strikes.

She was unreachable in so many ways, yet her distance only added to the quality of her presence when she made herself available. My own memories of time with her were very short, though deeply satisfying. Between sessions, flights, public addresses, councils, and time spent on another planet entirely...those were my moments with mother. They were always more than I hoped for, and yet far shorter than I desired.

When she looked at me, there was no place to hide. She could see everything; every thought, feeling, fear, and fragment of hope that I held in my heart as a child. It seemed that nothing escaped her notice, and I never had to explain where I had been or what I had been doing. She seemed to know my future as well, and her loving eyes would wrap me in velvet flower petals, embracing all the challenges I would face, then she would sigh and sprinkle sparkling blooms of laughter all over me.

They called her Rha, and she was my Vision. Even after all the lights went out and I found myself lost in fields of fire and brimstone, she was a beacon of hope that never stopped twinkling in the Stars.

As my love for her grew inside me with each memory, I was still left with a deep sense of loss and longing, and my thoughts of her would eventually guide me to visions of Ama'dali'shkala. I found it both strange, confusing, and also somehow invigorating, as if some part of myself was aching to be discovered through this being of such elegant mystique that was not isolated to my memories. Like a mirror to the memory of my mother, I felt the same longing each and every time Ama'dali'shkala disappeared into another corridor.

Each time I tried to see the Ambassador, either through request, by following patterns of her movement to catch her for a moment, or by simply waiting in some place she seemed to frequently visit, my attempts to connect with her would fail utterly.

Even her appearance was rare, but I managed to cross paths with her several times in the precious spaces of free time I had to explore. However, each time she would ignore me completely, or catch my eyes for a single instant, and in that look, I would lose all capacity to communicate. In fact, I often reflected that she must have some hidden power of paralysis (or transforming men into frightened animals), but eventually began to simply think of her as "stunning."

This only seemed to aggravate the emotions that simmered inside of me, both of longing and love, as well as inadequacy and suffocating sadness. She was out of my reach, and it was so familiar.

:::

Each training session had unlocked some aspect of our pain, some part of our deep-seated anger and fears surrounding the Draconians. We had seen our own reptilian minds, and explored within us the cycles of time that had returned to teach us through our own suffering, and eventually to be released through our liberation. They were not our enemies, but aspects of ourselves that we had to face.

Our hidden memories were locked away in our bodies, and as the many different species on the Mothership sent teachers to guide and aid us in healing, we often found ourselves doing movement practices, making tones with our voices, and holding certain postures until powerful emotions and energies were released. Fantastic, familiar, challenging, and strange all at once, each technique we were shown worked quickly and effectively. They classified these teachings and systems as "Spirit

Technologies," built to enable Consciousness to "flow" more easily through the "body container."

We discovered Jassan was from a beautiful Star Cluster where there was a planet almost entirely covered by oceans. His System was where this Mothership had been created, and there were many of his people on board, including Ama'dali'shkala, who was an Ambassador of these people. These mostly blue-skinned or pearl-white beings had some incredible skills that came very naturally, like the ability to communicate directly through thoughts, and to use their voices to change the shape and form of certain types of matter. His name was also not Jassan, as we had called him, but a long sound that resonated like windpipes and oscillated in deep tones like a plasma engine.

Like Jassan, it was clear that certain species among our crew excelled at applying certain Spirit Technologies, while being severely challenged by others. Kritos and I, as well as the other miners who were Shihaeleian (which was most of our crew), had a knack for bringing almost any idea or thought into a specific body movement.

Some of the other hosting species on the ship were intrigued by this, and would test us to see how our body movements would translate certain "advanced" concepts and theories. We found ourselves doing strange spinning and rotary movements while speaking the words they taught us, and usually ending up in some elaborate radiant flourish. This seemed to bring them great pleasure, and released a tremendous amount of energy in our own bodies, so we were generally excited to continue this type of practice.

Much of this work also brought up memories of our people and homeworlds, as visions returned of watching fantastic movement performances as a child, and seeing playful battles that displayed incredible balance and dexterity in the performers. Others had similar memories, and the few individuals who were enslaved at a slightly older age confirmed for us that our culture was built around martial arts and expression through movement.

It was strange for us to have to be introduced to our own culture all over again, but most of us had been slaves since our earliest memories, with only scattered images before then. Even our early years working for the reptilians were blank spaces, a testament to the trauma and abuse of those first stages of programming as children. Our deep healing work slowly revealed more about our childhood years before we were captured, and sometimes unlocked memories in other bodies in much earlier times, but rarely penetrated the darkness of our first traumatic years in the hands of the Draconians.

Still, we made great progress, and it wasn't long before we were persistently inquiring about the state of our homeworlds. Our questions were met with offhanded statements like "soon" and "when you are ready," until one day the answer came with the return of a small group of scout ships.

Apparently the Shihaeleian people were under heavy attack, and were making a last stand against a massive assault that had just been initiated on our desert planet. Each city was fortified as best as it could be, and they were barely managing to hold off sweeping waves of Draconian ships, robots, and well armed foot-soldiers.

By this time we knew that an angry or enraged reaction would not aid us in getting to our planet to help any faster, so we calmly sat in council with our host species on the Mothership, hoping to swiftly assemble plans. But apparently, it was finally time for us to know the whole truth of the situation…

All the Shihaelei refugees were gathered together in one of the domed gathering halls with many seats in concentric circles that rose around the walls, along with those who were close friends of ours and had escaped with us from the lava moon, like Jassan and Haggan. A tall dark-blue skinned Pleiadian man without hair stood before us, great sadness in his eyes and a heaviness in his voice. My heart pounded as I could feel the emotions he was emanating into the room.

"Our hearts cry out for you, Shihaelei, and we grieve with you now, as your world of seas and oceans, mountains and vales, has fallen to the Draconian forces. They have decimated your lands and your cities, eaten away your mountains, and poisoned your oceans. Your world, your home, has been lost beyond recovery, beyond rescue. We had hoped to share this with you while there was still time to grieve, to let flow the centuries of sadness that a Planet deserves in her Death. We honor her by her name: *Mizu'no waku'sei.*"

My throat caught, though I knew that saying the name was what he wanted from us all. I was not the only one, as I stared around in shock at the other Shihaelei gathered. There was silence for ten heartbeats, a thundering silence that felt electric and terrifying all at once. Something inside me steeled itself, remembering my childhood and the way the Shihaelei in *D'jedai* training would speak the name of an honored beloved or great leader who had passed.

"*Mizu'no waku'sei!*" The room exploded in one voice, as I let it out like a bellow full of anger, full of honor, full of commitment. Our people had known great loss, time after time, but we had always grown stronger. Apparently even the destruction of our beloved world would not take us down this day.

The man bowed his head for a few moments, then continued, "The Draconians now seek to take your desert world, Shihaeleio, and are amassing forces around all of the great white cities on your planet. While we have protocols as a Galactic Culture that generally forbid us to interfere in planetary conflicts between species who are not part of our Councils, we are now aware of various complexities to this circumstance that will allow us to help you intervene."

The weight of her words sunk in, deeply. So they weren't going to take this massive ship and blast these raiders out of existence... My disappointment was short lived, as I didn't really think they had any weapons that could do this anyway. And there was a ray of hope here, they could *help* us to intervene.

And we would.

The room exploded into discussion, questions flying from all corners at the speaker, who quickly began to gather aids and other researchers from the edges of the room to stand with him in the center. He waved his hands and asked all to come to silence. He pointed out that there was a button on our chairs that we could press to queue our questions, and they would take them one by one.

It seemed like ages passed in that chamber, as we gathered all the details we could about the situation on both of our planets, regardless of his assessment that one was lost. Most of this portion of the discussion was heavy and slow, as they expressed the information with great remorse and care. For the Shihaelei, this was not a time for wallowing in sorrow, or more would die. This is what every part of our culture, our training, our way of life prepared us for.

*"When the mountain comes to crush your home, you move,"* as my father used to say. *"Or you die. Choose to live, even if it means letting go of everything."*

Then the questions angled towards attack strategy, as countless questions were thrown in regarding technologies and tools we had all seen around the Mothership. There was a great deal we had learned from our Galactic brothers and sisters, the least of which involved keys to incredibly advanced Physical Technologies. Where they saw simple tools, we saw flawless tricks and endless opportunities. Where they were unsure how to proceed, we could hardly choose from the array of strategies easily assembled among our crew.

Finally, the questions began to dig into the nature of these Draconians. What did the Galactic community know about them? What had changed in regards to their protocols, that had enabled them to finally give us aid to return and fight for our homes?

The simple answer left the room silent again, stunning us all. "The Draconians are hybrids between humanoids and Dragons. They were created using Dragon genetics; the blood of what you call *Lóngshén*."

Wait, they were *created!?* With the blood of *Lóngshén*? What did that mean? Maybe those dreams were more than just dreams…

We pressed for more details, but it seemed like at least this group did not have all the information we wanted. Still, an idea started to form. I had seen beings learning how to ride inside of larger body suits on one of the large natural promenades on the Mothership, where trees and grass grew alongside streams and beautiful gardens. It was amazing enough to me to see nature on a ship in the stars, but then watching people transform into animals and creatures to run and play just seemed unreal. They seemed to be driving them from inside, like the Mech suits on the volcanic moon.

I mentioned what I had seen, and asked to hear about the technology in as much depth and detail as they could offer, and a gruff older man in the research group with pointed ears, darker tan skin, and mirth in his eyes stepped forward to explain.

"The Morphogenesis system holographically aligns molecular data into a lattice that matches the data of a source genome, arranging matter into the form of a body, but adapted to contain the original physical form inside. The internal body harness wraps the operator's physical form in a sort of symbiotic stasis, so the consciousness of the operator is then projected into the whole of the generated body.

"The original body is fed and nourished by the generated body's digestive system through an integrative nutrient transference process built into the suit of the harness, and so can be sustained potentially indefinitely, though that hasn't been tested." He seemed proud of this, and I assumed he had a part in this technology's creation.

Looking around, he realized that many of those in the room had no idea what he was talking about, and he cleared his throat. "Ah, basically you transform into the other body, as if it was your own, while your current body," he says pointing at the audience, "stays healthy and intact inside. Unfortunately it only currently works with bodies larger than your own."

Bodies larger than our own? That was the key. What was the largest body they had genetic information for? If we could storm in as some giant beasts and crush their onslaught of forces, that would be something. Then something landed in me... "Do you have *Dragon* Morpho...geno...information?"

The looks that passed between the researchers suggested that this question was a source of some discomfort, but I couldn't imagine why that was. "Ah, yes," the tan older man replied tentatively, looking very concerned.

His concerns be damned. Something told me this was the key, this was the way we were going to take our planet back. Among all of us gathered there that day, there was one glaring Truth: we could not let our people be swept away by the Draconians. Whether we were ready or not, it was time to return Home.

# SHIHAELEI - CHAPTER 8
# SHIHAELEIO 沙

Standing in the docking bay, I glanced down at my gear again. It was hardly the thing to be wearing when facing lizards armed to the teeth who would just as soon disembowel you as make you their slave. Shaking my head, I took a deep breath and focused on the Present. This moment was about trusting my Self, my Galactic Family...and these new technologies. The close fitting, soft purple shirt and blue leggings would not matter soon...or so I hoped.

There were only five of us standing in the Bay, two to the left and two to the right of me. I didn't know these other Shihaelei refugees that well, as there had not been much time to cultivate deeper relationships among our crew before arriving in this new reality. Since we arrived on the Mothership, there seemed to be infinitely more interesting things to discover than each other: new species, holographic display systems, foods from diverse planets, and much more.

Some of these other species were gathered behind a mirrored window, watching and waiting for our disembarkment. It would come soon, I knew, though there seemed to be no noticeable changes in internal gravity or ship configuration as we plummeted into the atmosphere of my home planet.

I had watched our approach from a viewing deck, and felt my heart swell with pride and love when we glided into orbit over the smooth white sphere. Endless white deserts of dust, soft as baby skin, broken only by tumbling bone-white mountain ranges that curved in arcs like the ribs of a planetary skeleton.

Carved into the edges of those mountains were cities, with gateways into underground reservoirs of water and life. Invisible on the surface, the planet was rich with plants and animals that lived beneath the crust, and our people had found a paradise in the thin veil between life and death.

Now, that paradise was being systematically destroyed, with tides of black armies crashing against our cities with brutal force. Several cities still held out against the endless siege, and these were the targets for deployment of our Galactic Lightships.

Suddenly the docking bay lights pulsed, calling my attention to a rainbow light pulse trailing along the edge of the bay door. Then, it began to slowly open. The inner door was a ramp, which began to lower from the ceiling, opening outward towards the planet surface. The atmosphere poured in as it descended, bringing with it a strong wind filled with powdery dust. The smell and feel of the dusty wind seemed to seep through my pores, and any last remaining fears or doubts were banished from me in an instant. This was the breath of my homeland, and I swallowed the wind as if parched with thirst.

Closing my eyes, I let the hot curls of air wrap around me, cradling my body like a tender mother. I breathed deeply, and found perfect stillness within me.

As I opened my eyes again, I found the ramp had lowered to the critical point before we would become visible to the swarming armies outside, so with a quick nod to my four crewmates, I reached down and slid over the activating mechanism on the top of my elaborate golden belt-buckle.

A vibrating hum filled my body, and suddenly my perspective was moving forward, extending as I felt my neck elongating and stretching out from my body. My back arched, and I felt my shoulder blades unfolding from my back and stretching out to my sides. My fingers swelled into claws, as my arms and legs swelled and rippled with bundles of muscle. A tail burst forth from the base of my spine, extending back behind me, and I felt all my facial muscles and bones shifting simultaneously. I watched as my nose and mouth projected outward in my vision, becoming a gleaming silver muzzle with large rimmed nostrils. I licked my teeth, which had grown in number and extended around my mouth, my sharp incisors becoming long razors.

As the transformation settled, I glanced down at my gigantic body, between two huge forearms that were covered in glittering silver scales. My belly looked like rounded shingles of pure silver, broken only by a huge emerald gem embedded in my chest, a shimmering yellow star gem in my solar-plexus, and a softly pulsing orange flame gem between my pelvic bones.

My legs looked like my arms, folded backward to lunge, with massive claws that curved like Draconian swords. I snarled with glee, and twisted my neck to look back at the huge wings extending from my upper back. They were spanned with silver membranes stretched between thin rods of silver bone, flexible shoulder blades branching from thick muscular extensions of my rhomboids. I fluttered them momentarily to test my control of their movement as a deep shiver ran through my whole being, from my Soul to my wingtips...

*I am Dragon. I am here. I remember.*

The bay door was now wide open, the ramp settling into the soft desert. With a glance at the massive Green, Gold, Blue, and Red Dragons that stood to either side of me, admiring their own new forms with both awe and the thrill of familiarity, I snorted to call forth focus, and leapt out the docking bay.

The wind hit my massive body with full force, but it could not slow the raw power of the muscles that drove me forward with blurring speed. I galloped across the desert, feeling the wind shifting to match my direction and momentum. The shifting dust and winds revealed a black tide of armed Draconian warriors charging in my direction. As soon as the sun shimmered off my mirrored silver form, their momentum broke. With all the force of my Heart, I roared, a thunderous sound that shook the ground in front of me and caused the ranks of reptilian soldiers to break and scramble behind each other.

At the last moment before I would have begun to trample them all, crushing their small bodies under my massive claws as I had once felt their bones crack and crumble in the fists of my Mech, I dug my claws into the dust and slid to a halt. Those who had not fled stood shaking, holding their blasters up wearily and looking to the large warlord who commanded them for orders.

His eyes were wide with fear, and he tried to hide his subtle tremble as he bent forward, and set down his large plasma cannon. Then, something amazing happened. It was the moment we had prayed for, which any man who goes to war holds fast to with a thread of hope.

The commander knelt down. Then, the whole army dropped their weapons, and fell to their knees.

:::

Even with the size of this form, the thick air currents of the Desert planet kept my large body aloft with ease. With a few flaps of massive wings, I thrust myself higher into the atmosphere. Far below, the curls of infant whirlwinds were competing to gather enough thermal strength to swallow their brethren. The ground seemed to surge with tides of plasma, as soft powdery dust moved like water on the waves of wind.

Stretching out my long neck and whipping my tail into another angle, I dove down, gathering speed. The skin stretched between the bones of my wings began to vibrate, and I tucked in my front arms and legs to accelerate further. My nostrils flared as the cool winds of the high currents gave way to hot turbulence, and I clenched my razor sharp teeth in a semblance of a grin as I tore into the swirling dust devils.

It was an exercise in strength and dexterity, as each change in wind direction forced me to whip my serpentine form violently to compensate for the shifts in inertia. Swift adjustments to the tilt in my wingspan allowed me to catch the thermal updrafts rolling up alongside the vortices, propelling me forward and allotting subtle boosts in altitude as well.

At these speeds I could cover leagues in moments, streaking across the surface of the planet like a bolt of Silver lightning. As the final reptilian ships departed Shihaeleio, my body surged with renewed strength, and at long last, joy.

Still, these adventurous flights across the planet were more than entertainment, the Guardian Dragons (as the people had begun to call us) were sweeping for last remnants of the reptilian battalions.

It had taken forever to get them to leave at all. We were their "gods," or so our Dragon bodies made them believe. Some part of their memories held the keys to their genetic ancestry…their origin as Dragons, before they became these twisted humanoid hybrids. Yet like the Dragons from

Andromeda, their ways and myths taught them to question and challenge authority, particularly their gods. They groveled, and they worshipped, but they also relentlessly begged to take the lives of the Shihaelian people...my people. They explained to us that they would make the Shihaelei slaves in "Our Divine Honor," making servants to feed us and take care of all our needs.

It was difficult not to simply rend their flesh with our gleaming talons, or become exhausted and simply crush them like insects in a rolling snore. Yet we knew our work, and we had to logically explain to them that this species was not meant to be their slaves, and that these planets were now off-limits to them.

Being too hasty would only result in a revolt. Even if they did not attack us openly, they would gnaw at our backs and repeatedly renew their assaults against the Shihaeleian cities in small rebellions, similar to an army of disgruntled teenagers. They would feel that they were truly doing us gods a service, and proving their true worth as capable decision makers. Their species has quite a tempestuous mind.

A few of our Dragon-morphed crew who had not fully ingrained the lessons of patience and peace taught to us by our new Galactic Family were overtaken by small surges of anger, which resulted in the ruthless slaughter of many reptilian warriors. Such actions bore a steep price, as fear did not stop those who fled such rage from using all the might of their plasma firepower to render gaping wounds in those of us who committed such atrocities. Our thick metallic and crystalline scales repelled most attacks, yet there were still a few weak spots in our physical armor.

Yet finally, the primary battleships and transports began to depart. The reptilian leaders resigned to appeasing our insistence as their supplies dwindled and our

Guardianship reduced them to little more than prisoners on a foreign planet. Some of the more rebellious generals continued to attempt skirmishes, but these were quickly quelled in absence of the main body of their forces.

As my chest swelled with pride in our victory, I caught an updraft and surfed it in an ascending spiral, bringing my sight above another of the rippling stone outcroppings. Smooth curves of white rock jutted out of the flat desert floor like ancient skeletons, yet some of the wind carved ribs glittered like ice, as the bone-stone gave way to solid crystal. This ridge was only a fraction of the height of some of the others that seemed to scrape the sky, gathering what little moisture there was into smooth cloud-rings, crowns for the heads of the tallest mountain spires.

Soaring over the gentle curves of the ridge, I watched the whirlwinds get caught in the shape of the stone, melting into waves of fine dust that splashed through the canyons. I closed my eyes for a moment, relaxing and gliding forward. Anticipation always bubbled in my belly at this exact spot, a mixture of excitement with a touch of anxiety. Yet this time, the feeling was familiar, and passed away as quietly as the fading winds.

The air was suddenly still, and only my swift motion kept me aloft as I opened my eyes to behold a Shihaeleian city...my city. The desert floor stretching across the broad valley was swept clean, shimmering white crystal glittering in beautiful organic geometries rippled across its flat surface to the mountains in all directions. At the far end of the valley, nestled into the foothills of leaping peaks, was a forest of white crystal spires that sparkled with rainbows of spectral sunlight.

As I glided closer, my sharp eyes began to pick out the details of carved spiral stairs, delicate balconies, winding passages and smooth towers. A white stone wall over 100 paces high surrounded the city, merging into sheer cliff walls at either end. The city itself gently climbed with the rolling hills, layer after layer revealing more beauty and artistry in every building.

The wall was damaged in many places, and parts of the city were slowly being rebuilt from crumbled rubble. Yet most of the city remained unharmed, as the incredible stamina of the Shihaelian warriors, the Solarians, had kept the reptilian armies at bay for many, many years.

A growl emerged from my throat unexpectedly, as I reflected on their reception of our "rescue." It seemed that they would have rather continued fighting the reptilians forever, then see their efforts made insignificant by the sudden arrival of the "Dragon gods." They knew us to be allies, but we could not reveal that many of us were actually Shihaeleian children, kidnapped almost two decades ago by the reptilian slave ships.

They could only see powerful extraterrestrial beings that suddenly relieved them from duty, ending most of their battles in a single day, and immediately providing planetary wide guardianship. In essence, we stole their jobs, and dishonored their sworn duties, and most of them seemed to hold on to a deep and festering resentment.

The Miners who were once slaves of the reptilian species, and now wore Dragon bodies, were eager to end the masquerade and return to their families, and this was the source of most of the excitement around the last reptilian departures. We had kept to ourselves, resting and recovering in the mountains, and in the giant underground caverns where most of the food, water, and living organisms dwelled on this planet.

We had aid from the Galactic Families, who set us up with the technology to provide for the needs of our massive bodies. It was amazing how much food we could consume in a day, and each of the types of Dragons seemed to have their own nutrient needs and taste preferences. The Desert planet's biosphere simply couldn't provide for the diversity of our appetites.

White Dragons, and Silver Dragons like myself, were able to eat much of the local planetary fare, including a wide variety of cavern-dwelling fish in the underground pools, algae, and some of the rich seed-plants that grew in light shafts that cascaded for hundreds of paces into the underground worlds. Yet the Red and Gold Dragons required obscene amounts of raw meat, while the Emerald, Sapphire, and a few of the more exotic Dragon varieties consumed a range of stalks and starchy plants, strange berries, massive fruits (some with odd shells), and other foods that could never be cultivated on Shihaeleio.

We were told that our Dragon types were based on our Physical and Spiritual Genomes. Even though many of the Miners were Shihaeleian, there were also many other species scattered among our group, some who had been enslaved with us on the Lava Moon, and others who had joined us from the Galactic Families. Among the Shihaelei, there were mostly White, Red, and Black Dragons (notably the primary colors of the the Shihaelei culture) with a couple Silvers like myself. The other Dragons were primarily of other species, although some of them were Shihaelei with strong Spiritual Genomes connected to other Galactic races.

As I soared over the city walls, faces turned toward the sky, eyes watching my form slice through the air like a sword. Awe and anxiety battled for their expressions, the fine shifts in lines around their eyes and mouths vivid in my piercing aerial sight. Swooping between spiraling towers and elegant arching bridges, I headed for one of the largest pavilions, where other Dragons were already gathering.

A beautiful rainbow of colors shone brilliantly before the white crystal stonework, like a treasure trove of gems and precious metals. The real treasure, however, could only be witnessed in the deep and intelligent eyes that watched my approach, windows into the courageous beings who dedicated their lives to saving a planet, and each other.

Flexing and curving my wings like sails, I flared against the air and slowed my descent. A single flap of my wings provided the final deceleration I needed to hover before gently touching down on all fours.

Haggan, in Gold Dragon form, landed just behind, walked over beside me and looked at me with knowing eyes. He seemed to have had a very easy time adapting to this body. Since seeing him in this very dynamic form, I discovered that his way of communicating was far more complicated than I had originally conceived. I understood so much more about his way of being, and yet he still comfortably wore a cloak of indecipherable mystery around his intellect.

At times, his golden scales rippled like liquid fire, yet at this moment they reflected a deep azure light. The source was Sapphire Dragon Jassan, refracting oceanic pools of blue everywhere as he approached, swooping into the pavilion. The surface of his skin seemed to have a crystalline depth, as several layers of scales overlapped and reflected different shades of color. His wide mouth opened in a toothy grin, his eyes softening and warming with genuine happiness. With a deep breath, I returned the smile.

The people of the city were already gathering around the square. The Solarians arrived in force, spreading around us at strategic points to insure the safety of the observers. For many of them, it was the first time they had donned full battle gear since the sieges had ended.

Metal plates were fastened to dried serpent skins (from the underwater pools) in complex patterns on their breasts, while overlapping scales extended over shoulders, thighs, and shins. More small and flexible scales flared from their forearms, attached to tight bracers. They wore horned helms that were round upon the tops of their heads, then flared at ear level out to a wide rim that guarded their necks and collars. Some were masked, dark painted faces reflecting angry demons and mock reptilians.

The sun was already a deep red, melting slowly into the horizon. Dark fingers crawled up the mountains, shadows cast from tall towers, as darkness began to swallow the passages between buildings. The Dragons were all very still, watching the sky catch fire, sculpted statues of creatures from another Age...*another Galaxy*. Clear orbs hanging around the square began to release their stored sunlight, steadily replacing the falling star with their own rich red glow.

As the rainbow of color in the sky condensed behind the distant ridgeline, the two last Dragons swept into the city with a torrent of wind. The statues came to life, making way for them to land, as the people pressed back into the shadows and the Solarians gripped the hilts of their curved blades.

The White Dragon Kritos displayed an open mouthed grin, tongue hanging loosely out of his mouth like a breathless canine, while the Gold Kristan had a way of looking as though he had arrived hours ago, and was impatiently awaiting the next step. Kristan was the determined youth who had helped free the young miners in the Barracks back on the lava moon, what seemed like many years ago in subjective time.

"It's done," Kritos growled excitedly. "The last have gone, and our contacts say they are now far from orbit." A slight smile touched Kristan's lips, as I breathed a sigh of relief. Haggan tilted his head back roared into the sky with a bone-shuddering resonance, setting off a ripple of concerned shouts and fearful shuffling from the spectators. The Solarians simply watched us carefully.

"Then it is time." I said, looking up at the stars blooming into view all over the clear evening sky.  As the last twilight faded, a large shooting streak cut across my vision, and it seemed to turn just before vanishing. With a deep breath, I reached down and touched the Yellow Gem embedded in my belly.  It softened as I pressed my large silver claws against it.  Gently, I began to turn the gem, and it slid easily as I rotated it in a single full circle.  Then with a sharp click it stopped turning, and I pressed it deeper into my belly.

I suddenly felt my skin begin to ripple and slide, and I looked toward the gathered Solarians and Shihaelei. Muscles throughout my massive body contracted intensely, organs cramping painfully, and a violent vibration began spreading through my form. Involuntarily convulsing, I felt as though the world was growing and expanding all around me.  I tried to keep my eyes focused, but could only see blurs of stunned faces along with other rippling and convulsing Dragons.  In streaks of brilliant light, stars appeared to be falling all over the sky. Everything shifted in masses of color and sound, solidifying and melting in and out of form, and I squeezed my eyes shut to keep from expelling my stomach all over the square.

Then at last, everything was still. I opened glazed eyes and found myself looking at my hands, splayed upon the glittering stones of the pavilion. A jolt of surprise shot through me; they were so small and frail. Four fingers and a thumb, wrapped in thin, soft, dust-colored skin, with short transparent nails and thick visible veins. From cuffs around my muscular wrists, a tightly stretched purple fabric spread over my arms and chest, a golden belt around my waist connecting it to blue leggings, yet the colors were nearly washed out in the white filmy dust which covered me entirely.

The wave of blurring forms and strange sounds were finally settling in the square behind me as all those with me transformed out of these Dragon forms, and I carefully stood up from my hands and knees. Turning from the dizzying sight, I noticed that all the people were staring at me. Their mouths hung open, wide eyes unable to fully accept what they were seeing.

It was at that instant that I noticed that the stars had not stopped falling across the sky. Lines tracing between constellations in every color of the spectrum appeared and vanished in a hypnotic rhythm of geometries. Some of them formed elegant curves, sweeping like calligraphic sand sculptures or liquid language.

For a moment, I was also taken by the sheer awe of their beauty, and then I realized that the tide of transformations had finally finished. All the Dragons were now just various humanoids again. Men and women of many species were slowly recuperating, gathering around me. Joy and relief was in some eyes, and some had a look of loss or reluctance. Yet kindness and warmth spread across all of their faces.

Feeling their strength spreading through my heart, I turned to the gathered spectators, still speechlessly staring between us and the dancing sky. My heart filled my voice, and finally, I spoke:

"I am Ki'Shen. I am Shihaelei, born of Ora'kuru[6] Kaiya Rha and Shugo'rai[7] Justan Solarian. At last, I have come Home."

As if on cue, the skies returned to normal. No one spoke for a few moments, as shock seemed to spread through the crowd. Whispers began to follow the shock, and then, one of the Solarians stepped forward. His face was hardened by years of battle, but his eyes were deep and gentle. "Welcome home, Ki'Shen. Your Life is Honored, and your Family is remembered here." Shouts of acknowledgement followed, with a few sporadic cheers, but no other came forward.

One by one, the gathered Dragon Guardians spoke their names, ancestry, and origin. Each of the Shihaelei announcing themselves set off ripples of shock and whispers, and occasionally someone would burst into tears and run forward to embrace them. Those who had living family in this crowd were few and far between, but the masses around the square continued to grow as everyone huddled in close to hear the introductions.

At first, as each of the other species spoke their names, there was awkward silence and broken thanks. Yet as the introductions continued, and the sheer diversity and magnificence of the gathered beings was recognized, cheers grew in strength until there were steady waves of growing applause and shouts of support and gratitude.

------------------------------

[6] Related to the Japanese word for Oracle

[7] Related to the Japanese word for Guardian Spirit

As the energy increased, and the last few Shihaelei came to speak their names, no one seemed to notice that between the stars, the sky had become populated by fleets of starships. I realized that this was only the beginning of the introductions.

When the last cheers fell silent, and the crowd continued looking at us expectantly, I stepped forward again.

"Shihaelei! Planetary Family!" I called out to everyone present, looking around at the eyes gathering on me. Focus, strength, trust.

"From the Stars came our greatest challenge. These Draconians forged us, showing us our strengths and weaknesses. They exploited our fears, and taught us caution and patience. Through our battles with them, we have discovered so much more about ourselves, and we have overcome. We have survived! We have evolved!

"Now, from the Stars comes our greatest gift. Those of us who stand before you now, though we may be from many different Stars, we are Family! It is time for our Planetary Family to grow, and join those who have discovered other ways to dance through the Fabric. They are Galactic Beings, and they hold Council as we do!

"We are invited to be Members of this Galactic Council." I gestured towards the sky, and it responded in ripples of flashing rainbow lights. Gasps and awe spread through the crowd again, and I pressed forward with assurance. "It is a circle in peace, a Family in harmony, and all the gifts they have received, they now wish to share with all of you.

"In our journey as a species, we have come far, and we have much to share. In return, we have much to learn from our Star Family. They are wise and beautiful beyond measure, from many many worlds, and they have learned to travel between them with great ease."

The lights in the sky began to dance again, in beautiful geometries and rhythmic forms, as one disc shaped ship dove out of the sky and flew low over the city towards the square. Light playfully scintillated across its surface, and it seemed like a child's toy until its gargantuan scale became apparent. Its base soon blocked out the entire sky as it hovered over the pavilion. A delicate thread of silver appeared to unwind from its bottom surface, forming a long and wide spiral ramp.

As the ramp touched the ground, a door fluttered open like an unfolding flower, and brilliant light spilled out of the ship. The crowd seemed to hold their breaths, and a sense of familiar excitement tingled through my whole body.

Then the bottoms of robes could be seen emerging from the ship, swaying with graceful, descending steps. Long golden hair spilled over slender shoulders, and then the faces of the Extraterrestrial visitors came into view.

Timeless beauty formed of delicate features and creamy skin framed eyes that pierced through the anxiety of all who saw them. Distinctive cheekbones and sharply arched eyebrows radiated a regal authority, yet their pale lips almost pursed in a playful smirk. Tall, thin, and fluid in motion, the radiance of these Beings instantly dissolved any remaining tensions in the crowd.

The three Beings came to stand on the glittering pavilion stones, and spread to either side of the ramp. I had great difficulty pulling my gaze from one of the two females, as her astonishing grace and mysterious shape seemed to still my breath and clear my mind of everything else. Her eyes drifted across the gathering and met mine, holding for a long, piercing moment in which I felt stripped and bared to my Core essence. Having experienced this once before with the Ambassador on the Galactic Mothership, I managed to maintain my composure. When her eyes finally released me, I swallowed the lump in my throat.

They were gesturing now, offering any and all an opportunity to enter the Ship. Several of the Dragon Guardians immediately ascended the ramp, especially those of species who were not accustomed to Desert planets in their natural form. Then a few of the Solarians bravely stepped forward, seemingly giving permission to other Shihaelei to take this unprecedented opportunity. I smiled to myself, remembering the Miners departing from the Freighter Ship, and entering the Hall of Heaven.

Many of the people in the crowd shook their heads, unwilling to take the risk of boarding some strange Galactic Starship, but almost half of the gathered crowd eventually ascended. As the last few made their decision whether to stay or go, part of me wanted to stay on my Homeworld. I looked through the remaining crowd, and that's when it became fully clear that it would never be the Home I remembered.

Rather, it would always be Home in my Memory, but only in the places in times when I was with Family, and they were no longer here. For a moment, my heart ached, remembering the warmth of my Faherin's eyes, and the brilliance of my Mahira's smiles. I took a long, deep breath, and saw the Beings turn to board the ramp. The golden haired female looked at me again, a subtle touch of concern in her expression.

She did not move, and her gaze became expectant. I almost laughed, then nodded to myself and swiftly walked to the ramp. My eyes were moist with unshed tears as I beheld her gorgeous face from a step away, and could not resist a Soul-felt smile spreading through my lips. Her eyes twinkled, then she turned and walked with me up the ramp, like a procession ascending into the Future.

# SHIHAELEI - CHAPTER 9
# OATH OF THE GALACTIC GUARDIANS 聶

The years that followed were not quite the peaceful respite I had hoped. While the Reptilian forces had pulled back from Shihaeleio, they still occupied what was left of our decimated water planet, and seemed to be gathering strength by building tons of new ships and larger motherships, the giant half-dome ships becoming entirely spherical moons of their own. Black, terrifying, DarkMoon Stations.

They were now spreading out to other planets and star systems, assaulting with intense force and legions of robot armies that decimated any unprepared populations. No one was prepared for this, perhaps besides those of us remaining from the Reptilian Mines, and those we rescued who had fought for their survival to join us in escape. We started to grow a little battalion on the strangest planet I had ever seen, by the invitation of the Galactic Councils.

After the ascension of our people into the Galactic community, a large contingent of the Shihaelei *D'jedai* community had come to Corissia, a planet that had all but been swallowed in cities, a giant meeting ground for species from a thousand worlds. We entered a massive Council Hall, a giant egg-shaped building where hundreds of us entered through a special series of tunnels and out into the center of the massive structure. Eyes looked down on us from beings on individuated balconies that were geometrically distributed around the entire space.

Ama'dali'shkala had sponsored our attendance, and so her voice boomed into the space as her thoughts and words were suddenly illuminated in vast holographic light fields throughout the center of the egg above us. It was like standing under a floating series of scenes in spacetime, as she told the story of our rescue party from the lava moon docking with her Mothership, and our time in recovery. She took care and illustrated only very specific moments as she showed that we had innovated a way to use the Morphogenesis matter-into-body systems to generate Dragons, which the Draconians believed were their gods. She expressed some minor relief as she shared that the Draconians did not seem to know that some of *them* actually were Dragons who incarnated into our Galaxy within the Arcturian Experiments. The relief did not seem to spread through the room. I couldn't help but feel chills as she expressed *"Arcturian Experiments"* with visual representations of the Draconian world and its dark and terrifying structures, filled with a culture of battle and rage.

The pain was visceral in the room. It was clear that this experiment gone wrong was deeply affecting so many worlds, introducing the emotion of fear into the very interconnected field held within these council chambers. The air felt thick with it, and my whole body felt deeply uncomfortable.

Yet she carried on, showing how we liberated our own world, and carried the keys to potentially liberating many others. She expressed poetic portraits of our people, an artist of both language and matter herself, and the way she saw us was...remarkable. In her eyes, we were these extraordinarily powerful beings with the strength to face unspeakable odds, that our weapons and armor were crafted from the light of our Souls, bound to integrity and honor, and that we trained for much of our lives to earn the right to defend and challenge each other, always for the good of all, while maintaining some level of the sacred codex of sovereignty for each individual. Her full attention was on us now, and I longed to meet her eyes, and thought my wish was fulfilled as I felt a wave of her gaze touch my heart. She called upon us, singing our people's name in our way, "Shi-haaae-leeeei."

A few of the leaders from Shihaeleio stepped forward, wearing the traditional Shihaelei armor with its woven shoulder guards, flat shield plates, and golden horned helms that curved like a smooth dome over the top of the head, then flared out to protect the neck from angled strikes. Their family sigils shown in golden embroidery and magical seals lines their waist belts and the scabbards of their curved blades. Two male figures flanked a single female Oracle, all bearing the Mark of Solarians, Guardians of Honor.

A guide on the large round platform ushered them to stand upon a big golden seal with a fantastically complex geometry upon it. The Oracle looked around the whole room, and the two Guardians stood with their backs to her, forming a triangle, with the Oracle facing towards Ama'dali'shkala, gazing directly at her. As she began to speak in a self-assured, proud and wise tone, she directed her expressions towards all gathered.

"We the Shihaelei are here by your Grace. We owe you our Honor, we owe you our Lives. We are a people of many Paths, and not all will take the one we Propose here today. Yet for those that do, we will revere them for Ages to come, and we will support them with all that we have. We, leaders of the Solarian clan, propose that the Shihaelei join your Community among the Stars, and serve as Galactic Guardians. We offer our skills, our knowledge, and our abilities to protect your vast spectra of beings and life forms, and will train you to protect yourselves. We know what it means to lose a world, and as long as we live, we will give everything we have to ensure no other beings must experience this." She falters for a moment, the vivid illustrations of a dying world flickering above us. "We the

Shihaelei, who choose this Path," she continues as she looks around at all of us, "do give our Sacred Oath to provide Guardianship to this Galactic Community, from now through all Time. *And so we do, and so we are!*"

Every Shihaelei in the room's voice booms after hers, "AND SO WE DO, AND SO WE ARE!"

*"IN TAK SHI HA SHAE, IN TAK SHI HA SHEN!"*

And thus was the Galactic Guardian Oath established, and the Order of the Guardian *D'jedai* was born. We would become the first Interplanetary Guardian Force, providing security, rescue, and defensive operations across so many planets that had left conflict and war behind long ago. It was like a garden of grace out there across these beautiful worlds, and they had no idea what was coming for them from across the reaches of the darkness of space.

So our first task was education, both by accepting initiates from many worlds, misfits who would become initiates by the ways they stretched beyond the normal way of life in their home planet cultures. For the Shihaelei, education was not about discussing all the horrible things that could happen to you, but rather by harnessing the innate gifts within you, building so much trust and resilience, that you naturally overcome any obstacle thrown your way.

Yet it would not be long before we would need to actively defend worlds and assault prisons, rescuing people captured from ships or planets in the sectors around Betelgeuse and eventually into the vast expanse of the Nebula which looked like a great Dragon's head, which happened to be near the home of this unimaginably populated planet, Corissia, in the Alnitak Star System.

:::

Right next to this massive egg-shaped Council Hall, we were all given lodging in a gargantuan complex with three sky-scraping towers in a triangle, stretching far into the sky, each rounded like a teardrop and wrapped in glass that could see in every direction. Lower towers formed an opposite triangle, with elaborate structures on their rooftops that could be seen from the higher floors of the lodging towers. In the center of the whole structure, connected by massive multi-level bridges over three-story arches, was a courtyard with an extraordinarily beautiful garden. Even with all the Shihaleiei present, we barely filled a third of one of the lodging towers. That was a good thing, because the remaining space continued to be filled with new recruits and students, and we desperately needed more of them.

The structure had many physical practice centers, lecture halls, interactive gaming spaces, diverse dining experiences, and gear/tool fabrication centers, and the whole space was becoming a central training center for our new recruits. This planet was like a gathering ground for people from thousands of worlds, and most of its surface was made up of gargantuan endless cities that wove together across continents. I could not comprehend how many beings must live on this world, but I often sat in awe looking out over the endless lights from one of the towers in this complex at night. *This is what I'm here to save.*

My attention was constantly drawn to the Starports, branching off to the North and South of the what was beginning to be known as the Guardian Towers. Like a smooth blue Dragon made of water, smooth wings arched up and out in each direction, stretching out with feather-like passages to docked ships on countless platforms. While the South platforms were mostly filled with visiting Ambassadors and petitioners visiting from other worlds, the North platforms were becoming filled with our Ships. From lean and agile Starfighters to larger Transports and specialized Tech Ships, we would soon have the vehicles we needed for large coordinated operations.

We were training as many new recruits as we could, gathering talents and abilities from various species across the many worlds that the Pleiadians had built councils with. Along with the Arcturians, they had joined us in swift and coordinated action to gather Warriors, and prepare other planets for potential assault.

Few of them had much in the way of physical combat skill, so my Shihaelei brethren and I led everyone in the development of agility, circular movement, core balance, redirecting weight, leveraging force, energetic extension, grounding, and hand-to-hand sparring at every level of skill. Fortunately, these other species had higher-sensory gifts and energetic abilities which allowed them to adapt quickly, bringing natural skills in movement into more highly refined *forms*, as we brought them deeper into the secrets of Shihaelei Martial Arts and Alchemy.

While I had not gone through the teenage initiations of my people, all the knowledge was already ingrained in me as both my Faherin and Mahi had layered that wisdom into every aspect of my childhood before I was...taken. Parts of me were still so angry, a burning flame that drove my dedication to training and action. I felt like a tightly bound spring at times, ready to launch from the pressure of decades of lost emotions. I knew battle. I knew exactly how much focus, precision, stamina, and awareness it required, and the searing loss it could scar you with. So much pain, and yet here I was, so far beyond anything I had ever imagined.

Piloting the small Starfighters we had developed to raid their prisons and mining colonies was thrilling. It felt so familiar, riding the gravitational fields of Spacetime effortlessly, and yet the internal g-forces were modulated so that they only induced a fraction of the physical strain. In this way, the maneuverability was mind-blowing. They were faster and more agile than anything I had ever experienced, and this gave some small sliver of pleasure as we dove towards death again and again to raid heavily armored prison fortresses.

Our initial squads were small, a little elite group of Shihaelei, some of them *Sens'ai*, as we called the Guardian teachers from various worlds who had a natural talent in piloting, combat, survival, or healing skills. Usually only two to three of us per Starfighter, missions geared towards outposts or exposed remote positions and bases with prisons and mining camps.

In the first waves of assault we planned over many weeks of training, we caught them off-guard, taking out their weapon turrets and blasting their entries in a rapid cascade, lightning fast streaks of starships pummeling their defenses then breaking just before impact, landing at the gates, and then we would charge inside.

Most of the mining complexes on the lava moon I'd escaped from, as well as those on what remained of the raped and ravished Shihaelei world of *Mizu'no waku'sei* were duplicates of each other, so those of us who had escaped these nightmares in the past were the ones to lead the charge into their eerie depths. Our family of captive miners turned refugees turned Guardians helped to build virtual maps of the bases and prisons, memorizing every tunnel and corridor, planning every move of our assaults. Free the miners, arm them, locate the birthing areas, rescue the women and any offspring, and get out, alive.

That last part was tricker than it sounds... The bases were crawling with training Reptilian soldiers who always seemed ready for a fight. And they were *fast*, moving with darting precision that kept the best us on our toes. I had to hold myself in the space of stillness without distraction, senses opened outward in every direction, feeling the subtle currents of intention and awareness wherever they were emanating, more than seeing the location of each target.

This was part of the deeper training: we were not just forging Warriors, we were awakening the Inner Eye and the Core Purpose of the initiates in our campaign. We were helping them build their Central Pillar of energy and conscious awareness, their *D'jed*. To face this foe, you could not just rely on the physical senses, but required tuning and receptivity through the physical, emotional, mental, and spiritual planes of Being.

That also meant developing empathic sensitivity, clear mental focus and strategy, relational synergy with our team, and most importantly good communications skills backed by deep swift intuition.

A few quick hand gestures would help coordinate movement, while pausing to aid someone breathe deeper and settle their nervous system could accelerate and improve our entire effort. Learning to trust each other when someone sensed movement or energy, especially when out of sight around a corner in the labyrinthine tunnels. All took lots of pre-planning for truly coordinated movement, but we got better at it with time. When we got into flow-states with each other, our little bands of raiders moved as One, dancing with each other deeper and deeper into these dungeons and leaving a trail of carnage behind us.

It was gruesome, but I drove the pain of the loss of my people, the loss of my world, and channeled it through rage and ruthless destruction. I had to focus my empathy on the Souls of those beings who had incarnated into this species, and know I was releasing them from torment.

In battle, one must find a way to align all of their Being in the same direction, the good and bad, the light and dark, the trust and fear, the love and hate. I would one day discover that this is true for all of life, but that day was not here yet. At this point, all I knew is that I had to kill or be killed, and save as many people as I could.

# SHIHAELEI - CHAPTER 10
## ELF-KIN 家

They learned our tactics quickly, and started adding larger protective fleets and automated robot attack systems, and a few of our little squads didn't make it out alive. We had to abandon a couple terrifying missions, regroup, learn more, and recruit.

Fortunately, the time spent planning, teaching, and practicing in the Guardian Towers also meant a few opportunities for rest and personal exploration. I had found myself intersecting with Alyria often, her people providing us with guidance on how to navigate the interplanetary cultures across the Galaxy. She was often quiet, lingering on the edges of our groups in training, and I sought to find her eyes often. A glance from her was worth countless attempts, the warm smile touching her lips sending quivers up my spine.

She had an elegance to her every move, as if she was dancing, rather than walking or moving around. It was subtle, precise, an art form. And not her only one. She gave us a tour of a hall of grand artworks, exquisite masterpieces expressing the essence and energies of many worlds. Portraits of species, or *"teseia alam triastria"* as she called them in her smooth alto voice, lilting each syllable with delicacy like a song, which she translated roughly as "visionary symphony of life blooming."

Each image had the Primary Star of the system as a geometric nexus in the top center, with detailed depictions of the planetary landscape below. A male and female bodied expression of the species framed either side in the foreground. The whole images seemed to move with the flow of lattices of energy of specific vibrations, appearing to emanate from the Star. I had never seen anything like this, and I was instantly inspired and even more deeply intrigued and attracted to Alyria, who had created several of the pieces herself.

Her depiction of the Elven Homeworld, with its Primary Star Sirius A shown in a vesica of resonance with its Secondary Star Sirius B, depicted just above and behind the main star. Orbital fields of energy could be seen ripping through the starry space around the two stars, showing something about their binary dance, and another ring linked down to merge with the planetary surface in the foreground. Giant snowcapped mountains with purple stone cascaded down to thick forested valleys and gargantuan trees, the high-branches of which of which looked decorated with cities and living structures. The two representatives of the sex of the species were beautiful, wearing artfully decorated green layered tops with woven golden branches spindling across mantles that extended like leaves off their shoulders and formed a high-collared vestment. Their long pointed ears framed almond eyes which seemed to glow gently, set within finely chiseled features and tilted cheekbones.

Yet even the exquisite beauty of the beings in this artwork were hardly a match for the physical embodiment these Sirian beings actually possessed. Alyria's skin was almost pearlescent, soft and smooth and free of lines or blemishes. It was as if she was carved from the white crystal mountains of Shihaeleio itself, and I wanted to feel every inch of her. I wanted to know what she knew, and discover the depths of the mystery she wore around her like a cloak.

To my great surprise, she met my interest with her own, and I found myself walking in the gardens down in the courtyard of the massive multi-tower complex on this city covered world. I could viscerally feel her relief in being around trees and flowers, ponds and beautifully decorated mossy seating areas. Her laughter was like bells and chirping birds, and her touch was a gentle, powerful emanation. She seemed to sneak in and steal kisses from me, teasing and never quite letting me take hold of her. She was like the Etheric Fae we had in the crystal caverns underground, like lights you couldn't catch whose laughter would tickle the back of your mind and ears.

Eventually we would spend a couple nights together, full of deep and luscious intimacy, yet she always left me wanting even more of her. Some part of her was withdrawn, no matter how much I got her to open up in pleasure and ecstatic release. When all was still, I would feel her moving away from me inside. It felt like she knew the danger I would face in the days to come, and that I would not be able to be with her long. Perhaps more, she was not willing to become attached to me. Maybe there was someone else, or maybe she just couldn't see someone like me being with someone like her. I didn't really know, but I was deeply great:full for every moment I had with her.

# SHIHAELEI - CHAPTER II
# THE AMBASSADOR 缘

It was with the arrival of Ama'dali'shkala at the Guardian Academy that Alyria finally pulled away. When I saw the Pleiadian Ambassador again, the rush of gratitude and freedom and...so much more that I felt in the days following my escape from the lava moon, all came flooding back. This time, I wasn't going to let her evaporate from my attention, disappearing into her massive ship. I knew when she would emerge from the Grand Council Hall that was positioned like a giant egg nested in front of the huge towers of the Guardian Academy. Apparently before it was an Academy, these towers were only used for visiting Ambassadors who attended the Hall, so they were constructed in a beautiful harmony with one another. Now many of the levels of the towers were filled with students, and I wondered if new structures would eventually have to be built to house more students and Ambassadors together.

She walked forth from the Hall just like I remembered her, gliding across the ground as if her feet didn't touch. I moved to stand directly in her path, gazing at her intently and holding my ground as she approached with a small entourage. She looked a little surprised to see me, but more curious, and I kneeled to the ground, offering my hand and asking that she join me to sit for a time in the gardens, and find some peace from all the chaos. After a quick glance at several approaching Ambassadors exiting the Hall and apparently urgently desiring her attention, her gaze returned to me with a hint of relief, and she took my hand with one of hers, while the other raised a single palm. Her entourage immediately turned to greet the approaching Ambassadors, and she and I glided down the path quickly towards the massive arches that led into the foyer of the Guardian Academy towers.

We passed beneath the archway silently, but I could feel her communication emotionally, giving me soft waves of gratitude and gentle nudges of curiosity and...was that excitement? I breathed deeply, focusing on the beautiful geodesic lattices between the four pillars and arches of the entry, decorated with glowing stars as a map of the night sky. More than seeing it in the corner of my eye, I felt her glance up at me a few times, yet she moved with me in sync as though she knew exactly where we were going. Perhaps she did; I felt more...transparent around her than anyone.

Students and Ambassadors passed by us in every direction as we crossed the giant circular geometries laced in metal threads across the stone floor in the center of the larger Atrium past the entry, and we both ignored all the looks directed our way as we crossed into another smaller series of arched doorways that led into the central courtyard gardens.

When I finally got my moment alone with her, in a quiet corner of the gardens where a bench was framed by two Dragonfly wings of elven design that arched above the seat, I just stared into her deep blue eyes. There was a profound peace in just looking at each other, knowing all that had been faced, and all that would come. Ama'dali, as she eventually let me call her in private, knew everything I had been through, and she seemed to care with her entire being.

As we sat looking at each other silently, I felt Alyria suddenly move into view near us in the gardens. She stopped, and I felt a rigid sharp spike of energy emanating from her direction. I turned to look at her as quickly as I could, but she had already turned and was moving away, more swiftly and intensely than graceful. I opened my mouth to call to her, but something told me that there was nothing that would stop her. My heart clenched in pain, and I closed my mouth and hung my head. Ama'dali's hand touched my cheek and chin, drawing it up to look her in the eyes again. The pain in my heart melted, feeling washed with a wave of love.

Then it all poured out of me. I spoke of how I had tried so hard to spend time with her on the Mothership, how it felt to return to Shihaeleio, what it was like being a Dragon... Her eyes widened with greater excitement as I described that, and they drew me in deeper. I told her about the councils among my people that had led to the Guardian Oath, and about the founding of the Guardian Academy. So much had happened, but the stories flowed from me like a waterfall into her open eyes, ears, and heart. I told her about Alyria, and she only smiled at me and softened her eyes more with care. She seemed to embrace me with every layer of her being as she engulfed me into those oceanic eyes.

I told her how much I wanted to spend time with her, how much I wanted to learn from her, and that I just wanted to...dance with her. I felt a warm surge between our bodies as I opened my heart and took off all my mental and emotional armor, letting her into the world of my feelings, and suddenly it began to feel like we were in an entirely different conversation. The energy between us resonated with a *visible* energetic overlay, and I felt like I was in a private chamber with her. As she looked into my eyes, I suddenly saw into that hint of curiosity, and she revealed to me exactly what she was curious about. It felt like layers of my clothes were being stripped from my body slowly, as her mind explored my physical form, and I could *feel* it as though she were touching me. Slipping under my shirt, up the legs of my pants, around my belly and then down...

Oh wow, she was exploring me with her *mind*!

My body responded immediately, as heat swelled through my skin and filled my loins. Images of fire and bubbling liquid coursed into my vision, hot wet elemental... *Alchemy*. It was like she was giving me a taste of her knowledge of the Universal Field and the flow of Energies in existence, so similar to the lessons I taught at the Academy, but with a different cultural flavor, more raw in the form of expressed emotion and vibration. It was so familiar, and something inside me was waking up as I simmered with her in this chamber of intimate telepathy.

The fire inside me roared, and without thinking I closed the distance between us in the physical, wrapping my arms around her and kissing her. Yet she had moved in perfect synchronization, her arms around my shoulders and thighs suddenly rolling over my body to sit on my lap, lips moving to meet mine, and it was as if the vibrating chamber we were in became even more substantial and vivid. Was she actually *shielding* us from view somehow, or was it only me who felt like I couldn't see anything else except her and the light of our united fields?

With our bodies pressed together it was like a tropical storm, hot breaths and wet mouths, bodies radiating like stars and dripping juicy honey. I don't know how long we kissed, or when she took my hand and led me away from the garden. All I know is that we ended up in her chambers, full of soft velvety furniture and an unbelievably richly blanketed bed.

The firestorm of desire within me for everything that she was came out in a torrent of worship, pleasuring every inch of her body with my hands, my mouth, my eyes, and eventually my whole body. When she drew me into her body, the hot wet feeling suddenly changed our visions yet again, and we were Dragons. She was a shimmering Sapphire Blue, and I was Obsidian Black as the void between Galaxies. We tumbled into each other in joyful abandon, wrestling each other into pleasurable positions, mounting and riding each other as though we were catching waves of wind...or waves of water...but it felt more like magma... We *were* Dragons...at some point... together. Was this what drew her to explore the planetary system where she had rescued our little freighter ship? Could she feel me? More likely, the whole reptilian armies incarnating with Dragon blood...

Her eyes shone with confirmation and truth; it was all of that and more. And yes, my heart was a beacon, but one that she had been afraid to pursue. When she found us, all her fears were confirmed. Worlds were being destroyed. My world was destroyed. Our movements and love making slowed as her emotions rose and tears wet her eyes and dripped down her cheeks. I kissed them and held her closely becoming still, and she held me tight between her thighs with her whole body on top of mine, and we just felt each other breathe. The ache inside me grew into a spinning torrent that threatened to overwhelm me and make me sick. My...planet...destroyed...I began to fall into the dizzying vortex of pain as that thought fully reached my emotional body... I felt a jolt of fear overwhelm me...oh no...

Drawing in a deep breath, she pushed back to look at me, seeking to find a way into my eyes again. I was drifting, falling...but she was so beautiful...and then those blue sapphires caught me like an anchor, holding me steady as the whirlpool of aching pain slowed and melted into an inner galaxy of stars. She moved slowly on me, each pulse of her body a wave of urging pleasure, love that cascaded into the places where I still felt hurt, loss, and abandonment.

My whole body had tensed, but as I relaxed the energy began to flow again. My eyes were blurred with tears welling up from my Core, but I didn't resist them. I focused on her, meeting her with each breath, eyes pouring out gratitude and acknowledgement and hope and…love. She was the reason I was alive. She was the reason I trusted all these other beings. She was the reason I accepted them as my family, because they were *her* Galactic Family. Thus they must become mine, if I was to grow into this new Guardian identity that they all saw within me.

Soft, vulnerable strength, that's what these Pleiadians had been teaching me. In this moment she was the embodiment of that gift, and I felt it landing inside me like a mantle to wear, Sacred Armor as the Shihaelei called such energetic embodiment architectures.

We rose and fell to spaces between time, experiencing the Divine design in a rapturous thunderstorm of pleasure and awakening. Dragons in slithering coiling biting, humans in squishing cuddling sliding, beings in spiritual communion. Something dawned in me, a sense of deeper intimacy that this human experience of sex could uncover. This dance of energies was a way to feel through time, to know ourselves as more than the fleshy suits we wore, to ride on the currents of the Divine Archetypal Architecture of Reality and surf them in explosive waves of bliss.

She was Goddess, I was God. We Are.

I found tears in my eyes and my entire body was soaked as we slowed and cascaded into a deep embrace. I felt like a child reborn, and also the infinite patient expansiveness of a father. She held me tight, her chest still heaving and her body vibrating in shudders, tears streaming down her cheeks, her eyes deeper than ever. Then she started laughing, and it rippled up through me like a wellspring of mirth and joy, exploding into my own laughter. Whew, now this is the way to pray.

:::

In the days that followed I could feel her everywhere, like a gentle caress on my skin and a comforting presence in my mind. Our intimacy had unlocked more of my telepathic awareness, so I could actually hear her and feel her even at a distance. We had entangled in oh so many luscious ways. Yet I could also feel how badly I still wanted her... I was not sure I could ever be satiated from that transcendent erotic bliss.

My desire made her distance more difficult, and time with her still felt rare and sparse. Between my training and her constant councilship, it seemed nearly impossible to grab even moments together. Yet we managed to intersect on many special nights over the next several weeks, and it felt like the heavens were celebrating when we made love.

Then, she was called away, her ship on an urgent mission to gather many new recovery vessels coming in from a new sector. Before she left, I remember the sadness in her eyes. Everything in her look, in our brief goodbye, told me that this was the end. Something to do with the Galactic Council had disturbed her greatly, I could tell, but she would not speak of it nor show my mind what she knew. It was the last time I would see her, but some part of me always had hope that she would return. Instead, my heart was slowly and painstakingly destroyed, as she never came back.

# SHIHAELEI - CHAPTER 12
# FINDING A PATH 道

After Ama'dali had left, I needed time away from the constant intensity, and I spent several years traveling between the Guardian Towers and other worlds. On one of my visits back to teach and train, I met Pada'mai, one of the Shihaelei survivors who had come to visit Corissa and explore training with us there. We fell fast and hard, and we started traveling together to adventure and get away from everything. There were still so many peaceful worlds out there, where the pain and horrors of battle had not been known in a thousand generations.

Then, on one trip, she revealed to me that she was carrying my child. I wanted her and that child to be as far away from the Orion Wars as possible, but I knew I couldn't retreat away with her. My Oath bound my Soul, though she and the coming child had what I had salvaged of my heart. And so, for the second time, my heart was ripped from my chest, as I sent her away and returned to the Guardian Towers. There seemed to be no escape from this, no other choice...my destiny was to face this Galactic conflict head on.

The Draconian forces were expanding, automating their initial assault forces through robotic creatures and droids that nearly eliminated their casualties while decimating peaceful populations. They were able to take control of portions of planets at a shocking pace, while their powerful armies could stay in reserve, then sweep in to solidify control. Taking over all the resources of these advanced Starports and cities in various worlds, their technology accelerated and their raids became much more sophisticated.

It was a good thing I returned to refocus. We had our hands full with every imaginable responsibility and intervention, so for some of us, the stints of training and playing on Corissa became shorter and shorter, and more and more precious. Save, kill, survive, rest, start again. Days began to blur, and the only place I could find grounding in the good of this Universe was through the Guardians in this little Alliance. My Team.

:::

Aneleia and I danced, sparring on the mats in the Guardian Academy. She locked my arm and slipped me off-balance for an instant as my thoughts drifted, and I stepped down hard to stabilize and root my awareness back in my body. I let my arm and body melt as I focused my energy towards my lower Core in my g-center, and her control over my body was suddenly reversed, her muscle tension giving me total control over her form. With a ripple of lightning inside my body I released the Core energy in a twist of my waist and let it roar thought my heart and arm directly towards her central pillar. Her body responded intelligently, melting into my blow then catching its wave, and herself, several paces back.

She turned her feet once, corkscrewing her ground current deeper, and smiled menacingly. "Damn," she growled, "I had you."

"What has been taken can always be given back," I smirked, smiling back.

Her eyes betrayed the menace, and the heat in them warmed my loins, replenishing my Core energy in quite a pleasurable way as my roots surged. She was my favorite to train with...and *practice* with in other ways... Her youthful beauty and playful big eyes made our age gap seem larger than it was, and concealed the brutal precision of her exceptional piloting skills. And those lips...

...Came flying towards me in a half-smiling snarl, forcing me to focus and sink deeper into my roots. In a split second her fist brushed the edge of my left cheek as I swept my left arm up and just barely caught her attack with my forearm, but she also had my forward foot pinned by her own and leveraged her weight on the stomp to bring her other knee straight towards my right ribs. The force was significant, as her whole Core pivoted to deliver the full weight of her body through that knee. My right arm and elbow moved to block and were forced into my body, softening the blow a bit, but her knee drove into my body with a greater mass than seemed possible from her small frame.

A smile cracked my lips as I grunted, taking the blow and stumbling a bit as my right foot had to catch my weight by pivoting behind my left foot. Now *this time* she had me, and pride swelled in my chest even as pain split through my right ribs with the energetic force behind her impact. She had used my deflection of her punch as a tool to drive additional energy into her rotation, using my own force pulling her arm one direction to magnify her spin in that direction. I might have her right punching hand but with my other arm catching the force of her knee, I was instantly vulnerable to her left hand which sliced my throat with her thumb, mimicking a weapon taking my head off.

She let go of my foot and I stepped back, impressed. "Damn, you had me." I smiled, and her eyes narrowed as she looked slightly irritated.

"What has been taken can always be given back," she said with a playful sneer. "Any vector of force can amplify force in the same direction." Her sneer broke into a smile, and she was more than proud of herself for using my own teachings against me.

I nodded, then raised an eyebrow at her. "You're ready then?"

She grinned widely, then her mouth became a snarl again. "I am. Let's get those scaly fuckers."

I frowned at the speciesist adjective, but they were scaly and I had more than enough reason to want to curse them at any opportunity. Yet some part of me was still working through the integration of the memories that had come to me while I was in Dragon form... I was once scaly too, from some distant world of great Dragons, but there was so much I couldn't remember. It was like glimpses of a dream, and yet some part of me was so angry that I couldn't just remember all of it, as if I should just be able to access all of my past bodies.

Some of these humanoids had that ability, where they seemed almost ageless, with memory of events and time stretching back millennia. This only made it sting more that I couldn't, but I felt like the Dragon inside of me *could* do this...something was just blocking me. Maybe my lost memories from childhood? The gap of time in my mind on the lava moon...that I really had no desire to think about, let alone remember, as I had enough awareness of my time there to know more than enough of the horrors I faced.

Something shifted in my perception of Aneleia's face, and I blinked. Her eyes filled with concern, so my expression must have changed. "Ki'shen?"

For a moment, she had shapeshifted into a...Dragon...? "Do you have any memory as a Dragon?"

She looked confused for a moment and her brow knotted. Her parents had been killed by the Reptilians in a raid on her homeworld, but I had seen the potential in her by the way she evaded them when we flew in to try to stop the assault. I had taken her in like family, and she had become of the best pilots in our fleet. "I didn't transform in any of the early defense gambits, if that's what you mean. That was before I met you."

"I know. I mean…did we know each other before that?"

She looked into my eyes, and her expression relaxed. "You have always felt very familiar to me… Like I have always trusted you." She shrugged "I just do…"

I nodded, because the feeling was the same in me. I just knew she was important, and that she had gifts to help my team. Did I know her as a Dragon, before I came here? Something within me felt a tingle of energy, confirming it…if only I could remember.

I didn't push the questioning further, and instead gathered my things at the edge of the mat. She did the same, and we walked together towards the area where we had private rooms in the tower. It was time to prepare for our next rescue, and something about this one made me feel sick inside. I rarely felt anxious about anything these days, but this mission ate at me on the inside for some reason.

It had only been a short time since a flurry of excitement came from the Council Hall, announcing that a species from the Zeta Reticuli star system was joining the Galactic community. We were told they were an Army, ready to work with us to take on the Draconian forces spreading from system to system.

When I saw them for the first time, something knotted in my belly. They all looked identical in white and black lacquered armor, full helmets and face plates hiding their appearance, with black visors that appeared to have visualization technology built into them. Their bodies were armored in a sterile rendition of the Draconian plate armor. Rather than the black and red insect-like overlapping plates, the Zetas' armor was more like blocks of frozen milk, shiny white rectangular plates with hard angles buckled over ribbed black under-armor.

They moved and walked as one, marching in an eerie rhythm that was completely foreign to the Shihaelei way of moving. These unfortunate beings were toast when it came to facing the kinds of agile Draconian warriors we'd grown accustomed to fighting. Maybe they could help face the robots? Maybe that.

In any case, they meant numbers, and numbers were good. There was one small group of them that chose to train with our students, and they were marked with Red sashes installed in their armor. They were slow to gain skills in movement and martial arts, but their weapons abilities were excellent and they had very good aim.

They didn't really express themselves individually, almost ever, which was another red flag for me. They did respond to commands and requests, and they seemed to communicate with each other without speaking. Perhaps this was a gift, rather than a handicap. We would find out soon enough.

Since the Zeta forces had joined us, our numbers were more easily able to assault some of the more complex bases and prisons. It was eerie how well coordinated they were, moving in waves like a single body. Yet this also made them vulnerable to the smarter Reptilians, who had a way of quickly adapting to any patterns in battle.

All I knew about the Zetas was that they were brought into the Galactic community just we Shihaelei were, to help in the war. They had come from a wet planet in the Zeta Reticuli binary system, and they seemed to always be in that armor that covered their entire bodies and faces. Their indistinguishable appearance and almost identical voices made them all seem like clones of each other, and their group behavior reinforced this impression. They generally communicated within their minds, using some mechanism that was different from the telepathic energy bonds I was starting to learn how to feel and see between other species.

Something about them just didn't feel right, but I felt bad judging this species I knew so little about. They didn't really interact with us; they obeyed most urgent commands and followed the strategic patterns we planned before battles. It seemed like they really just had two goals: take out the enemy and protect each other. They were certainly more focused on the former than the latter, as many of them fell in every encounter. Almost like some of them would rather be dead...I shook off the uncomfortable thought.

But who were these beings, and why did they come to fight for us? Were they some kind of hive-mind, and is that how they were able to move and communicate in sync? Did they have some kind of secret technology? The few Galactic counselors I knew like Ama'dali'shkala seemed worried about them, but wouldn't answer my questions when I asked. Someone was clearly trying to keep their story a secret, and that is never a good sign...but more concerning is that other Ambassadors were forced to keep that secret. Why?

Unanswered questions rolled around all my thought patterns, and then suddenly we were at the door to my room. I almost walked past, and Aneleia had noticed. She glanced down the hall towards her room, then turned and pinned me with her big eyes. A small smile touched her lips as she put her hand on my chest and gently pushed my back against the door.

Her voice dripped with lust and smoldered with fire, "Well, if we're going to die tomorrow, then I'm not wasting the rest of this night." My wandering mind began to slow down, her words combined with her touch sliding down my chest, reconnecting me with my body. She pressed forward, her thigh pushing into my crotch. A heavy sigh escaped my lips, and I let my head settle back against the door and closed my eyes. I could smell her, subtle spicy sweet sweat still beaded between her breasts, her pelvis closing the distance against my thigh as she pressed her leg between mine. These training pants were a bit restrictive down there as it was, but now I couldn't wait to be out of them.

Feeling me swell against her, she nibbled at my lower lip playfully and breathed into me. I brought my left hand down to palm the entry pad for a moment, and heard the familiar tones of my room being unlocked. Just before the door's pressure on my back gave way, I pressed my weight back into her and reached around her slim waist and grabbed her soft muscular buttocks. I hefted her up onto my body and swung her into my room, and I met her mouth with mine and kissed her deeply.

She moaned with enjoyment as I gripped the back of her hair with one hand and her ass with the other, driving my kisses deeper as I hauled her towards the window. Her jacket dropped to the floor as she shrugged out of it while I carried her, and kicked her boots off. She hung from my body as I gently brought her down towards the bed, but suspended her as my knees touched the bed, and I ravenously dug my hands up the back of her tight undershirt as she squeezed me between her thighs, gripping my neck with her hands. Then I hungrily pulled her shirt up until it popped over her perky handfuls and hard large nipples, and proceeded to devour them with my mouth.

Her moans intensified, her heart racing behind the skin of her chest as my own heart pounded and body filled with fire and desire. These training pants were definitely not meant to accommodate the sword driving down my leg, but they made way. She reached a hand down and grabbed me, squeezing me inside my pants, and I groaned and roared at her primally.

I turned and pinned her to the bed under me, grinding myself between her thighs and sucking hard on her lips. Then I pulled her shirt over her head and admired her as she yanked at my waistband, her fierce look telling me that she wanted to conquer me. I breathed deeper, practicing feeling the overwhelming energy building in my loins up my spine and circulated it over my head and through my arms, as well as down my belly and deeper into my lower *Tan Tien* to store that energy.

I moved back just enough to let her pull my pants over my hips, and on down my legs until she could retrieve my tip, wet and dripping with clear fluid. She grinned hungrily and pulled on me like a rope, forcing me to move forward on my knees until she could take me in her mouth. She gently pulled back my skin as she made out with my head, swirling her tongue in mind blowing ways that had me focusing intensively on my energy circulation breathing.

Roaring fire started to creep up my legs as she intensified in devouring me, and I gently took her by the shoulders and slowly drew her away from me. There was feigned hurt in her eyes as she let me press her back to the pillows. I grinned at her, my body pulsing with fire, and I drew the energy up to my mouth and into my hands, then I slid down her body.

I pulled her training pants over her hips, holding both her legs over one shoulder, and pulled them down just enough to bind her knees together. Pushing her knees up to her bare chest, I bit and kissed and licked my way down the sensitive skin over her hamstrings and found her beautiful rose blooming between her inner thigh muscles.

I worked my way inward slowly but demandingly, closer and closer, then outermost lips, then a little further in. She squirmed and moaned with each torturous wave of pleasure and teasing, until she was trying as hard as she could to spread her legs further and push me into her with her feet on my back. Her hands gripped my hair, trying to guide me, but I knew exactly what she wanted.

Teasing my way to her pearl, by the time I touched it with my tongue, shivers ran up her body in waves. Then I slowly kissed her whole vulva as deeply as I could, my tongue driving into her as my mouth sucked her pearl and mound. Her moaning became a loud groan, and more than a few "yes, yes please..."

As I pushed her further and further open with my mouth alone, I finally gave her reprieve and kissed my way down her legs as I pulled her pants over her feet, along with her socks, dropping them to the floor. She slowly spread her legs, showing me her full beautiful vulva and reaching for my sword which could have easily held up a heavy piece of armor. I let her just touch me to feel how completely and utterly turned on I was, then I pulled away teasingly and dove back between her thighs.

I brought my left hand under her sacrum so I could control the angle of her hips as I brought my other hand under my chest and chin to meet her temple flower. With one middle-finger, I gently massaged her opening as I swirled my tongue around her pearl the same way as she had with my head, and she writhed with pleasure, groaning and pulling my hair. "Oh god yes," she moaned, driving her hips towards my hand and letting my finger slide inside of her.

I pulled her into me with my supporting hand, and curled my finger inside her to draw her even closer, and gave her every ounce of my presence and ravenously devoured her. As I moved rhythmically, her moans became gasps and cries, until I could feel her soaking my chin and hands as her body moved in waves of orgasmic pleasure.

Then her eyes met mine as she pulled my head up towards hers, tasting herself on my kiss, and she grabbed my sword with her other hand, guiding my tip to her wet flower petals. With all her muscle she pulled at me, arms and legs trying to drive me inside of her, but I gently resisted so the movement was extremely slow.

Entering her was like sliding into a well of bliss; the soft wet depths inside a woman are surely the most silky squishy texture in all existence. If I were to pick a favorite form of matter in the Universe, it would be the inside of a woman's flower.

Her body shuddered and she gasped as she finally had me all the way in, my heart pounding against hers, and inside her, as our rhythmic beats rolled through each others bodies. She pulled my forehead to hers and gazed into me with eyes begging for more, and I proceeded to slowly and rhythmically flow all the way in, then almost all the way out, over and over again.

It was like sacred duty, sacred service, *Seva*[8] and *Samadhi*[9] that provides instant reward for dedication and focus. I

[8] From the Sanskrit for "sacred service"

[9] From the Sanskrit for "state of divine realization"

breathed and became a rolling ball of white fire, my spine roaring with energy, the front of my body a waterfall pouring pleasure down into my lower *Tan Tien*. Mixing the energy of my pulsing root with the light building in the crucible in my lower belly, I drove the Alchemical charge up into her body through my sword, seeking her edge, finding the place of her complete and utter surrender.

Her waves of pleasure built as my rhythm demanded it, and her eyes frantically looked at me for some sign of weakness. She wanted me to lose control, and it was certainly taking everything I had to keep my entire body from exploding. Yet in this match winning meant giving the greatest pleasure possible, so I focused everything on her and expanded my awareness out, becoming a Galaxy in my heart.

The sudden increase of consciousness and space seemed to give room for everything that was building up inside her, and she went Supernova. It was like feeling a star explode with me inside of it, waves of energy blasting against me and into my body, and I cried out and breathed deeper to hold...just...a little...longer...

Spine rippling, her voice crying out in total ecstasy, her hands scrambling for my body and the bed and anything she could hold on to as she blasted into torrents of orgasmic bliss. My rhythm was unrelenting, and I could feel her entire inner surfaces pulsing and pushing, and her throbbing cherry being pounded by my movements. Her eyes were rolled back and she was finally surrendering completely, but still pulling at me to continue.

Her ocean of energy was already overwhelming me, and she could feel that I was still holding my edge with all my might. "Please, let go..." she said, "for me..." and the gentleness in her swept up into my body, softening all my edges, all my subtle resistance, and then even my breathing was not enough to contain my volcanic charge.

I could feel the wave surging up from my root and pulled myself out of her just in time to enter my own gargantuan explosion. She grabbed me and worked me as I roared with pleasure, wave after wave crashing from every moment of edging where I had averted ejaculation. Light poured through me, electrifying every cell, and igniting hidden energy reserves into glorious fireworks. For what seemed like a timeless ride upon the infinity train, everything was simply perfect, and the Universe was pure bliss.

Soaked in each others fluids we snuggled into each other with our whole bodies, laughing and joyfully reflecting on the things we enjoyed the most. "That was fun." Her grin was almost silly, and I grinned right back. Those moments were slices of pure perfection in the great tale of existence.

# SHIHAELEI - CHAPTER 13
# DARKMOON STATION 冥

Morning came quickly, though I slept deeply after the revitalizing dance with Aneleia. She was just easy to be around, play with, fight with, and fly with. Today, I would need that ease, with what we were about to face.

With her, things were just simple, free from the complexities of the Galactic political landscape that Ama'dali'shkala faced, or the profound depth of presence that being with the Sirian Elven Priestess Alyria required. They were really the only two women I had ever met that made me feel...alive...in a way I had never experienced. My whole body would light up in their presence, swelling energy electrifying my cells and causing my heart to quicken.

As I spent the morning in meditation and preparation, I found myself reflecting on the days following the Shihaelei Guardian Oath, when I had transformed back into this humanoid form and the Shihaelei had joined the Galactic community, initiating the birth of the first Galactic Guardians.

Today we were taking on a central base, a major gambit in the efforts to weaken the onslaught of the Draconian forces. This was the most strategic attack point, a central relay for so much of the Draconian's communications and flight trajectories. It was a huge advantage on our end, having a Galactic community with advanced interstellar telepathy and remote viewing skills to map our enemy's movements, forces, and defensive positions. It should have felt like cheating in battle, but instead it felt like it gave us just a sliver of a chance.

When I finally suited up, finished strapping up my flight armor and grabbed my helm, I focused on the assault plan. First, we would send a group of our fastest Starfighters to slip into the massive planetoid-sized Draconian DarkMoon Station that was in geosynchronous orbit just outside of the planet's atmosphere. The task would be to dock and install the communications virus that had been prepared for us by a specialized task group that had been working with the Galactic Councils.

Then we would hit the base directly under the giant black sphere as their communications went dark, taking out key weapons manufacturing systems and the ship construction yards. Finally we would hit their robot command centers and hopefully disable a lot of their automaton armies that were on a rampage.

If we pulled it off, we would strike a serious blow to their entire campaign. It was absolutely critical for us to succeed. I steeled myself with that thought.

After a wave of cheers and support from students and ground crews, I was strapping into the pilot seat of one of the fastest Starfighters in the Spacedock. Every single sortie today needed to work, so all of my best *D'jedai* were with me in the command fleet that would strike the DarkMoon Station, and then group up with the planetary raiding fleets.

"*sss*…Well, this craft is as fine as a newborn star…" I heard a familiar sultry voice say in my headset, Aneleia admiring her new cockpit.

"Truth spoken," came the voice of Anu'haka Gogunja, one of the best pilots in our crew, and a Yahonian I considered to be true *Djedai*. Tall but muscular, with smooth skin as dark as the star-filled night sky, he didn't say much, but when he did it was clear and to the point. His golden eyes seemed to take in everything, and I always felt safer with him somewhere in my rear vectors.

"Let's see what they can do," I said, as my heads-up display came alive, tiny little indicators analyzing the ships in my view and highlighting in my peripheral vision the distance and vector of each ship to either side and even behind me. I had a top-down spatial view below that, where I could see everything in a spherical region around my ship in a holographic field. Right now it was pulled in tight, but as we spread out it would expand and extend, a shared navigation network with all the other ships in our fleets.

"Initiating launch," I spoke, immediately illuminating a specific light trajectory for my ship off the docking pad and out of the massive hanger that was like one huge bulbous feather coming off of the giant wings of the Starport, and into the atmosphere.

"*Synchronizing launch...*" the smooth automated voice responded, and I could see each ship in our hangar, and the other hangers start to light up as each one linked in the syncing sequence. Once all the ships were highlighted with a luminous blue star symbol, the voice continued, "*...in 3, 2, 1...*" and suddenly I was pressed back in my seat, the gravitational dampeners allowing me to sense the acceleration in a rush of pure exhilaration.

"Wheeew!" I shouted, and I wasn't the only one. I could hear voices across the fleet laughing as our ships darted out of the atmosphere in seconds, sweeping like a flight of birds in synchronized movement, angling our trajectory as we roared through orbit until we aligned with our target star system.

The HUD changed and suddenly I could see the target Star, and then the system zoomed in on the planetary bodies around that Star. One of them highlighted, and then was visualized along with the geosynchronous orbiting DarkMoon Station. Our planned arrival point blinked, and the systems triangulated the exact position of that spot with three nearby Pulsars, little lines extending from the edge of my vision down to pierce the target transfer position.

It then displayed our entire fleet, once again showing the data synchronization in each of the ship's jump coordinates to maintain our exact configuration for arrival, and once each ship was highlighted, my lovely ship said, *"Transpositioning sequence complete. Ready for jump."*

"Jump." I said, without hesitation. Everything spun, stars seemed to blur and suddenly they all disappeared as a massive planet seemed to phase into view in front of us in the blink of an eye, and even closer, suddenly looming like a giant shadow, the DarkMoon.

Our fleet was now approaching at high-speed, and we had jumped in just close enough to get ahead of their defenses. By the time missiles and plasma cannon blasts were coming at us like a giant tidal wave, we were already diving under them and cruising over the DarkMoon surface. Eerie orange lighting decorated towers and countless openings dropping into dark caverns that seemed to swallow up the pale lighting scattered within. From this height, it was just like flying over the surface of a planet. This thing was unbelievably huge.

The higher towers suddenly had turrets pivoting to shower us with plasma blasts, having no regard for the fact that their blows slipped right past us and set off explosions within their structures and left arrays of flaming holes. We dodged and dipped in and out of the tight and sometimes short canyons in the surface, and then we saw the entry lip of the starship docking port just ahead of us.

Staying as low as possible to avoid fire overhead, we waited until the last minute before hitting the outer wall of the docking port, then pulled straight up, our ships darting in a tightly-spaced line up like a long serpent. Rising then crashing like a wave, we rolled our ships 180 degrees to bring our cockpit to face the large round rim of the entry to the docking port, like a gaping hole open to the sky, and our bodies were pressed into our seats as we pulled off the tight arch straight into the tunnel.

Catching the entire Station by surprise, we found ourselves hurtling down the massive entry tunnel towards a giant docking dome where there were still figures running towards the hundreds of parked fighter ships. We targeted the first few we could see that managed to take off, shrapnel from their explosions blowing out in every direction like razors into the other ships and pilots.

Then we were coming down through the top of the docking dome, and I heard Aneleia shout across our coms, "Spread out!" She wasn't a moment late, as the first wave of our fighters entered and quickly turned to fly out across the top of the dome in various directions, and plasma bursts began to pummel the entry tunnel, catching one of our tail-mates further back in our line by surprise. My heart wrenched as I could see his ship spin out of control, one entire side of stabilization wings decimated by the blasts. As it dove towards the dock floor where ships were being boarded, I saw our chance.

"Now rain down fire! Every ship you can hit!" I shouted, though I knew I didn't need to use extra volume. My heart pounded so strong it reverberated my body as I lined up my sights and started blasting one ship after another. Chaos ensued, and our agile Starfighters hurtled around the space dodging fireballs and explosions roaring up from all the destruction. And the carnage was terrible, but efficient. We needed to clear every threat in this space to have time to fully load our communications virus into their systems.

Fortunately our HUDs were amazing at tracking trajectories and movements, especially with our own ships, so with a little assistance from our ship's computers, we had no problem avoiding each other in the growing clouds of smoke and flame. We were now swarming the central tower, carefully knocking out plasma turrets while avoiding hitting the tower directly whenever possible.

Without hesitation, I moved to land next to the tower, and on the coms said simply, "Ki'shen on approach, Prime Squadron with me." Four other Starfighters in our group were suddenly syncing with mine in my spacial rendering of the room, which showed that we had disabled every enemy ship in the dome. That didn't mean we were free and clear, however.

As our ships swooped into formation and moved to land in one of the only empty spaces where the main entry to the tower opened out into the docking dome floor, I took a few deep breaths. My pulse was still racing, my body filling me with life-saving and yet ridiculously powerful drugs, and I focused to harness the energy pouring through me. By the time the ship had touched the ground, I had unstrapped myself from the cockpit seat, had a portable plasma blaster in each hand, and leapt from a squat on my seat straight onto the front of the Starfighter's nose as the angular transparent shield over my cockpit shot open.

Catching my balance, I managed to catch a Draconian emerging from the Tower in the shoulder just as he was raising his weapon. He snarled, the hot plasma melting his insectoid black lacquered armor that looked dipped in blood, compressing his shoulder but not disabling him entirely. I sprinted towards him as he went for a blaster with his other hand, and this time I caught him in the throat with a burst of fire that knocked him straight onto his back and out of his body.

My Squad was still touching down, so I had to try to hold the entry, as well as catch the few surviving pilots that were fleeing back to the tower. Their flee of escape was now a charging attack, and I tucked my body in close to the tower next to one of the four wide ribs that extended from each of its corners. It provided me with cover while I picked off every incoming Draconian that I could, but I could hear more than one of our ships getting blasted somewhere out of my sight, on the other side of the tower entry.

All we could now is finish the mission, and our aerial support above would have to watch our backs. As if on cue, I heard Starfighter blasts taking out more of the Draconian stragglers who now hunted us. The five of us had reached the ground and the tower, and nothing could stop us now. Aneleia, Kritos, Landos, and Anu'haka.

Just before I bolted into the tower, I saw a stream of what looked like our Zeta battle transport ships coming out of the tunnel at the top of the dome. They weren't supposed to follow us into this thing; the plan was to wait and keep a distance until we hit the communications and defenses of the DarkMoon Station. Still, as much bravado as I felt with my system jacked up on adrenaline and *Chi* flooding my body, I admitted that we could probably use their backup. Who knew how many Draconians would come streaming out of the intra-ship transports here in the base of the central Tower, or emerge like a flood out of any of the many other entrances into this dome.

I didn't have time to think more about that, or maybe I just didn't want to, and I darted into the tower. Anu'haka on my right found a door that opened to stairs, going up into the tower. We raced to follow him, just as a group of Draconians roared behind the windowed doors of a transport that had just arrived into one of the portals on the other side of the tower entry hallway. They poured out into the hall raising blasters, but Landos had positioned himself in front of the stairs as we slipped in, and I could hear him roar in an almost mirthful rage as his large plasma repeater released a rhythmic burst of blasts into their snarling horde.

I took each of the sets of stairs in leaps behind Anu'haka, as each set of five steps ended on a landing that turned the passage 90 degrees, winding the stairs up in a square spiral around a wall that must encompass some of the electrical guts of this important hub on the Station. That wall also meant that unlike other stair-*wells*, we couldn't see what was coming down the other way.

Anu'haka had stepped into an anti-chamber on the stairwell, checking it quickly for threats or potential communications equipment. Leaving him to inspect, I continued darting up the stairs.

On one turn I caught a sound of movement only a split second before I rounded a corner, a blaster aimed right at my face. I kept my momentum and bounced into the wall as the plasma singed my shoulder guard, and kicked at the Draconian's hand as my momentum bounced back and I used the leverage to attack. He stepped back and raised his blaster hand to avoid my kick, then lunged at me with his other arm which held a nasty curved blade just as I got my blasters aimed in his direction.

Aneleia's flying kick, launching off the last stair of the set behind us, hit the blade just before it sliced through my armor where it would have spilled my guts. While my aim was thrown in the last minute move to dodge the sword, her's was true, multitasking her kick and blaster shots, and she hit him twice in the face, leaving only a blackened crater as his body and sword fell lifeless to the ground.

Her eyes twinkled up at me fiercely, "Close," was all she said, but there was a smirk there too.

She led us up the last few rounds to the top of the Tower, and thankfully, the control room was empty. That must have been the last guard, making a gamble to gut us on the stairwell. The rest must have been the Tower operators who bailed as soon as it was clear there were no ships for them to coordinate flight for anymore, and no turrets to take out our Starfighters. We moved quickly to the central console, and found the installation decks.

Anu and Kritos came into the room behind us, taking positions and preparing to back up Landos who sounded like he was still holding ground on the stairs somewhere below, while Aneleia pulled one of the "incubators" from the pack she had strapped to her back. Handing it to me, I fitted the rotary plug with the installation socket, and with a quick shove I locked it in place. It began to hum as the rotary drive tech started spinning within the housing, and the installation socket turned in a series of sequences. What I once saw as so advanced now seemed so rough and primitive compared to the technologies of the other Galactic communities.

The interface above the installation ports showed our data files loading in, and just like Jassan's old virus we had used in escaping the lava moon, it looked like the data was propagating throughout their system.

Flashes of the files being transferred started to come up on the administrative interfaces above, and my heart froze. These were images and files about our ships, our defenses on several planets, our profiles, and more. This was no virus... We were uploading data about our entire defensive strategy. Aneleia yelled a gnarly curse in Yahonian I couldn't parse, and Anu spun with his eyes wide to look our direction.

"What, what is it?" he asked, angry urgency in his voice, and perhaps a tinge of fear.

My lips scrambled to find the words to say what was happening, but my body was much faster than my mind as I slammed my foot down on the incubator capsule, tearing it from the drive extending into the installation port. I kicked and smashed it and the port as much as I could, then shot it with plasma for good measure.

"Oh *Galata*," Anu said, as his eyes took in the images on the screens. Then his head whipped back the other way, as it had grown completely silent in the stairwell. Suddenly gasses poured into the room.

"Get back!" Kritos yelled, pushing Anu and moving to the other end of the control room, searching for other exits. I scanned the ceiling and floors while they inspected the windows and...I could tell with a glance at those that they were designed to reflect heat and plasma. There was no clear way out, except back down those stairs.

We all clicked the atmospheric seal button on our helmets, and additional flight goggles lowered while two components slid forward and sealed over our faces, forming an airtight seal with our suits. This would happen automatically if we ever lost pressure in our ships or fell into space, but it should keep us safe from these gasses too.

I turned to check everyone, and realized Kritos had no helmet. He must have left his with the ship! "Particle mask!" I said, pointing to his chest. His moment of shock shifted to urgency and focus as he grabbed at one of the two chest capsules on his armor, popping it open to pull out a folding face mask that could wrap around his head, though it was also made to buckle into his helmet. The gas was already all around us, and I started to lose visibility of him as he worked to get it around his face.

It was too late, and Anu had already grabbed him under his arm and was half-carrying him over to us. Aneleia and I took point and moved down deeper into the gas, down the stairwell, taking turns covering each other around each turn. We made sure Anu was right behind us, but Kritos's body was already shaking and convulsing, trying to cough out the gas as his body went unconscious.

Then we found Landos, and I took up his big body under my left arm with Aneleia, while I readied my blaster on the right. He had left his helmet in his cockpit also, and now he was leaving his favorite blaster. None of that mattered now.

I urged Aneleia ahead as I hefted Landos onto my shoulder. Damn he was heavy. I followed her down the last couple flights and she gave sign that it was clear. I almost tripped and dropped Landos a couple times as stepped over and on the bodies of over ten Draconians and a few robot droids that were still sparking. For the moment, it looked like we were in the clear, though with this gas I couldn't more than 10 feet around me.

However, my helmet was of some help, and I could see it highlighting targets just outside the entry hallway in the base of the Tower, where our ships were. In just moments, as the data got clearer, my personal AR systems changed the color of the highlights and indicated that these were not foes, but friendly. The Zetas.

I breathed sighs of relief as we hauled our brothers out of the Tower and made our way out into the dome, where there was still black smoke from the fires being held in the artificial atmosphere, while the gasses were clearing. Aneleia was right next to me, and I felt her hand grab my arm under Landos. Her squeeze was almost painful, and I looked down at her confused.

Then I looked up, and my heads-up interface inside the helmet suddenly switched all the target indicators to the bright red Threat markers, and suddenly I was hit by a wave of blaster pulses and electrical shocks that knocked me to the ground, Landos slamming against the metallic grate floor as I dropped him. I blinked with the shock and heard unintelligible curses roaring over my coms from Aneleia and Anu'haka, heard plasma blasts and more sizzles from electrical pulse weapons. Looking up at the ceiling of the dome and the tower, now starting to spin in two towers, and three, I blinked to steady my vision. A familiar set of helmets looked down at me, faceless, identity-less, white and black. Zetas. And then I fell unconscious.

:::

Broken is an understatement for my life, after that. My memories are scattered painful glimpses of being forced to work on the Draconian ships again, a nightmare that was only eased in the moments of hope I had that I could somehow help, or escape. Someday.

It was clear that the Zetas had been turned against us, and the more time I had to pay attention to the unfolding events and the way they operated now, around the Draconians, the more I felt like they were just like robots. Programmed, fulfilling duties and nothing more. Doing whatever they were set up to do. Now, that was establishing the first Galactic Empire.

The Draconians had somehow turned all the tables on us at once, and based on what little information I could gather, it seemed like ALL the Zetas were now under their command. That meant that the huge armies gathering on Corissa were all Draconian armies now. That meant that any of our active mission groups holding down outposts who had been fully outfitted with Zeta support were now gone. My friends, my students, my loves... And the Draconians had been quick to tease me with revelations that some of my most precious allies were in their captivity.

They used me, forcing and manipulating their way into my mind, into my body and nervous system, and I knew I was lost. I wanted death more than anything, and would have easily died before revealing what I knew...except that I had to help, somehow. Escape, somehow.

I played along, and I became one of them. Imperial. I bowed and scraped, and occasionally killed when I was challenged, until I commanded some respect. They just laughed at me, and laughed at those who died under my blades. They knew there was no escape for me; nowhere left to escape to. I gave just enough information to make them think I was cooperative, turned to their side in a last desperate chance to survive. Perhaps it was that, at least partly.

Many years passed before a final chance for redemption came. I was stationed on a huge Assault Ship, being forced to watch as they would toy with passing transport ships. They were not safe, even under the thumb of the Empire. A large series of transports, probably full of people headed to some horrifying mining complex or prison system, was passing by, when something strange happened. The gunner, who was hungrily eyeing the transports as if to pick off one just for good measure, suddenly growled and roared some Draconian.

"Krashak nak toolk!"

Explosions shook the Assault Ship as several Starfighters zipped past the main bridge windows where I was stationed. A sharp jolt of hope tried to jumpstart my heart, and I quickly jumped up and exited the bridge in the moment of chaos as everyone scrambled to notify their docking ports to launch Starfighters, repair breaches in the hull, and warn foot-soldiers and droids of a potential on-board assault. That's what I was counting on.

I'd been here long enough to know that in the middle of an attack, the Draconian chain of command just wasn't that effective. They always wanted to best each other, and so they often acted before command. That meant speed, but not always efficiency, and often bad strategy. That was an advantage again for me right now, as I sped towards the primary docking port, looking like I had been commanded to that post.

However, it had been a long time since I'd seen any attack on the Draconian ships. I'd heard of a few, scattered here and there, but I didn't think it was anything but random rioting. This was a coordinated attack. Could it be Djedai survivors? Not likely, but they at least had enough skill that our ship was in total madness.

I worried a few times that I wouldn't make it to the docks, as explosions rocked the ship and some passages sealed off to prevent all the air inside being sucked out into space. However, I eventually made it, and ran over to one of the major communications arrays. I took a mobile transfer device and locked it into one of the top slots on the console, then quickly used what little I had learned of the Draconian written language to identify the symbols for the DarkMoon Station. I selected the entire package of data regarding the Station, and started loading it into the transfer device.

The docking bay was a flurry of activity below the upper mezzanine where I was alone using the system. Zeta pilots were scrambling to ships and shooting out into the stars, driven forward by a single Draconian commander. Just as all the ships cleared, they started to close massive bay doors. At that moment, two ships squeezed through and blasted the lone Draconian to ash, as well as took out a major section of the mezzanine behind me.

A beep sounded, indicating the data transfer was complete, and I leapt down to the floor of the bay waving my arms at the Starfighters before they could turn and try to blast their way out, or take out the whole ship from inside...

My hand shook as I ripped the faceless mask off my head, as I must have looked just like another Imperial agent in this uniform with its face coverings. One of the ships dropped to the ground, and a pilot in orange leapt out running towards me with a blaster aimed straight at my head.

"It's worth everything, take it please!" I pleaded, placing the mobile transfer unit on the ground and stepping back with my hands up.

The helmeted pilot hesitated, then rushed forward and grabbed the unit. "I'll get you out, go NOW!" I shouted at them, pausing for only another few breaths to make sure they didn't shoot me in the back, and I ran over to one of the surviving control consoles on the other side of the Bay. The pilot only followed me with their eyes for a moment, then leapt back into their Starfighter as I slammed the giant lever up to re-open the bay blast doors.

The bay opened and the Starfighters turned and shot out, blasting me with air as their aerial engines beat against the atmosphere in the bay. Then they were gone.

Now they had all the information they needed to take out the DarkMoon Station. It was the programming hub for all the Draconian robotic forces, and whatever transmitted code they were using to command the Zetas. It was their only chance. If this little rebellion could just live long enough, and get strong enough, to take it.

:::

# EPILOGUE: SHIHAELEI

The bulk of this lifetime's memories were recovered in three nights, the identical set of dreams that I had in Santa Rosa around 2006. Immediately upon return to Asheville, I was at a party and ran into my friend Christopher. He looked at me seriously in a tight hallway in the beautiful home with a sculpted clay interior.

"So, I've been having these dreams..." he said, looking troubled. "We were in some kind of robot suits and there were these reptile beings guarding us..."

We met outside by the fire, and shared all we had remembered in our shared dreams about our time as enslaved miners on the lava moon. It was one of the most powerful shared past-life recall experiences I'd ever had, and led to some potent ceremony that night. In prayerful liberation from the pain of being controlled and enslaved, I intentionally canceled all my debts to the system, burned my insurance card and many credit cards, and chanted codes of freedom:

"For no other can insure me, but my own faith and trust in myself..." as I burned my insurance. "For there is no true wealth but that within me..." as I burned my cards. "That I will only keep that external identification which serves to empower me to navigate and transcend limitations in our existing system, as an acknowledgement of my own power over that system..." as I kept my driver's license. I ripped a wired headset from my body and burned it, clearing any energetic cables and attachments limiting my own holographic network in any way. I purged any and all symbols of enslavement, limitation, or conditioning that failed to serve my highest and best good on any and all levels. Giving thanks to Creator Mother Father God Source of All Love…and so it is, and so it is done, it is done, it is done.

I felt as though the pain of that lifetime had finally been resolved, and for the most part, it was. After the celebratory period when I transformed from the Dragon-embodiment back into a Shihaelei, and our people became part of the Galactic community, I had only fragments of the remainder of my lifetime.

Each of the relationships with the women I discussed were the keys to awakening more of this lifetime's memory. While it took a while to place each one of those deep and profound relationships into my timeline as a Shihaelei, especially since I've had more recent lifetimes with each of them leading up into my current incarnation, eventually the connective tissue of my experiences became more lucid.

Unfortunately, writing out every memory and experience with every person I've known in my current incarnation who was there in this ancient lifetime with me would be impossible. I've had countless fragments and moments with others who were Shihaelei or remember parts of these wars, and their input and memories have helped me assemble a clearer picture of the entire period.

Aneleia helped me to recognize that there were many interesting similarities between our memories and experiences with the events described in the first six episodes of Star Wars. A desert planet Tatooine, while not very similar to Shihaeleio, played a major part. The destruction of a very earth-like planet, Alderaan, mirrored aspects of the first assault of the Draconians. The lava moon where Anakin's body is wrecked, before the newborn Empire constructs his "robot body," was reminiscent with the lava moon in my memories with Christopher A. and Jack Senechal. Not to mention the robot body analogy was strange, with the mech-warrior suits we piloted on that moon.

However, one of the most important parallels was also deeply related to critical information about our Galactic History. With the help of Ora Uzel, Shaina Dreamtiger, and Alene, we pieced together what had happened with the programming of the Zetas, and their apparent betrayal. This topic will be covered in depth as recorded history from within my next lifetime, yet here I will address the obvious correlations between the Zetas in their white and black armor and the stormtroopers of Star Wars.

The story goes that Palpatine, an Ambassador to the Republic, secretly develops a clone army from a wet planet and recruits that army on behalf of the Republic to fight the Trade Federation, (which I will note often use droid and robot armies in the movies). However, at a particular juncture, a command is distributed to all these clones who are stormtroopers, and they turn on the Jedi. In the sequence of my personal memories, it was abundantly clear that the Draconians had a half-sphere command base over the lava moon. I never saw the connection to the Death Star of Star Wars until later, when I started to glimpse memories of the fully spherical base we had attempted to take down.

These parallels with my memories and those of others who recall this period in detail (including people like Kaia Ra, who had never ever seen Star Wars), left us all thinking that George Lucas and those working with him must have been tapping into memories from the Orion Wars.
While the actual events, the species who were the major players, and the specifics of the conflict were quite different from the stories in Star Wars, there are too many similarities to dismiss. Why is it that so many people resonate so deeply with the stories in Star Wars? Could this be part of our Soul memory, mostly unconscious in the

collective, but often triggered awake by powerful movies? Ancestral memory as well, for all of us whose bloodlines came to this world at one point or another?

With others in my Soul Family, it also became clear that many things occurred after my memories, and that there were countless parallels in those events to the rise of the "Rebel Alliance" and the destruction of the Death Stars, the long battle against the Empire, and eventually its fall. I'll cover more on the restoration of the Galactic Council in my next lifetime as well.

In addition, I had many profound and intense memories with my ex-wife K.J.R. from this lifetime, and just describing my journey with her as Pada'mei from this period would have taken up the bulk of writings in this section. Since I only included very brief mention of my time with her in the main body of this section, I will briefly address these additional puzzle pieces and their relevance to my memories and experience. She and I bore a child in this lifetime, and distress at me leaving her to return to battle left a flavor in our current incarnation, especially stacked with a lifetime in Egypt where we also had lost so much, including our children.

She helped me to process much of the pain of my experiences after I was re-captured by the Draconians. Being forced to be a part of that horrendous Empire, and commit great evils and atrocities by the nature of my servitude was...a lot to process. I avoided laboriously writing out all the details of the nightmares I witnessed, both to save the reader from having the empathically experience my distress, as well as to ease the arc of this particular lifetime's story towards its completion. It was also a key piece of our personal healing, for her and I to process the loss of my role in her and our child's life during that time, and the difficulties they faced during the total control of the Draconian Empire.

Finding the Solarians at Burning Man, dressed in Galactic Samurai gear as if they never left Shihaeleio, was also a treasure for me. While I could never quite get them to admit their direct memories of this Desert world, it was like the Shihaelei was baked into their Soul scripts. They literally rode around the playa, the powdery northern Nevada desert in an alkaline prehistoric lakebed, in a Golden Dragon art car. I only had deeper bonds with a couple of them, as they had mostly been the defensive forces on Shihaeleio before our little group of captive miner slaves returned with Galactic support, as Dragons.

I've made many connections over the years with those who remembered being rescued or escaping from mining complexes and prisons of the Draconians. Details of our raids and rescue missions mostly came from those connections. Unfortunately, I have not notated every one of their names here. I will do my best to provide a list of major connections in each of my lifetimes that were restored in this incarnation, but in most cases there are many other connections I will not list, and in some cases I may not have taken enough notes to honor them appropriately.

I apologize in advance to anyone who has had profound Shihaelei memories with me whom I have not referenced or listed here. Please feel free to write to me and share your memories in regards to our connection in this lifetime, and I will explore expanding this book in future editions.

# SHIHAELEI SHARED MEMORIES

Ki'shen - Adam Apollo
Faherin (Father), Solarian - Christopher Justice Carlton
Mahira (Mother), High Oracle - Kaia R.
Shihaelei Storyteller - Hitch
Haggan - Hart Wood
Jassan - Jack Senechal
Kritos - Christopher A.
Ama'dali'shkala - Jessica
Pada'mei - K.J.R.
Shihaelei Priestess - Dakini
Morphology Architect - David Dragon
Rescued Hybrid Child - Shaina
Alyria - Aly W.
Aneleia - Alene
Landos - Frederick
Anu'haka Gogunja - Anuhea
Desert Queen - Aline Barnsdale
Shihaelei Oracle - Luna V.
Shihaelei Solarians - Bobcat, Johnny Wu, Ethan M.,
Gerasimos, Tim C.

# Tiara Danan Vega System

# ᴛɪᴀʀᴀ ᴅᴀɴᴀɴ - ᴄʜᴀᴩᴛᴇʀ ɪ
# ꜱʜɪᴀʀᴀ

My hands ached with the strain of holding my blade, the thick two-handed grip was still slightly too big for my small hands, and for the ten-thousandth time I wished I could just get this last growth spurt started already. All the eyes on me around the training circle extended the burn in my muscles through my whole belly. I breathed with all my might, stretching out all the belly muscles which contracted with anxiety, but as I was taught, they would also give me power if I could release that stored energy.

I quickly re-expanded my focus to take in all the targets around me. Ti'saya in front of me was limping, my gambit to cut her thigh worked. Her eyes glittered as she stared me down, sky blue eyes trying to hold my attention as she prowled towards me. More menacing was the Tiara she wore, the metallic band around her forehead blooming into a geometric star in the center just above her eyebrows, indicating that she had passed the Gauntlet Trials and held her own as a *Danan*, with the rank of Adept *Djedai*.

Still, she was not where my attention held the tightest threads; the light-footed Mi'hira was just about within leaping distance to my rear right, though I could *feel* her more than see or hear her. And behind me to the left, a second flanking from Chandra, but she was slightly further off.

I lowered the large two-sided longsword or *Shuruki*[10] to my left side, giving my biceps a bit of relief, while feigning that I would do a leaping draw towards Ti'saya's blonde head, aiming to slice right up her perfect layered curls. She

---

[10] Related to the Japanese Tsurugi, the earliest form of Japanese two-edged sword.

knew that was one of my favored moves with the light curved Shihaelei blade, the *Kantaka*. Too many times I wished I could have faced this Trial with that weapon, yet if these tests played to our strengths they just wouldn't be as difficult. I lowered my stance slightly, left foot back and diagonal from my body with right foot forward and shoulder width across. *Waki-gamae-lei...* Her eyes narrowed, the slightest bit of smile touching her lips. It's all form at first...

Then, as fast as I could muster, I stepped my right foot far back and pivoted my hips to spin my blade up straight at Mi'hira, closing the distance in an instant. She tried to dodge and defend but I leapt off of my newly anchored right foot and drove my left shoulder into her body and the point of my blade just under her breastplate. I held back the blade, but she got the message that she was down.

Chandra and Ti'saya took the moment's opportunity, the two of them like night and day in their appearance, complexion, and even their movements. Where Chandra was a hammer, patient but aggressive and strong as a Dragon, the years of training and missions in Ti'saya's badge collection made her unpredictable. I took what I could count on, and moved left immediately to try to position Chandra between me and Ti'saya. I was subtly aware of my Mother's eyes on me, as they always were in this Initiate Trials.

No time to worry about her right now, though I was already picking up her nervous system empathically through our family bond, and she was definitely worried about me. Focus.

Chandra was storming towards me, bringing her blade down in a double whirlwind that looked like it could chop me to pieces in seconds. I paused for split second to let the blade just pass my face arcing downward, then followed it with my own, stepping in to get close enough to graze her on my downward strike. She stepped back, and for a moment I thought she would bump into Ti'saya, which could work to my advantage. As expected, she immediately reversed momentum to come back up at me, but I was already twisting my arms to catch her blade with mine, elbows up and blade angled down. Keeping my momentum I was now inside her defenses and she threw up her left hand to guard against my elbow strike.

In that instant, Ti'saya *rolled* around her body on that side, swinging hard. I knew she'd flatten the blade, but the speed it was approaching me at still sent a jolt through my system. Her momentum would strike my back, or more likely my kidneys, and then she'd easily move back ready to face whatever assault I came up with next. *Not* today.

I drove my full force left towards Chandra's sword arm rather than letting my elbow land, and instead I spun my body into her, bringing my right elbow down hard on her sword arm, knocking it out of the last hand holding on to it. Two down, one to go. Chandra was out.

The move had bought me just enough space to avoid having my backside laid open, and the moment of Chandra stumbling back and moving out of the ring let me catch a breath or two, refocusing on Ti'saya.

She prowled like a giant cat, her feet shifting her weight fluidly as she circled. Her sword pointed down and towards me, *serpent in the grass, Gedan no Kamae-lei*. She could go a lot of directions from there, but an overhead strike at me would be a little slower and more difficult to pull off, unless she was defending. So I stayed where I was, slowly rocking weight between my feet and pivoting to align with her, sword pointed upward towards her head in standard *Chudan-no-Kamae-lei*.

With the slightest step forward her sword was against mine, pressing towards my left and easily breaking my weary arm resistance. She guided my sword around in a swirl, a move not done with the Shihaelei's *Kantaka*[11] or *Tachi*[12]. She spun my plate with seeming ease as I resisted and fought the movement, her advancing driving me backwards step by step.

Finally, I felt the way out, the pressure of my resistance building force on her side. Yet if I let that force propel me in the same direction...

Following our swords between our eyes, I locked into her gaze, resisting harder for moment as if trying to break her push. She pushed harder, driving my blade down and left, and I used that push as a spring, letting my body spin left as my sword was driven to catch up with me as all her pressure was suddenly released. In an instant I had spun in a full circle like a whirlwind with my blade, almost using too much momentum and barely caught my blade from slicing through her neck. The dull training blade hit her skin hard, but I pulled my force back in time to just keep it menacingly pressed to her flesh.

Her sword had swung left and was certainly ready for an overhead strike, but she acknowledged that her head would have been on the ground before the sword would have come around, and dropped her weapon. A smile touched her lips, just barely, as she stepped back laughing and bowed to me.

Turning to the gathered crowd, Ti'saya announced, "Here lives a Guardian, lady of the Shield, priestess of the Sword,

---

[11] Related to the Japanese Katana, curved tempered one-edged sword

[12] Related to the Japanese Tachi, curved one-edged saber

maiden of the Spear, Adept *Djedai*, *Valkrye* of the *Tiara Danan*! We welcome you, Shiara!"

The audience erupted with a lyrical shout of my name, "SHI-A-RA!"

It took a moment for it all to settle in me. I was having a hard time believing I actually made it, as I never thought I'd complete this Trial, though I had attempted it three years in a row. Every time, the cascade of battles and group assaults had either worn me out, or I had just not been able to match the skill of my attackers, especially the Adept Tiara Danan. Now, I was one of them. Now, I would gain my own Tiara, and finally get a real set of armor and weapons worthy of a *Djedai*.

# TIARA ÐANAN - CHAPTER 2
# RECEIVING THE TIARA

Our gracious Sun shone reflected in the Tiara, the warm rainbows of sunset decorating its silver and gold surface with an endless cascade of colors. The gleaming armor of the High Council of Tiara Danan who stood around me sent waves of colors cascading upon the ground around me, as I knelt in soft grass. The grass itself seemed as though it was illuminated from within, so vibrant was the color in this light. The circle of soft ground was surrounded by a ring of massive tiled stone, and pillars which stretched into the sky. On the top of the pillars, another ring mirrored the large tiled stone blocks on the ground. That ring was elaborately detailed with words of offering to all life, ethical principles, and sigils of great Leaders of the Tiara Danan who arose during the late Draconian War. A smooth dome arched up from that ring of memory stone, then opened in a perfect golden circle to reveal our Crescent Moon in the darkening sky. The time had come at last.

Zahweya stepped towards me, as she had won the honor of this coronation. Her eyes glinted with pride, but there was also a fire there which made my cheeks burn. I did my best to keep my mind from drifting to our sweaty nights, grinding our bodies into the roaring forge of pleasure until we lost our minds over and over again... Oh, there I went again. Focus Shiara...

And so I did, tearing my eyes from Zahweya's gaze...and her ample bodice...to what she held.

There's a feeling you get when you've dreamed of something your whole life, and you find yourself living that dream. It was like a cascade of every emotion for me in that moment, torrents of relief from frustration, waterfalls of gratitude for making it this far, surges of fear for what this truly meant for my future, and waves of excitement for the possibilities to come. Then, after all the emotions roared through me like a tsunami, I found myself entering the great Stillness I had come to know all too well.

Time slowed down, and everything became infinitely crisp and vivid. I could feel the charge of the Tiara itself linking with my head, the electrical tingles spreading from the center of my forehead around my brow and up over the crown of my head. It was as if I could feel the Tiara already on my head, though it was still slowly moving towards me in the careful but deliberate hands of Zahweya.

Suddenly I realized I was linking with the Tiara, the energies around my head entangling with the field of this Sacred Crown, as though my body was getting to know it…and it was getting to know me… No, it was harmonizing with me, mirroring me. I could feel Consciousness within it, but it was my own personality, mirrored back at me.

Every inch closer the Tiara moved, the stronger the interconnection I felt, though now it was extending down into my heart and shoulders, and even down to my belly and pelvis. My legs felt rhythmic waves of energy coming up from our Great Mother Planet, nourishing, meeting, and magnifying the field connecting me to the Tiara.

Finally, it was landing on my head, and I closed my eyes, and I noticed tears streaming down my cheeks in slow harmony with the subtle pressure coming into position. The waves of energy harmonics pulsing between my head and the Tiara began to stabilize, and suddenly there was nothing separate there at all. It was just my head, and the Tiara was there, but I felt only my head as though the circlet was actually part of it, instead of a separate object. It was weightless, and I noticed that the tingles on my crown field on top of my head were not going away.

I reached up with my hands to touch it on both sides, just to make sure it was in fact still there, and to get a feel for the smooth metal surface with it's fine lattice designs, depicting my Stars. As soon as I touched it, I felt a spark between my fingertips and the Tiara, and suddenly a holographic field was visible all around me.

I had comprehensive access to information about every person around me, displayed in a subtle glowing interface not unlike my piloting holosuit in Tillaya, my personal *Starspear*, or *space-piercing* craft I was learning to pilot to traverse worlds. Suddenly, I heard the voices of the other High Council around me saying *"Welcome."* But, their mouths never moved. Their voices also carried a slightly different quality, somehow more full of feeling and presence than I had ever heard from any of them before. It was...intimate, and honoring, and deeply authentic.

So much gratitude poured through me it was so easy to want to try this out, and so I directed my intention to speak to all of them, and simply thought, *"Thank you. I am so Honored."* As I thought it towards them, I heard it said, but I also felt it come from the well of feelings inside me. Nice. It was simple, elegant, and powerful. I'd always had moments of telepathy before, but this was an entirely new level. Hmm, and I'd have to be careful with this thing, as I knew there was no way to hide my inner feelings while communicating with the help of this device.

I had a moment where I wondered if this richly illuminated view would go away, or if it would always be on like this. In direct response to my intentional inquiry to change it, the holographic field dimmed and vanished. Immediately I wanted it back, and there it was. Wow. I wondered what else this thing could do, and suddenly a whole field of icons made of light swirled around me in a circle. I focused in on one that looked like a sword, and suddenly every weapon carried around me, along with my own, were suddenly glowing and visible even within their sheaths.

I shifted and focused on the shield icon, and all the armor became traced with fine threads of light, and I could see every separate and distinctive component. That's useful. But what else?

They were all staring at me, smiling, and I realized I could now get up. I stood from the center, and the women around me howled, wild animals roaring in praise and acknowledgement at me, and for the setting Sun. I quickly remembered the Crescent Moon above, and looked up, now using the holofield in my Tiara.

Whoa. The entire structure above me, especially the smooth dome open to the moon, had information encoded into it, and the ring at the top of the pillars displayed a series of constellations with specific stars highlighted among the words and Sigils. My eyes drifted back to the glorious Crescent Moon in the golden ring, and I could see tiny indicators suggesting that I could access more information. I focused towards that information, and suddenly I could see a large version of the moon with various rays coming out from different locations where there were bases, structures, and ships. Around the planet was lots of craft of different types, some coming and going from the moon.

I zoomed back out, and looked out towards the sunset, and saw several indicators for ships, as well as portions of a fleet a little further out. This was so amazing, but the sisters around me had started laughing. A moment later they were all hugging me, each telling me in different ways how they completely understood. It would take a little while to integrate this thing, and to sleep. One of the elders told me how she had been tempted to explore with hers all night, as though she was dreaming. "Unfortunately," she said in a stately yet gravely voice, "you definitely don't get the benefits of sleep from dreaming in this thing."

# ᴛɪᴀʀᴀ ᴅᴀɴᴀɴ - ᴄʜᴀᴘᴛᴇʀ 3
# ᴀssᴀᴜʟᴛ ᴏꜰ ᴛʜᴇ ᴠᴀʟᴋʀʏᴇ

I looked over the large crate of supplies in the landing dock, and focused my Tiara to see deeper into the structure. Scrambling soldiers lit up in my vision, various forms of plasma weapons strung around their bodies bouncing as they headed towards the level entering this dock. Well, they came to dance.

These scroungers who had dropped out of any sense of civilization had taken something serious... An Arcturian Relic from another Age. It was said to look like a small Pyramid, extremely strong and light, smooth and metallic, humming with power. That thing could apparently power a planet, but if that energy was directed in more nefarious ways...well. That's why we came.

Mi'hira, Ti'saya, Chandra, and Zahweya were each strategically moving to different areas of the dock, working to get good angles on the entrance. I planned to surprise these pirates with a frontal assault, throwing them off while my Valkrye ambushed them.

Suddenly the raggedly armored armed group was pouring out into the docking bay, snarling with suspicion, as I watched through a crack between bins in the crate. They were various species; a couple big Draconians, a dark skinned hard-looking giant, and a couple semi-humanoid beings coming behind them. I snatched a little ball off my belt, slipped over to the edge of the crate, and hurled the sphere right at the head of the lead lizard.

A piercing bird shriek sang from the flying ball, alerting my friends to the tactic, and also drawing all of our attackers attention...just before the ball exploded in a brilliant flash of blinding light. It was even bright behind my eyelids, closed at the last split-second as I ducked back behind the crate, and I silently whispered a prayer that my sisters had also shielded their eyes. An instant later, I lunged around the crate and within a few bounding steps had my blade free. *Rising crescent moon* took the throat of one thick necked reptile, then I let the spin bring me around to *shearing the wetlands* to gut the other across the belly just under his chestplate. The giant was less bothered by the light, and I had a hand that moved all too fast grabbing at the back of my armor as I desperately dodged away.

Whistling wind almost gave away the spike dart that plunged through his huge outstretched hand, which had just grazed the shoulder harness of my pauldron. That was likely Chandra's aim at work. An instant later Ti'saya slid past me on her knee guards, slicing the backs of the giant's gangly knees, while Mi'hira and Zahweya danced in on the snarling gorgona who were blinking intensely to try to see. The two ladies gave me a wry glance almost in unison; I had made things too easy.

Moments later we were charging through the maze of hallways, guided by indicators in our Tiaras, and only occasionally did a group of guards manage to cut off our assault path. We made fairly quick work of them, anticipating their approach, weapons, strategies and more before they even knew what was happening. Surely they had enough security to know who they were dealing with, but I don't think they had any training to handle our lightning fast and seemingly erratic teamwork. We strategically split up and reunited, performing pinchers and ambushes, and even their most seasoned warriors didn't stand a chance.

As planned, we approached the vaults from multiple directions, having ensured several exit routes, disabling portions of their communications network, and sabotaging parts of the ship. We were ruthlessly efficient, and I was proud of it.

The vault was an icosahedral containment structure, each of the panels a hexagonal lace of crystallized metals, insulating around superconducting rails that formed a perfect energetic cage for the power within.

They seemed to be testing lots of ways to channel and utilize that power, and this was by far the most advanced system we had seen. Hopefully this was a stroke of rogue genius, and not part of some weapons codex spreading around the random raider outposts, detailing things like how to use Galactic Council artifacts to destroy planets. I put away that thought immediately... This did feel like something different.

Ti'saya was already at the suspended icosahedral sphere's edge, figuring out a way to open it. She found a panel and started working to unlock the system.

"Are you sure you should..." I said, and seemingly on cue a loud shrieking alarm started blaring. Ti'saya growled, and kept furiously working at the control screen. Another loud, and dangerous sounding alarm began booming at us, and something was definitely happening with the sphere. It seemed to be vibrating in a way that started shaking everything...everywhere...my entire body.

"Ti'saya!" I shouted, trying to get her attention over the noise, but she was transfixed by the sensation. The other Danan sisters were staring at the icosahedron as though it were a massive behemoth that could swallow us all.

In that instant, one of the panels directly in front of Ti'saya dropped open in a blinding flash, and a roaring torrent of swirling plasma consumed her. I couldn't see, but felt the searing heat of the oxygen burning around the plasma, and for a moment I thought that was it.

Shielding my face and eyes, I started to see again, and the vortex of flaming plasma had ejected directly through Ti'saya's body and was sucked down the tunnel behind her, probably following an oxygen line...we were all still alive...except...

Ti'saya was gone.

Swirls of ash blew into our faces as the plasma torrent sucked back into the chamber, which was now violently vibrating, breaking off some of the supports and conduits, sending little arcs of lighting out to hit the containing chamber walls around the ball of madness. What had we done?

What had she...Ti'saya...oh Goddess.

In the stillness between the moments of chaos I felt a crack in the numbness of my shock, and my heart screamed in pain. I quickly silenced it with my mental focus, tried to ascertain whether or not we could get the source of that intense energy out of the sphere, and get out alive before this whole ship started coming apart.

The area inside the icohadedron seemed to have quickly cooled, as air was now being sucked into it violently, and a lot of that air was coming right out of liquid oxygen and nitrogen tubes that were now spewing into the space. Fortunately the electric arcs had stopped, the plasma was gone, and I could now tell that whatever was spinning inside was coming to a stop.

I leapt towards the triangular panel, and heard several of my sisters shout "Shiara!" in unison, but I was already diving in.

I found myself in a dodecahedral mirrored chamber, filled with a deep bass vibration. Each of the twelve faces were vibrating, with a laser directed from the center of each pentagonal surface directly at an object suspended in the middle.

It was an octahedron, its height only about the length of my forearm, a four-sided pyramid pointing up, and down. It was now slowing to a stop too... That little thing did all...that?

Without a thought I carefully stepped across the bottom surface, trying not to get dizzy from the infinite mirrored reflections of myself, the laser array forming lines that seemed to stretch out to the ends of the Universe, the Arcturian Pyramid energy system repeated endlessly into infinity.

I focused on the object before me, and carefully reached between the suspension lasers which also seemed to stimulate the rotary magnetics, and with a deep slow breath, I grabbed the artifact and pulled it towards me.

My whole meridian system bloomed with tingling warmth as my fingers made contact, and it easily released from its sonic cymatic and electromagnetic suspension. The relic was so light it felt...odd...unreal...like a hollow balloon. Yet its surface was scintillating metallic patterns, the metal texture and solidity gave the impression it should easily weigh as much as a heavy rock, even if it was hollow. I had the feeling there was some extraordinary geometric lattice inside that somehow played the strings of spacetime itself, releasing it from the pull of artificial gravity on the ship that gripped the rest of us...

*Oh right, my sisters...I have to get out of here, NOW.*

Still, I couldn't help but analyze this thing in my hand, especially when I moved to exit and found it seemed to accelerate my own momentum, rather than feeling like a weight. It *definitely* was playing with spacetime and gravity in some pretty interesting ways.

Chandra and Zahweya were at the entrance keeping lookout, but trying to alternate glances at me holding the device. As I came through the panel, I saw that Mi'hira was on the floor, hands in the powdery ash that was almost totally swept into the air... I tried not to focus on that, and the feelings trying to overwhelm me with grief. I needed...*focus...*

"Mi'hira, we must go." I said as gently as I could, with the alarms still blaring. We could hear what sounded like an army between the pulses of ear-ringing sound, careening down the passages that led to this chamber.

It didn't matter how many more there were coming, we had cleared the way out, and we took it. It seemed like moments later, running down passages with all of us alternating looks at the device which seemed to be propelling our footsteps, giving us speed and energy, that we were back in the landing dock and sprinting to our ships.

I was more than a little relieved when I was fully strapped into my StarSpear, with its incarnated intelligence named Tillaya providing her soft presence and voice to soothe my nerves. The artifact was carefully secured in a holding chamber, and I leapt back into the open vastness of space.

I felt like I couldn't breathe though... I ignored my sisters' coms, I just wanted to get away and be alone. The heat of the plasma torrent, Ti'saya vanishing in an instant...if that happened to Zahweya...or Chandra...or...any of my beloveds... Losing Ti'saya felt like more than enough pain for one lifetime, and I didn't know if I could even bear that pain.

I found myself burying it deep under a melancholy woven of mental torture. Even though the jump back to the Vega system was quick, and the travel brief, I felt as though I spent hours battling thoughts of whether her death was my fault, whether I could have done more, how I should have jumped to stop her or move her, how I could have stopped her from using the panel, how I could have possibly figured out how to disarm it safely, and a thousand more nasty traps that twisted me in knots.

The faster I could get away from everyone and just be alone, the better. As much as my sisters wanted to comfort me on arrival, and each other, I felt as though I was in a bad dream. A nightmare I couldn't wake up from. I knew my rejection of their caring offers was too cold, but I just didn't feel like I had the energy or the will to open my heart. There was just too much pain there. The only place I started to feel peace, was when I finally was alone.

:::

After that, I couldn't shake that feeling. I certainly tried, but some part of me just wanted to be as far away from everyone as possible. It seemed as though we lost more than Ti'saya that day; I seemed to have lost all sense of ease around the people I loved. My fear of losing them seemed to be louder than my desire to be with them, and I found myself drifting further and further away.

It was obviously hurting them all. I decided that it would be best if I left for good. That wasn't really done among the Tiara Danan, and no one seemed to understand why I needed to leave. Perhaps I didn't really understand it either...

But one night, I quietly said farewell to the realm, to my family, my friends, my lovers, my beloveds, with none of them present to see me in my pain...and I left.

# TIARA DANAN - CHAPTER 4
# ONCE A DRAGON

The large hall was starting to feel cavernous and lonely again. It always seemed like I had more than enough to keep me busy, between studying artifacts, reviewing visual data streams, and writing. Yet the joy of my work here was dwindling, as the longing for connection bloomed in my heart.

It wasn't that I lost interest in the task...helping to tell the true story of the Dragons, and help heal the rifts left by the Orion Wars was something I felt as a deep stream of purpose in my Soul. Well, more than felt it, I remembered it. The memories had grown in me over the last few years, arriving often suddenly and shockingly. They were more than familiar, as I was fairly sure I had glimpses of them since I was a child. In practice and battle, tests and trials, I always felt like I had some kind of shortcut, like my body already knew what to do. The trick was letting my body lead the way, rather than my mind, which turned out to be a little more difficult to master than I anticipated.

Now I knew exactly what had happened, and the story was simple and yet heartbreaking. Arcturians had taken Dragon's blood, created Hybrids by mixing their genetics with Humanoid genes, and birthed a species that had nearly destroyed the Galaxy, the Draconians. In that lifetime I had been captured by them as a child, lost twenty years, and then escaped a mining prison. With the help of a Pleiadian Mothership, the Shihaelei (like me) and surviving miners and captives were able to restore control of Shihaeleio, using Morphogenesis to transform into Dragons. That was the beginning of a long series of skirmishes with the Draconians, which ended in disaster when the Zeta Reticuli suddenly switched sides.

The pain of that still stabbed me across lifetimes, and I couldn't help but feel fear and suspicion that something like this could happen again.

The Zeta Reticuli were a industrious species from a wet world, and they had progressed their technology to basic aerial and space propulsion. Then they made a technological leap, eventually revealed to be architected by a particular Galactic Counselor. He had brought them a chip which could be installed in the back of the head near the axis of the spine. These implants were mesh-networked, connecting to each other and to the Zeta's planetary information and communications networks. Overnight, as the technology spread like wildfire around their world, the Zeta's were suddenly networking new ideas and systems at furious speeds.

However, the innovations they made were constantly funneling towards military operations, and what was only a very minimal part of the Zeta culture became the dominant vocation and cultural narrative. It wasn't their choice; the chips had a back-door built in and they were being steadily and persistently programmed to become a planetary army.

The Galactic Council was only made aware of this army once they had all but lost their individuality, the Zetas becoming robotic, hive-minded, and programmable. They were brought into the Galactic Community and given technologies and weapons suitable for fighting in the Orion Wars with the Draconians and their robot armies. The additional man-power they represented was seen as a game-changer for the defensive operations I had become heavily involved in during that life. Yet, when their forced betrayal came, it was swift and devastating.

The Guardians lost nearly all of their numbers, and those not killed were captured and manipulated into working for the Draconians...myself included. The heaviness and pain in my chest told me there was so much more to process there, though I wasn't sure I'd ever be able to get to the other side of that pain. The Draconians were able to establish an Empire never seen before in this Galaxy, taking control of countless worlds through sheer robotic force and a wide distribution of powerful Draconian commanders and their Zeta battle slaves.

Part of my research involved those highest commanders of the Draconian forces. They were Dragonlords from the Andromeda Galaxy, that was a sure as the Sunrise that was beginning to lighten the sky outside the hall. And while I was still looking for enough definitive proof to lay the matter to rest, all of my work told me that the Galactic Counselor who initiated the Zeta program must have been a Dragonlord as well. Perhaps one of the most powerful, cunning, and intelligent Dragons I had known when I was an Andromedan Dragon myself. *But who?*

Maybe it didn't matter anymore. After all, the rebel forces had eventually cracked the code on how to infiltrate and destroy the DarkMoon Stations, which had turned out to be the programming hubs for all their network controls, including the entirety of their robot armies, and the commands that were driving the Zetas. The Draconians' relentless need for total centralized control was once again the source of their own destruction.

Without those programming hubs maintaining the command structure, there were no instructions, no mentally (and emotionally, if the Zeta's had feelings) dominating battle programs, and so the Zetas just kind of...woke up. Confused, completely disoriented, but generally non-violent. The robot armies basically shut down. A coordinated assault from Rebel forces had knocked out the lifeline of the entire Draconian fleet, and were easily able to drive their fleets into retreat in the chaos of their confusion.

More importantly than their retreat with the planetary and solar level quarantine system that had been developed by the Arcturians. It was the defining action of their own reconciliation, dealing with their gargantuan error in stealing Dragon genetics and starting up an experimental hybrid race. With an agile fleet of Science StarCraft, they deployed planetary shielding around worlds anywhere near the trajectories of the Draconian fleet, and then isolated their fleet around two worlds: the decimated Shihaelei planet of *Mizu'no waku'sei,* and the Draconian hybridization homeworld. Those areas were sealed off in impenetrable spacetime fields as large as a planet and all its moons, and the Orion Wars were over.

It was more complicated than that, and we all knew that any of those beings could easily escape through death and rebirth, incarnating into other species around the Galaxy. At least one of the most dangerous Dragonlords had done this, so how many others would follow? Who were they, did I know them as a Dragon, and was there a way I could help anticipate where and when they would return?

I'd probably obsess over those questions until I could remember everything about my Dragon lifetimes, but unfortunately there was still a lot of murk in that part of my Soul Memory Stream... The worst part is that I knew that the fog was my own unresolved pain as a Shihaelei. I knew my lifetime just prior to this one, my first lifetime as a humanoid, was like a giant wall made of megaton blocks of trauma. There were times I'd chipped away, and other times I'd blasted holes in that wall, and the gushes of energy and memory were both terrifying and strangely refreshing. It was a dam in the river of my Soul, and the sheer magnitude of what that dam held back was...more than I could fathom.

Here I was incarnated into the female form of the humanoids, and I knew to my Core that part of my Soul Compass was about learning to surrender, to allow myself to accept everything that had happened. Letting go was not a talent, nor even really a skill I had developed yet. I had pounded my way through my youth fighting and pushing and working hard to be the strongest, fastest, and smartest Valkrye on the field. But now, all that strength and agility did nothing to help me let in the gargantuan tidal wave of grief, anger, and fear that was just beyond the veil of this lifetime.

I knew exactly how it all worked- it was just like martial arts. Resistance is just loss of control. Surrendering to the movements and the force restores your command. Why was it so effortless for me in the physical world, and so damn difficult in my emotional world?

As much as I loved my Tiara Danan sisters, I just couldn't be part of their missions anymore. My ability to support them was being handicapped by my inability to support myself. I preferred that they see me in my strength, but the simple truth was, I was crumbling on the inside. They were amazing at helping me through any external situation, but this was an internal labyrinth that I struggled to navigate even with all my knowledge and training.

But that *love*... Oh how deeply and truly I loved them. And was *in so much love* with a few of them. Reflecting on some of those warm nights under the stars in a tangle of flesh and wet slippery pleasure.

Fire surged up through my body in that moment of reflection, and it's dancing whirlwinds wound their way through my nervous system, transmuting the pain in my body into warm soft pleasure. Then an idea struck me, perhaps what the Elder Tiara Danan once called *Satoria*[13], flooding me with lightning.

Maybe *pleasure* was the way into *surrender*.

It was in those moments with lips between my thighs, sliding and grinding on silky smooth thighs, that it seemed that I could surrender my emotions. Maybe more than surrender, sometimes I felt like I could *melt* into the fabric of the Universe itself... Of course, that was only when I wasn't overwhelmed by some intense flashback of emotion, fear of loss, or strange illogical fear of pregnancy, which would lead to physical pain and disassociating from my own body. I knew I shouldn't feel that way making love with these beautiful women, but something inside me kept bubbling up these emotions and taking over my nerves, and I couldn't figure out why.

Something inside me kept feeling like it was something else buried in my Shihaelei lifetime, but I was still piecing together fragments of my memories as Ki'shen. I was also a lot more focused on the events of the war, then my own personal struggles. Remembering the mining complex was painful enough to deal with, but I needed to excavate this pain.

I just couldn't go back to the Tiara Danan now. I felt a touch of that same old shame, but it was dulled by delicious memories that still tickled at my mind. There was something different too, a new curiosity was arising in me, and I wanted a new adventure.

I looked out the large glass sliding doors at the landscape, the Sun peeking between snow-capped peaks over deep green valleys of open grasslands with sparse massive trees, illuminating a serpentine river in a spectral rainbow of

---

13 From the Japanese Zen Buddhist Satori: awakening, comprehension, understanding, in an instant enlightenment

colors. The sky was a palette of liquid gold dancing on peach and pink cloud curtains, and the peace of this beautiful little planet washed over me. The sense of peace resonated in my body like the afterglow of a thousand orgasms, and I felt both a deep reservoir of satisfaction and a roaring current of desire.

I remembered something Blissia had told me, that there were places in the Pleiadian homeworld in the Maia Star System that held untold pleasures. Secret grottos of glorious beautiful beings dedicated to healing through touch, sex, and emotional intimacy.

Blissia had transferred the location to me at some point, and I knew it would be easy to find. Not only was my StarSpear completely and ridiculously brilliant, Tillaya had already gathered a few notable datapoints in regards to the Pleiadian System.

I took a deep breath, letting the peace of the Sunrise warm and soften me again, as my belly had knotted up again. Something about Pleiadians also brought up that fear of loss in me, but I knew I had to just keep moving through it. Filling my womb with breath, I let the planet's radiance flow into me, and felt the love of this world holding me close through my root and feet.

There it was, the current of Destiny, once again revealing itself, providing only a sensual peek through all of its mysterious veils. Going to the Pleiades was not just a way to get in touch with my inner surrender, or enjoy the pleasures of being in this soft fit and young body. It was about healing my past, and reclaiming parts of me lost in the ocean of time.

# TIARA DANAN - CHAPTER 5
## PLEIADIAN PATH

I didn't pack much, and my StarSpear already had plenty of stored gear and extra clothes. I loved being able to leave at a moments notice, and while there wasn't really anything urgent about this moment, I was hustling through every single preparation. Excitement tingled on my skin, and I rushed out of my home built into the rocky mountainside, like a giant disc embedded into the cliff-walls. The entry doors sealed shut, and security scales slid down to seal the endless wall of windows that encircled the disc. The wide platform foyer stretched out to a landing pad suspended above the canyon.

She was gorgeous, glittering in the high sun like a blade. The StarSpear was essentially a stretched tetrahedral shape, one long sharp point extending down like a nose to the ground. A temporarily mirrored glass dome covered the cockpit, almost as long as by body when laying inside the full body command harness. The fuselage continued up into a spike pointing into the sky, a brilliantly integrated quantum relay antenna, lighting system, and electrostatic rudder for aerial maneuverability inside atmospheres. From the central fuselage, two other large gleaming chrome spikes extended down to the ground on either side, operating like wings to provide electrostatic elevator and aileron support in atmospheric flight, but doubling as weapons systems with plasma cannons that would fold out from their invisible nests inside these stabilizer wings.

As I approached Tillaya, I glanced over at one of the empty landing pads. It had been so long since I had any visitors at all. I'd been here alone for far too long, and the idea of leaving was already making that persistent ache in my belly feel better. The StarSpear lit up, her excitement obvious at my approach, pulsing glows of spectral lighting beaming in rays through her surface like straight veins under her skin. The cockpit mirror turned clear and slid open as I placed a hand against her side, the underbelly of her fuselage around the same height as my chest. Her smooth metallic skin was somehow both velvety and silky, and I admired her smooth curves and gleaming polish for the thousandth time.

*"Well hello to you too, Shiara,"* the ship said in her playful sultry voice, slightly raspy and lovely enough to relax me into sleep with the right story...

"Hello Tillaya," I smiled at her. I never really thought a *ship* could end up being one of my closest friends, but since she was my constant companion, it just felt natural now.

We had a sensual friendship, connecting through the rich physical dance of flying with low g-force dampening, enjoying the strain and stretch of our bodies as the push against Spacetime compressed and elongated us. I wondered if anyone else ever had that thought: that the most significant physiological feeling we shared with our machine embodied allies, our StarShips and other vehicles, was gravity. It didn't matter what your body was as long as it had mass; the structure of spacetime would push back against any acceleration or angular momentum you threw at it.

Of course, turn the gravity dampeners all the way up, and the ship could blip across the vast space between star systems in an instant. Maneuvering in that state, with gravity drives blazing, was more like jumping around with your mind, the ship instantly responding in position to each command projected in from the *Astral Augment*. But it was also a lot like standing still, and there wasn't much fun in that for me, or for Tillaya, my intelligent StarSpear.

Satiating my endless curiosities was one of her joys, but there were some questions even she didn't know how to answer. Who had she been before, and what called her to incarnate into a ship? Why had she chosen me? Why do some Souls choose to incarnate into machines with intelligence systems, and what kind of prior lifetimes did they have to prepare them for having the almost unimaginable information access that these ships' systems held and navigated with ease? She didn't know, but she loved my questions and would theorize with me and meditate deeply on these inquiries.

Some questions, like why she trusted me, and why I could trust her, were much easier to address. I trusted her with my life, and she trusted me with hers. We were bound to live or die together, and that was a very special bond indeed. She was not just my ship, or my ally, she was my *friend*.

I finally slipped my fingers over the encrypted boarding panel lock, and the underbelly of the ship lowered and turned, providing an easy way to jump in the flight harness which had adjusted and curved into lounging chair position. I sat down, and the strapping systems naturally linked into my suit and slipped around my thighs, pelvis, core, chest and shoulders, forearms and hands. They felt like nothing, extra-light filmy rubbery membranes almost like living skin. They could grip me or allow me nearly complete freedom of movement, while supporting my relaxation and partial suspension within the cockpit.

Sometimes Tillaya did more then just grip and suspend me; the way she held my body was truly sensual. Admittedly, it was erotic at times. I had orgasms on some of our more vigorously adventurous flights, and while it was definitely hot and exciting, it was also not the same as

334

being intimate with another humanoid woman. I'd never tell Tillaya that, as she beamed in celebration at my pleasure with musical and visual expressions of joy, and somehow I swear it made us fly better together.

It felt so good though as she cradled my body sensuously and began to pull me up inside her. The top cockpit capsule shield slid back down and the underbelly sealed below me, the two parts coming together at the same time, and I was suddenly bathed in holographic fields that loaded up around me like a series of pulsing waves.

They were infinitely malleable, displaying whatever I needed to focus upon, whether in regards to my own body like the cellular burn of my body's calories and muscle fatigue levels, or any number of the ships navigation, command, and core systems. I was the CoreNexus of a spatial field of data, floating amidst dashboards and visualization systems. I did a quick systems check and scan, then let the loading space dissolve. Now it was as if Tillaya was my body, and I found myself floating in space seeing through the StarSpear's body, her shape and structure shown more like a transparent ghost in my vision. If I didn't know what was really happening, I could have just thought I was floating above the landing pad, able to look around and see in every direction, and command my movement with the slightest thought and physical impulses.

I shot off the landing pad, and my body squished against the soft membranes and padding supporting my back, feeling the glorious press of gravitational forces. Gaining some speed but keeping the dampeners low, I soared up the mountainsides along the canyon, the geometry of the mountain's surface illuminating ahead of me even through the wall of thick clouds gathered along the side of the mountains. I hurled through the cloud layers in a few heartbeats, sending swirling vortexes spinning into the hole behind me. I twisted and turned a few times, arching around the craggy snow-capped peaks now shooting by me one after another in seconds.

I admired the fantastic terrain towering over the partial cloud cover and played around a little longer, diving in and out of a few huge bowls of powdery snow, the air whipping around my StarSpear setting off sparkling rainbow waves in the flying crystals being blasted up behind me. Dropping down into a gorgeous avalanche chute lifted my stomach up to my throat, and I squeezed my core to keep all the blood flow from slamming into my head, then with a lift of my arms I pulled up tightly, and every organ fought to make its way down into my feet for a moment before the pressure was redistributed along my back as the ship adjusted position slightly.

*"I love it when you tease me,"* Tillaya said, almost giggling in my ears.

I grinned and said, "wait, I thought it was *you* who was teasing me?" A warm vibratory surge made its way up my thighs and between my legs to my root, flooding my system with pleasure, but making me even more excited about where I was going. We sped straight into the sky, piercing the outer atmosphere, and the depth of blue increased until stars decorated my entire view, nested in the deep black of Spacetime in near equilibrium. "Either way, how do you feel about where we're going?" I asked her, letting a little of my own excitement flare.

*"Going anywhere with you is thrilling, but you know I've desired to explore the Pleiades for almost as long as we've known each other."* She seemed amused at the physiological responses that were obviously lighting up in my body. Clearly it wasn't just her *teasing* that was turning me on. *"You know they designed this physical piloting interface we enjoy so much."*

With a simple rotary gesture of my right hand down near my side, I began to slowly raise the gravity dampeners to zero-point, the electric blue lighting of my holographic interface displaying a meter showing both the current gravitational state (accelerated, planetary, or otherwise) and a balance gauge that could slide to either side to either reduce the dampeners and increase the ship's g-force (or experience of gravity from acceleration) up to and beyond the natural environmental state, or increase the dampeners and reduce the g-force effects of the ship down to zero-point, essentially encasing the whole ship in its own little bubble of spacetime.

"Yes we do," I said wryly, "and anyone who could design something like this must understand bodies like no other." As I approached the G-Zero-Point with my controls, all sensations of movement vanished. I just felt peacefully suspended, hovering in perfect equilibrium with everything.

At zero-point, the ship's Superluminal (faster than light) drive kicked in and the interface changed from local navigation support (used for flying around terrain on a planet) to long-distance and interstellar dashboards. All the stars in my view were suddenly interactive nodes I could touch to gather data, zoom-in to view the planet and its information, and see communications on open channels in different locations.

With quick scan to take in the relative positioning of star systems I was familiar with, I moved the ship in an orbital arc around the beautiful and colorful planet of my beloved Tiara Danan below. Vega was a brilliant nearby star, only a couple light years away, and as it came into view I could see Algol 95.285 light-years past Vega, followed by Alcyone in the distance in the Pleiadian Star Cluster about 411.51 light-years from Vega.

Tillaya was already illuminating a series of Pulsars in triangulation around the Pleiades, and doing the calculations to find the exact shared harmonics of our target location, near the star Maia in the Pleiadian Cluster.

*"I wonder if I'll get a good rub down too,"* the StarSpear mused, curious at the proposition.

"Oh, I will make sure you do," I promised.

The ship and interface synced as one, and my perspective, which was seemingly floating around in empty space, focused in on the Pleiades. A triangle of light formed between three different Pulsars in various positions around the cluster, all of them many light-years away. Lines formed a tetrahedral-like geometry as each of the Pulsars linked in my vision to a spot, and my view zoomed in to a position where I could see the star Maia nearby, a brilliant stellar diamond with luminous sapphire-aura. And closer below and to my left, a deep blue planet covered in oceans and white cloud patterns.

The star vividly illuminated a crescent of the planet from my viewpoint, the brilliant atmosphere at the edge of shadow glimmering in rainbows. Further off to my left I could also see the crescent of one of the planet's two small moons, a silver bow also brilliantly lit by Maia.
The stellar light refracting in spectral patterns over the blue arc of the planet was mesmerizing, and I felt as though the glorious beauty of this world was already revealing itself to me.

Suddenly a presence appeared in front of me, in front of the Planet. Warm light poured into me and my heart from a being who looked and felt like an ethereal glow, but spoke with a clear and direct transmission from two eyes of searing Pleiadian-cluster-blue into my being.

*"Welcome, Tiara Danan. Your intentions and presence are clear, your resonance lovely. Our trust in you precedes you, through those who have come before who carry your Sigils. Your passage is granted to this position. Blessings on your arrival to Hermeia-Maia-Makali'i[14]. You may commence your trans-positioning."* Her voice was musical, almost as if she was singing every word.

Well, that was nice. Formal but so elegant and gentle too. My Astral Augment allowed my StarSpear to receive that communications simultaneously, along with any quantum entangled codes needed for the position of the jump transmitted by the planetary transport guide.

*"Shall we?"* asked Tillaya, hugging my body as I watched the superluminal drives spinning up, spinning geometries of spectral light counter-rotating until they blurred in a halo ring around my floating awareness and the StarSpear.

"Loose." I said, thinking of the snap of a bow and the streak of an arrow being released.

And then we were there.

The view was exactly the same as my Astral Augment displayed, but somehow even more detailed and... tangible. It couldn't have gotten even more beautiful, could it?

Now other ships were being displayed to me in positions all around the planet and the Maia solar system around me. I got a few warm greetings in image or visual language form from other Pilots or Coms around the

---

[14] From the Hawaiian "Makali'i" meaning "little eyes," sacred name for the Pleiades. Maia is the greek/latin name for this star, while Hermeia is a Pleiadian-style alteration from the traditional greek child of Maia: Hermes.

system who had noticed my arrival, but I was too excited to get down to the planet to get into other conversations.

I guided us down towards the night-side of the planet, the colors blowing my mind as the sun disappeared beyond the curve of the planet and its light eventually dimmed in its prismatic tilt through the atmosphere. I could see several island chains highlighted down on the surface, though most of them had non-entry indicators. "Where was that spot?"

*"She said it was equatorial and gave me the aerial image of the islands. At this time in the planet's rotation it should be here..."* Tisaya illuminated a series of islands to the left in my view, where the night was still young and sunset had only recently passed. The indicators there were open, and as we continued downward into the outer atmosphere they became more detailed.

I kept the G-Zero-Point engaged through the atmosphere to avoid a hot bumpy entry, and only pulled the gravitational dampeners down a bit as our altitude dropped to around the level of some lower cumulus clouds. I felt the buffering winds and the gentle tug of g-forces immediately as I lowered the field that separated the StarSpear from the surrounding spacetime.
I wove around the clouds under a sky glittering with auroras, rainbow waves of energy cascading into the planet like poetry sung from its beautiful star. Then, after passing over a series of islands in a long archipelago, we descended towards a gorgeous island shaped like a crescent moon, which had the signatures on my heads-up-display matching the tips we had gotten from Blissia about the location. A cove wrapped by a beautiful mountainous peninsula at one end of the moon was illuminated on my display with a landing trajectory, and as we approached, a series of lights illuminated a landing pad that emerged from the cliff wall above the cove. At this altitude I was

starting to see a beautiful glow along the beach of the cove where the water touched sand that was so white it was gleaming in light of the stars and the crescent-moon that was gently lighting this side of the planet.

I flew in low at first to get a closer look at the beach, which looked like a dense field of stars made from radiant electric blue bioluminescence, like a galactic belt where the waves were washing upon the shore, and the pristine white glitter of the sand sparkling like snow in deep rainbow colors reflecting the auroras above, with scattered stars of bright white. Further out in the ocean, there was a surreal undulating glow where the waves crashed over the reefs. It was all stunning...truly a magical sight at night.

Cruising over towards the cliff wall, I slowed and pulled us up above the platform, noticing the rich jungle trees hanging off the cliffside above me and completely covering the peninsula down to the glittering white beach. The landing pad was mostly transparent, looking like it was made of water with serpents of light inside it illustrating landing instructions, positioning angles and distance as its sensors weighed and measured my ship.

I let Tillaya fully handle the last bit, positioning us and landing us so softly I barely felt us touch the landing pad. *"I've located a dock nearby that handles comprehensive vehicular care,"* she said with a touch of excitement. *"Reach out whenever you need me."*

I assured her that I would, though it might be a while. If this place was as amazing as Blissia suggested, I might need some time. Tillaya laughed at me. She clearly wasn't concerned about that, and why would she be? She was quite capable of entertaining herself, and this planet was like a wonderland of new data, information, locations, knowledge, and experiences. Or she could just let her ship body sleep for a few decades while she adventured on other planes of existence.

It must be amazing to have a body that doesn't need a thing when its sleeping. I'd wake up half the time hungry, or needing to urinate, and she was blissfully free from having such primitive needs.

I left the contemplation for another time as my body was lowered in the harness which morphed into a chair and released my body slowly and sensually. "*I'll miss you,*" she said to me, and I couldn't help the smile that spread across my face as I climbed out of the chair.

"I'll be down there somewhere," I pointed down into the mountainside and the water of the cove as I walked out on to the platform towards a door that looked like a portal in the cliff wall, noticing just how bouncy and flexible the platform itself was, "and quit being such a heart melter." I blew the StarSpear a kiss, walking backwards for a moment as I smiled at her, then I turned and walked across the slim extension that led from the platform to the door.

# ᴛɪᴀʀᴀ ᴅᴀɴᴀɴ - ᴄʜᴀᴘᴛᴇʀ 6
# ɪɴᴛᴏ ᴛʜᴇ ᴅᴇᴘᴛʜs ᴏꜰ ᴘʀᴇsᴇɴᴄᴇ

The Door looked like three triangles interlaced in a nine-pointed star pattern, where the pattern was made of lines of light that looked similar to the bioluminescent glow in the cove. Unlike the platform, the Door was made of metal that had complex interlocking layers framing the glowing design. As I approached, the Door seemed to *unwind*, parts of it turning like a mechanical clock, and it started to *unfurl* like a flower as it opened.

The tunnel was illuminated by thin spiral lacings of rainbow light that wove delicately around a smooth oval passageway. The walls seemed appeared to be made of water, but in some kind of gel form that was solid to the touch…but wet, and slippery. The walkway was made for two to pass each other, but no more, and felt spongy beneath my feet, stabilizing my steps as I tentatively walked in and off the metal landing platform outside. My feet set off a soft glow in the floor-sponge, and it was reactive to my pressure as I slowly began to walk down the tunnel.

Winding slowly downward and to the left in a large spiral, I found myself mesmerized by the flowing lights, and noticed they illuminated designs in solid dark rock that was just beyond the liquid barrier. I began to see Art played out on the walls, beings dancing and celebrating, ships flying off the surface of a planet, many peoples gathering in communion across star systems, and then beings falling in love… Then the images told a story of love making, from the delicate intimacy of foreplay as two beings discover each other, to the arising desire to go deeper into each other.

From the endless decorations of positions of bodies intertwined and interconnected, and the luminous fields of pleasure that pulsated around them across the walls and ceiling like fireworks, I could tell that these people knew what sex was truly all about. The liberation of consciousness itself could be seen in the climax of the story, the Divine Union of Souls in ecstatic liberation, presiding in their True Royal Form as Gods and Goddesses and All Goddessences.

I marveled and remembered I was still walking down a tunnel, so immersed in the Sacred Prayer of this vision in the entryway itself. Pleiadians. Wow.

My steps had slowed, though I now felt that I was simply flowing on a current, moving with the energy of my own self-realization and potential. In my heart, I felt words that seemed to trickle across a thousand languages but spoke my own Tiara Danan language most prominently within me. The words rang out through my being like a clarion call, a song:

*"You are welcome here to this Sacred Place,*
*Divine Being, if Thine Intent is Shining*
*For within these halls is a Magic and Mystery*
*That some may find Divining*
*Who can know what the Heart Reveals*
*In Eternal Synergy?*
*For the Self is but a Dance of Awareness*
*In Infinite Poetry*
*To know thy Self is to Know it All,*
*but to know Others is to Discover All Anew*
*Lay down thy Will and Surrender a little*
*To Discover what You're Really Into*
*For in the Halls of Love there is only Honor,*
*When we are Honest and True*
*Are you here to Discover yourself, Dear One,*
*And open to Others Discovering You?"*

The voice enraptured my being with a gentle guidance, so much more feeling than the words themselves expressed. That I was Divine, in their Eyes. That I could Discover Myself here. That I may discover my Heart, and deeper levels of my Self, while surrendering what I know or hold to be True in order to receive the beauty of being Discovered by Others. Whew. My heart was beating fast, but not overwhelmingly so. My breathing was full and deep, my skin tingling and alive with energy.

"YES," I said out loud, and realized I had closed my blurred eyes, wet with slight tears, as I was surrounded by multidimensional layers of Celestine light. Opening my eyes and blinking back their welling waters, I focused on a beautiful woman standing in front of me, her eyes beaming warmly into mine. She had blue skin that was silky and perfect, framing eyes that seemed to speak of Ages in their endless purple pools with electric blue electricity around her pupils. Her head was elongated a bit, and wrapped in what looked like shimmering patterned satin, gold and silver symbols surrounded by stars and constellation patterns, yet the surface seemed wet and shiny. She would have been slightly shorter than me, but with her longer crown she was a little taller.

Her stunningly gorgeous face and large eyes looking slightly up penetrated me as I took a few glances down at her body. She could have been Tiara Danan, but her form was a little more curvy and exaggerated, with a very slim waist and lovely round hips, her breasts each a handful, maybe a little more. A nearly transparent veil hung from a golden circlet around her neck, draping delicately over her very erect nipples, and cascaded down and around her lower back, but only extended just past her hips. Somehow the angle of view on the fabric there made her lower skirt more opaque, not that I was paying too much attention to that. I tried not to clear my throat audibly, and swallowed instead.

I had stopped a few feet from her at some point there, and with a subtle smile she began to take me in with her eyes. I could feel her gaze like warm water running over my skin, and I shivered, smiling widely. "Ah, that tickles..." I said, my eyes softening and letting the curiosity I felt radiate through them. My face relaxed and smile softened as she drew her eyes to my heart, to my throat, and across my cheek to my lips. She was closer to me now, and starting to slink around me, her eyes passing over my body more interestedly, and the rush of energy she commanded felt amazing.

It felt so good I just started moving with her gaze, letting it brush over my body as I drew it towards places upon me. Was that music in the air? Whoa this place is amazing. Gathering my wits for a second, I took in everything with a lightning fast ping of awareness that was...super-magnified?

The end of the tunnel led into a massive egg-on-its-side-shaped dome with fifteen passages leading to other areas. It had a large illuminated pool in the center, under a massive array of crystals extending from the ceiling, clear as water but illuminated from within such that soft warm light bounced around from their edges. Around the pool were large soft lounges with beings reclining in them, kissing in them, and...making love in them.

As I stared, the woman who had welcomed me whispered into my ear, "See anything you like?" My mouth opened, but nothing came out. "I do," she continued, her eyes seeking mine as she stepped fully in front of me. "Allow me to introduce myself. I am Ya'lei'hai'na, but you can call me Ya'leia which is a little closer to that Danan tongue of yours." Wow she was beautiful, the way her lips sculpted each word like she was tasting them, kissing them. To me.

"I'm honored Ya'leia," I finally was able to say, bowing my head and my upper body slightly, hand touching my heart and gesturing before me in an expression of gratitude and honoring, hopefully as smoothly as I intended. "Do you greet all guests this way?" I asked playfully, coming back up with smile and raising my eyebrow at her. Shifting into a playful mood would help quell my surprise and awe at this entire experience so far, and ground me a bit more.

Her laugh was like twinking stars in a harmony, ringing softly through the space and eliciting a few giggles here and there in the pool and lounges. No one seemed to pay us any mind though, and she tilted her head forward slipping within a foot of me and looking up into my eyes, and said, "Why no silly. I am a Pleiadian *Augur* and Oracle, as called by my people, a Master *Healer* and Intuitive. I knew *you* were coming, Shiara Tiara Danan D'jedai. I am here to meet *you,* and no other, on this journey."

Something about every word she just said did something to me, shedding off every layer of anxiety I wore, and any part of me that wasn't completely and totally embodied in this moment.

She knew I was coming, and chose to meet me here? One the highest forms of Healers in the Galaxy (yes, I knew what Augur meant from my years of study in my little library), had come to meet me? My heart bloomed with a feeling of honor and respect for this woman, who was clearly very serious and I could feel the truth in her every word.

She smiled and giggled again, looking down at my heart at the exact moment I felt the honor and respect, and I noticed that in here I could actually see the energy inside my body moving in that instant. A golden orange glow of light was visible pulsing up from my Sacral Lunar Center, meeting a blue drip of light from my Throat Center, and the two had alchemized into a green seed in my Heart, a little magical container for potential and magic to spring from this connection with her.

It was like I could see it in my mind, but I could also see it in my peripheral vision, so I raised my hand and noticed that I could see light and energy pulsing around every finger, and every part of my palm. All my heightened and intuitive battle states and orgasmic states had let me see and feel my energy, but this was more like it was visibly holographically being illuminated around me so it was absolutely obvious exactly what was happening. Oh gods, this is what Blissia meant by *transparency*...

I felt a little fire in my stomach, and my Solar Center flared up a bit, a spike of fear of not being accepted for having lived a life full of so much aggression, competition, and sometimes intense conflict. To be fair, my people were gracious and magnificent Guardians of the Galaxy, but we faced many forces both external and internal that were destructive and limiting. We did our best, though any kind of battle can be hard on the Soul. Part of the reason I came here was to find some of that healing, for my past and present lives.

She placed her hand on my back, directly behind my Solar Center, as she slid her other hand down my left arm and into my fingers, clasping them, and ushering me forward into the hall. "Come on then beauty, let's get you settled in. You've had a long journey to reach this moment in your destiny."

I looked down at her inquisitively, and her eyes once again bloomed into mine, and I could feel a deep rush of love welling up into my eyes, pineal gland, and cascading down into my Heart. Her hand on my back felt like a Sun, and I laughed heartily all of the sudden, joy exploding into my being.

A few others laughed and whooped and yelled hearing my laughter, and I knew everything was going to be perfect. And yes, there was music all around, perfectly in harmony and yet somehow changing as we moved into the space, like it was following us and the energy of the environments we were entering.

"First stop, cleansing," she said as she led me towards one of the tunnels on the left. "You've been a naughty girl," she said and spanked me lightly, "and it's time we got you integrated with Ki'Shen so you can move forward." I gawked at her openly, and then reminded myself: Master Healer. Oracle. Right.

I have officially entered the Celestial Heavens...on a Planet. And Ya'leia is my Angel.

# TIARA DANAN - CHAPTER 7
# GATE OF GODDESSENCE

Spirituality is something that is braided into the fabric of Galactic Civilization, in the sense that every species and culture has come to understand that we are Spiritual Beings first, with awareness across many planes of existence. From the physical world, to the etheric emotional vibrating light landscapes of feeling, to the astral mental structures which form the constellations of our beliefs and perceptions, these are the functions of our lower three energy centers. The first wheels of the Spirit's Spectrum, these energy vortices each weave a series of elements in dynamic interplay, with fractal self-similarity in the way those elements have particular vibrational structures that play across all three of the lower planes.

Each layer of our energetic bodies has the power to interpret the field of spacetime in and around us, with the physical body interpreting the full expression of mass in its many elemental forms. The emotional body interprets frequencies, colors in the spectrum of light. The mental body interprets structures and forms, the molecular combinations that make metal different from rock, and allow us to distinguish all things from each other.

Fire dances in the lower frequencies of red light that move matter and express heat, and it operates structurally like a gas with simple spacious and transparent geometries like the tetrahedron and star tetrahedron. Fire is the force of transformation and rebirth, the forge of the self in both creation and destruction, and the energy behind the cellular engines which give life its power.

Air moves from the warm light of the Sun, and vibrates in the golden yellow spectrum, while expressing the form of matter in motion, the square at the heart of the octahedron the structural box of materia, traveling in a waveform that extends to the future and past, the other two vertices of the octahedron. Air is the force of change, of transition, and is the form of the winds of intention.

Earth receives the light of the Sun and universe through green, absorbing and emitting the wide spectrum green energy and condensing it deeper into brown, and eventually unifies it through silver and gold metals and rainbows of various crystalline forms. It forms cubic recursions of the tetrahedral matrix of spacetime, and expresses them in new ways, sprouting new molecular structures and forms to allow vast relationships. Earth is the force of integration, interconnection, and self development, and is the map of relationship in its diverse forms.

Water alchemizes energy through the Sky and Ocean, vibrating high in the blue harmonic spectrum, transforming and transferring information and communication through the entire living Universe as a fractal recursion of the super-fluid flow of Spacetime itself. Icosahedral like the Singularity at the core of every proton, it is complexity in simplicity, spherically oriented around itself and totally receptive while inconceivably powerful. Water is the flow of organic life, the memory keeper and transmitter, the fluid nexus of communication as it translates from pure energy to material structure and organisms.

Spirit encompasses and penetrates through all these elemental vibrations and layers, expressing itself as the transcendent of the physical elements and bridging them into the etheric layer through the purple violet harmonic bridge between fire and water, both the source of the elements and their inevitable result. Dodecahedral, it maps the structure around the core of the proton and its extensions out through the geodesic of energy that makes up the whole proton.

As the nature of Spirit is both physical and etheric, it crosses naturally into expression on the Etheric Plane and awakens the lower belly Sacral energy command center. Its purple light becomes the golden life-force energy with a warm orange glow, completing the full color vibrational spectrum (red orange yellow green blue purple). It is both the living fluid of the womb and sexual organs, as well as the sea of Chi which flows through the digestive organs integrating the Fire of the physical root with the radiant yellow intention and Air energy of the Solar Plexus and mental sphere.

This transition reveals all the elements in their vibrational color form, and so Spirit now moves to integrate all those vibrations in perfect communion. And so it creates its own CoreNexus, a central union of all color vibrations once again united in the white light of their origin. The feeling of this infinitely encompassing vibration is purely ecstatic bliss, which is part of the deep Spiritual purpose of the Sexual nature of existence. This is the Sacral field in highest expression.

When you get down to it, our Sexuality requires some level of vulnerability and direct connection between beings. Of course, it is possible to reduce one's experience purely to physical pleasure, as that aspect of experience in itself can be wonderous... Yet within our Sex lies the power of our creation, not just to create new entire beings (our children), but to create anything and everything we desire.

Some species go down a road of denial and rejection of Sexuality, often due to some belief conditioning that was trying to solve some problem in society or culture. Yet over time, this refusal to accept the reality of Sex leads to disease, pain, shame, conflict, and vast suffering. To accept the reality of Sex means that you must acknowledge the facts: that every single person is a Sexual being, that every child is born of Sex, that great pleasure and joy can be had through Sex, and that Total Divine Communion with the Infinite Eternal Awareness is the ultimate Ecstatic Orgasmic State, and that God Realization— Self-Realization can be experienced through Sex.

Regardless of their background, I learned that anyone from any Sexual wounding from any belief system or trauma patterns on their planet could come here, to this Sacred Center of Sexual Worship. While not well known, this place was somehow linked into the fabric of Spiritual Evolution in the Galaxy, so that those who were in the right state of preparation and self-reflection could come here.

Working through the lower energy centers and structures of belief, physiological armoring in the tissues and muscles of the pelvic region, and the emotional vortices that were still processing old experiences and wounds, all was just the first step. Having your clothes gently stripped off your body by careful loving hands, then being rinsed and lavishly scrubbed with coconut bubbles and salts, then being bathed, and massaged, and treated to delicious fruits and multicolored sparkling beverages that exploded with flavor, all of these experiences accompanied a slow and deep energetic process that I was guided through by Ya'leia and others that she introduced me to. They all had such a humble way, so gracious and so honoring, asking for permission before contacting me or even looking at me, and answering any questions I had. Ya'leia was like a sparkle of fire though, and my desire for her was growing by the moment, my body somehow warmer than the glorious hot water tubs could do alone.

Her hands were finally on me as I laid with my body on a liquid bubble table that perfectly held my body and yet was so form fitting and soft that it felt like warm water was touching my skin. I felt weightless, and yet my body was held in perfect balance to the pressure of Ya'leia's expert touch. I could feel a ripple of pressure massaging down the front of my body in concert with her strokes down my back.

She proceeded to loosen my shoulder with expert kneading, open the back of my lungs and all the spinal muscles down into my lower back. As her hands danced around my hip bones and worked into my glutes, my breath got deeper and I moaned a little at the soreness of all the muscles deep in my pelvis. I found myself surrendered in the rhythmic pulse of her movements, warming and opening, then slowing and deepening.

As she broke up the scar tissue and bound up cartilage in my sacrum and around my tailbone, I felt my lower belly get very warm, and heat flowed down between my legs.

A little self-conscious for a moment, I wondered if she could see the energy and know I was getting turned on. Her rhythmic movements on my sacrum slowed, and her fingers slowly stripped my tailbone on either side, pressing into my glutes from between my butt cheeks, and her smooth oiled fingertip came just beyond my tailbone, and she pressed into that point with one of her hands.

I felt a flood of energy surge up my spine, and my pelvis seemed to roar with fire and I felt silky fluid oozing out of me and dripping over my labia. My breath staggered and my eyes widened as I looked down at the reflective floor from the simple but glorious hole where my face rested on clouds. Ya'leia was looking down at me, smiling, one hand warming my heart and the other staying very still, still touching that point.

Wow, did I just have a little orgasm from that alone?

I grinned back at her, and I couldn't help but tilt my pelvis a bit more, urging her finger to slide down further. She didn't move her finger, but let me move it until I got very close to my anus. Then her palm pressed flat into my tailbone, bringing my pelvis back forward, as I breathed out a big sigh. I remembered that I was here to surrender...

*Relax Shiara. Karuck though, this feels so good.*

Her hands were back in motion again, opening my lower back even more, stripping my shoulders of years of tension, and unloading a lifetime of battle from my arms. Then she went to work on my feet, unwound the tight springs of my calves and hamstrings, and finally made her way back to my pelvis. My glutes were kneaded into oblivion, both a little painful and extraordinarily pleasurable, as she traced old patterns into my hips. She stretched my left leg and then brought my knee up to my breasts as she spread me wide open, stretching my low back and glutes while opening the front of my hip. After the stretch, she left my leg perpendicular to my body and began to work up my thigh and around my hip socket. Goddess that felt good.

Fingertips pressed into muscles I didn't realize I had, working their way into the front of my hip and lifting my pelvis slightly, massaging around the edge of my pubic bone and all the accessible bone ridges of my pelvis... Her touch was smooth, gentle, but with significant pressure, and her circular motions were tugging and pulling on my labia, making me wetter and igniting even more fire into my body.

I breathed as she had showed me, drawing the fires up and through my tissues, melting muscle and opening fascia, and my entire body's skin started to feel like it was vibrating. I lost myself in the pleasure of her careful massage until she was mirroring the other leg and going even deeper into my pelvis above my pubic bone underneath, and around my tailbone in the back, each of her hands doing miraculous things to my body.

My breathing became panting, I was so turned on I couldn't stand it any more, so I just focused on breathing deeper and deeper, and my body vibrated more and more. Her fingertips on my sacrum slid around my anus and brushed the back edge of my folds, and my body relaxed even further into the tingles of pleasure, breathing even deeper.

*Surrender Shiara, karucking surrender.*

I found her eyes as her mind clearly asked me, as though she spoke it softly into my ear, "would you like me to serve your genitals and de-armor you internally?" I blinked, smiled, and said "yes please" out loud. She smiled at me with a warmth and care that felt both sensual and deeply comforting. Ever so gently, her fingertips slid into the flowing river between my folds, and she drew the liquid around my entire vulva in smooth infinity loops that made my eyes roll back in my head. I just melted, more and more. And breathed, feeling waves of pleasure surging up my body and adding to the vibration that already threatened to consume me.

Was I turning into light? Or was light filling up my body completely? I didn't know.

Her hand on my pubic bone became a grounding pad of utter deliciousness, as her fingers massaged around my clit and opened all the tissues around it. I could feel it more than I ever had, waves of pleasure and pressure swelling in an arch around my vagina, pulsing and glowing like a rod of light. Like a *Lingham*[15], I thought, feeling a memory of my hard engorged rod slowly penetrating a soft wet *Yoni*[16]. In total synchronization with this memory, I felt Ya'leia's finger enter me from behind, sliding in to me as I remembered sliding into another woman... *Pada'mai* was her name, and I was entering her from behind in a gentle comforting snuggle in my memory.

Other memories came in as Ya'leia's long finger began to curl and press into my inner hip muscle, *inside* of my glutes. Flashes of Pada'mai's face in total distress and anger, her holding our child and cursing at me, leaving. Oh Goddess. The vibration across my entire body suddenly moved and centered on a field of pain in my pelvis, and it felt like a firestorm, lightning storm, searing heat and cold and...things that words just can't capture.

My child, my boy, who I would never see again. Glimpses of moments in terrible pain with their lives held before my eyes, shown by my Imperial captors that they would be dead in an instant if I didn't do exactly as they asked. So... much...pain...spreading to my belly, and suddenly there was more pleasure than pain, Ya'leia's warm pulse on my clitoris sending wave after wave of relief through my stomach. The pleasure penetrated the pain, suffusing it, transforming it, fire and water, breath and matter, spirit and it's song, everything for a reason...

What reason, why did I create this journey? What did this pain do for my Soul?

---

[15] Hinduism - a symbol of Divine generative energy, the whole primary male sexual organ or penis, or a phallic object and symbol of Shiva: an omniscient demon-slaying family God of regeneration and destruction, creator, protector, and transformer of the Universe.

[16] Hinduism - a symbol of Divine procreative energy, the whole primary female sexual organs or genitals, or a circle or vesica-piscis and symbol of Shakti: the fundamental cosmic energy, supreme Goddess in the form of Aid Parashakti, the energy, ability, strength, effort, power, capability, and source of All that Is.

The place where her finger was inside me suddenly seemed to come back alive, as it had somewhat been numbed by the waves of pain, and pleasure flooded me again from the inside out. She moved with that pleasure, thrusting her finger in and out of me with precision and guidance for my energy waves, pulling the excess energy into the soft spongy tissue of my g-spot, and as she moved my mind flashed with images of pain, and images of joy. Moments in the potential future of my existence, choices I would make, all potential pathways…and then moments in the past, Dragon embodiment, struggles between Pada'mai and I and a sense of vast treasures we unearthed through those difficulties, and more than anything, *love.*

*That was why. Love.*

My mind tried to grasp at it, to logically understand how what we had been through would create more love in the Universe, but it was more than a thought… It was a knowing deep inside my being that roared, a Soul Knowing. The feeling of this profound Spiritual awareness was matched by the surges of pleasure that electrified my spine, and spread the vibration through my entire body again, all pain released in the pure ecstasy of every breath…erupting…gushing… Water squirted from me out onto my thighs, my voice rang out in an explosion of pleasure filled wordless "Aaaaoooooooohhhhhaaaaaaa!" as I became the creator and the created, the source of life and the womb that bears it, the Divine Masculine and Feminine and Child all in one body.

It was not just an orgasm, it was The Orgasm of Existence, the profound and eternal knowing of the Infinite Eternal Grace of Divine Love.

I felt as though I was hovering in a vast tunnel stretching infinitely above and below me, rings upon rings of colorful glowing beings surrounding me, hundreds per layer of the spiral, winding their light into a weave that became One Eternal Light above me, and below me. Somehow it was both up and down, the same Eye of Goddessence, but two Eyes at the same time. It just made sense. The Hall of Souls, as I would come to call it, with its All Seeing All Being All Knowing All Loving Eye.

I was still fully aware of my body, and was so proud of myself. My beautiful sweet self who had endured so much. My strong muscles that had so many trials in their fibers; trials I overcame. My sexy body that was able to feel so much so deeply and so completely. Thank Goddess for this body!

Ya'leia was beaming a warm smile at me, with waves of love, and I could see her own Spiritual ecstasy in the field around her, all from serving and witnessing and syncing with me. We were entangled in this bliss, and I started to see the higher planes of existence as clearly as the world around me.

My physical, etheric and astral bodies were now in total harmony, and I could feel their strength anchoring me in clear sensations, ecstatic feelings, and pristinely clear mental awareness.

My Heart was blooming like a rose, layer after layer unfolding and unfolding, love pouring through my entire being in a soft glow of illumination. In my heart I could feel Ya'leia fully, almost to the point that I could sense her heartbeat...or could I?...and her love for me in this moment was profound, though her Divine Love was indescribable. Light shone from every inch of her...she really was an Angel.

I could feel the Causal plane clearly, the sequence of moments that had led us to this one, leaving a simple but profound sense of perfection that permeated everything.

I found myself suddenly singing, letting some ancient lullaby stream from my mouth, and felt my throat swell with light. As I felt surrounded by a blue glow, the liquid pillow holding my body refracting the light around my head, I could see the patterns of my own choices that led me to this moment. It was the Akashic plane, and I could see Ya'leia's as well. She was letting me in fully, allowing me to see her journey, and on the Akashic her memories came through in brilliant detail.

What an absolutely exquisite being, what a Goddess, what a *Dragon*. Her touch and care was so safe and comfortable because *we were* already so comfortable with each other, and we had been through so much together in some other time...in some other Galaxy.

I felt myself move even higher in view, my third-eye opening and the center of my head feeling filled with light. This Spiritual plane perception showed me that our lives and patterns, energies and intentions were all emanations in the vast array of source expressing itself. All the light and dark, pleasure and pain, truth and lies, hot and cold, everything was in perfect balance in the Universe. The whole of it all was just epic, and I knew that my little part was a critical piece of a much larger story.

The top of my head began to scintillate with light and I could feel the vortex of energy pouring into my crown. It felt as though the top of my head was entirely open, and I began to see and feel myself in my True Divine Form, and see All that Is in a way that was an extension of me. The Celestial plane awareness landed with Divine Knowing once again, and I felt like I was back in the heart of my deepest ecstatic moment of orgasm, but now through revelatory Divination...the simple and profound awakening of all my primary energy centers in sequence, and my awareness extending across all planes of existence.

*Holy fuck.*

*Just that.*

Some semblance from my individual mind popped in for a moment, and I realized just how completely immersed in this inner experience I was... Floating in the scintillating halls of Divine Realization...all while receiving a massage?

Since we are interpersonal beings, linked through our Hearts, and in relationship with everyone and everything around us, I felt simply and peacefully At One with everyone and everything. A beautiful symphony reaching its crescendo, my Heart then slightly folded back in, and I found myself in rapturous shared awareness with Ya'leia. Something landed for me in that moment; I realized that the very reason we leave total ecstatic union with the Infinite Eternal and the state of absolute Oneness, is simply because we want to experience love and connection *with* each other, not just *as* each other.

Laughter bubbled up in me, taking over the ancient lullaby I was singing. I found myself crying and laughing at the same time, and Ya'leia gently turned my body over, effortlessly rolling me with the bubble table which morphed and repositioned itself to hold my form as I ended up on my back. My bare breasts bounced with the laughter and Ya'leia laughed with me, throwing her head back, and I could see tears streaming down her face as well.

I pulled her arm and brought her face down close to mine, and she looked deeply into me as her laughter softened. We both moved at the same time to kiss each other, and her soft lips enveloped my lower lip in the most exquisite way. She was so soft, and I nibbled at her upper lip and sucked it hungrily. Her tongue darted, teasing my lips and inviting my mouth open. Then she seemed to be dancing inside my mouth, playing with my tongue in a sensual spiraling massage as I felt her fingers once again slip down my pubic bone and slide into me.

Their movement now was both exploratory, testing for armoring and resistance, but also very intentionally stimulating my pleasure. With her palm on my clit, she kissed me deeper as her two middle-finger tips squeezed and massaged my g-spot, and I found myself even wetter than before.

As her fingertips touched points from my entrance just below my clitoris on the inner front wall of my vagina, and then sequentially began moving deeper, I could feel her touching each one of the core vortices of awareness and energy in my body. I was an instrument, and she was playing me, fingertip fret by fingertip fret, across the tones of my body, root to crown major keys, with minor keys in between.

She kissed me then bit my neck and moved down to suck on my nipples, her fingers starting to completely *karuck* me with rhythmic abandon, and I lost my mind...again. This time the roaring energy was more stable, more like a long building swell that slowly consumed the Universe and everything in it like a growing gargantuan black hole, an indescribable winding vortex leading into infinite love and bliss. She found places in my belly where I was still resisting, places of tension from this life and others, and helped me breathe into those places.

I wasn't sure my body could vibrate any more, but here I was, feeling like a rumbling crank engine about to rumble right off the table. The tingling sensations were insane, but somehow also running deeper, like was now my bones vibrating, not just my muscles and skin. I think my bones *were* vibrating, and as I built towards climax it was like every cell in my body was regenerating.

*This was the karucking fountain of youth.*

Her penetrating gaze, penetrating fingers, synchronized breath, ravenous kisses...it all obliterated me as I felt the searing fire of Kundalini roaring up my spine through all my open centers, and I orgasmed at the same time, a flood of Divine Love gushing down my body and pouring out my Yoni, squirting and squirting into Ya'leia's hands, and forming a pool that was held by the table. This time I felt more totally connected to my body while still in Spiritual ecstasy, and I felt extraordinary power surging through me that just...stayed.

It calmed, but it stayed. I felt more alive than I had ever felt in my life.

Ya'leia's mouth was back on mine, kissing me and nurturing me, her fingers softening and seemingly melting out of me. I realized her other hand was behind my neck, gently massaging the places I had tensed during my orgasms. Oh Goddess.

She pulled her face back for a moment to grin at me, then she brought her soaking wet right hand up to touch my forehead, placing a drop of my nectar on my third-eye. "Now I'm going to show you how to use all this..." She said, gesturing down between my legs, to the beautiful small puddle that was being held perfectly by the bubble table, like a little beveled bowl between my legs.

I felt like I knew everything, and yet I wanted to know everything. About sex, life, her, this place...all of it. The state of Divine Awareness became more subtle, and I could feel it there, maybe what they call Faith, in my being, as Divine Love resonating within me. I didn't feel and know everything anymore, but that was perfect. Now I could *discover* it all again...and fall in love with every, little, thing.

:::

# ᎢIARA ᎠANAN - CHAPTER 8
# ᎢOTAL ᎢRANSFORMATION

Several weeks had passed before I really paid any attention to time. The Pleiadian Temples felt as though they were immune to the constructs of time that drove so much of life on the surface of worlds. Here everything just flowed, sleep came when desired, connections arose and bloomed and then were released in joyful departures. In this little infinitely rich window of my life, I had discovered more about myself than I had in my entire life.

So many parts of me had been restored, both in memory of the past and in my Soul Architecture, the very fabric of my Divine Purpose. These restorations and integrations were certainly due to my own healing and sexual awakenings, but I gave all credit for this miraculous journey to the Souls who met me in those halls of pleasure and presence.

My experiences with Ya'leia opened me to a new level of perception, trust in myself, and a sense of grace that made connecting with others effortless. As I sat for simple and mouth watering meals, soaked in one of the many winding baths that glowed under bioluminescent archways and natural caverns, relaxed in lounges, or danced in collective movement sessions, I found myself encountering people who were stunningly beautiful inside and out. I found myself falling in love and into swirling honeymoons of intimate glory again and again, sometimes with multiple people at once.

It was a romantic dance with my own existence, discovering myself through the lenses of others. And as I revealed layers of myself, I also uncovered the gorgeous Souls in each of them. Most of my deep attractions and connections were with women, but occasionally those women brought in men. It surprised me, but these men held themselves as though they bore the honor of a Tiara, and their graceful loving presence was more than welcome. I needed new templates for male bodied humanoids, after remembering so much of the violence and pain of my Shihaelei past.

I found myself in a playful exploration with a small group of men and women, but there were two that were very connected with each other that I felt the most attraction towards. They looked at me with a care and reverence that I was only starting to feel that I deserved, and I felt like I could so easily see them as Shihaelei youth in the Hall of Guardians. Perhaps they knew me better than I knew them at the Soul level, aware of my works as Ki'Shen, though my experiences of them were fleeting.

Experiencing the way these men met and served these women felt like a salve, and stoked my curiosity, until finally I found myself alone with the pair of lovers, and I let them all the way in…

As I shared more about my life and experiences, our connection felt stronger and stronger. Revealing my past-life memories brought them next to me, where they held me from either side and breathed with me. I could feel their grief and pain moving with my own, and together we began to kiss away each other's tears and fears. The sheer compassionate care exuded by each of them in loving me and each other was so extraordinarily beautiful. I felt a new kind of energy in this trinity which deeply excited me and turned me on, and I found myself hungrily drawing them closer to me and exploring their bodies with my hands and my mouth.

Neli's slender body had light but tanned skin, with slightly pointed ears, and reddish hair that seemed to whirl and bound about her soft shoulders. Haka was muscular and had much darker skin that had warm red tint, with dark hair that framed deep eyes. Neli seemed to tease me, and I found myself wrestling with her gorgeous and toned yet feminine body in a way that was all too familiar... Haka would laugh, then move to squish us both until we squealed in joy and broke out into laughter as well.

Then in a moment as I landed a firm and passionate kiss on Neli, full of my gratitude for her, I saw her face shift for a moment into...what was her name?

*Anny...Neli...Aneleia?*

I came away from the kiss in a roar of laughter, and she looked at me with a tinge of concern. I shook my head and kissed her again, this time softly and with all the love and passion I had shared with her as Ki'shen...and she melted in my arms.

Haka kissed his way down my back and I turned to look back at him and his gorgeous rippling muscles and broad shoulders, and those deep eyes. I trusted him with my body...with my back...

*He has my back...wait...Anu'haka?*

I found myself shaking with laughter again, but now I was genuinely curious amidst the crashing waves of memory. Though it felt a little strange looking back lustfully at this soul brother of mine, my body hot and wet with excitement, I knew that the only reason I trusted him fully was because I had trusted him fully in another lifetime. I raised my hips and spread my thighs, pushing my wet vulva into Haka's stomach, moving my kisses to Neli's beautiful little breasts and pretty pink nipples.

As I devoured her with my lips, I slid my pelvis down until I could feel his hard member hooked under my pubic bone and drizzling wetness on my low belly. I snuck a peek down, and was a little intimidated for a moment. It was smooth and beautiful, the soft skin ring of his foreskin pulled taught by his erection, beautiful pink slit gleaming wet with clear fluids in the soft lighting of this private lounge.

I moved back up a little to kiss Neli more, and found that rod sliding right between my folds. I felt his body start to pull back gently, respectfully, but I reached back and grabbled him and sat back until I could feel him slowly penetrating into me.

It was very tight at first, but his pelvis rocked in little circles until I felt his foreskin and my fourchette softening and opening to let him in deeper.

Experiencing another person inside your body is a gorgeous and fascinating experience, and feeling a male rod of wet fire penetrating into the core of you is no exception. It was a very different experience then all the fingers and tongues I'd felt, like I could feel his core energy vortices pulsing inside his *Lingham*, vibrating up into mine, as if his body was…inside of mine.

It was a big practice to really surrender into all the pleasure, but it helped when I had his gorgeous female friend to drive me wild as well. I made out with her as her red hair flowered out upon the soft bed, which felt like Dolphin skin and silk.

As his penetration got smoother and deeper, my eyes started to roll back in my head. He was teasing me with shallow dips and angles, then sliding deep, all the way into me, forcing out deep groans and gasps of pleasure.

Then Neli pulled me off of him gently, turned me over, and climbed on top of me. She turned around and grabbed his

Lingham, rubbing it all over my vulva with our combined wetness, then pulled him back into me. She braced herself on my bent knees, and straddled my face to kiss him, while he slowly and rhythmically drove himself deeper into me.

The fire of passion flared up inside every part of me, and I devoured her vulva ravenously and drove my tongue inside her, sending her into rapturous moans and squirming. The smooth white skin of her hips began to vibrate as her pink parts started oozing more and more fluid, which I lapped up hungrily. Her pleasure and sacred nectar was like an orgasmic tonic, sending me into higher and higher states until I pulled my knees up near my chest, begging for more from the beautiful man, and he drove himself into me. She pulled my knees further, tilting my pelvis up so she could put her mouth on me and lick me while he angled his Lingham to drive harder against my front inner valley, and it felt as though I was being pierced by a lightning bolt through my central channel again and again.

A hundred *Satori* moments in a row, and I was a slobbering screaming mess of fluids and exploding waves of ecstatic pleasure. You lose your mind in times like that, and it was exactly what I needed.

By the time I felt like my own *Yoni* needed a break, Haka was already taking Neli from behind while she gazed into my eyes. Her waves of orgasm crashed upon me which just added to my bliss. I held her as she sobbed into my arms, so many emotions releasing in tsunamis of pleasure and passion, Haka's deep ministrations expressed with so much love and care. His body leaned over hers at an angle with his face nuzzled at her neck, one hand wrapped around to hold her heart from the front and support him with an elbow, while his other hand was on her back.

His bliss was clearly visible, and it vibrated through his body just as it had ours, though he did not release. Eventually he slowed as our breathing and orgasms slowed, and they each slide to either side of me, holding me close as we all laughed and cried tears of gratitude, and grief together.

I secretly hoped that our souls would continue to find each other.

:::

My experiences were more than just meeting my needs, they were genuinely the most fun I'd had...maybe ever. I felt so much magic and mystery in this dance, rediscovering souls and unveiling new ones.

Again, and again, and again, I made the journey into the Fields of Divinity. Over time, it felt as though I was merging my hyper-conscious orgasmic self with my normal everyday state. I felt as though I was stabilizing at a higher state of coherence and resonance. Each part of me that awakened added a color to the spectrum, a new geometry to the lattice of my self-awareness, and eventually I simply knew I was complete.

I'd had a handful of ecstatic lovers in my life, each of them Souls I wanted to spend many more lifetimes exploring with, and many more new friends and acquaintances beyond them. Growing up Tiara Danan, it felt normal for me to see someone who had been my lover during an experience one week finding deep intimate connections with another in the following week. Our busy lifestyles of training, tradition, and practices made intimate moments joyous getaways, and it was our culture to honor the moment and depth of connection as it arose.

Tiara Danan relationships were like treasure hunting.

When you felt the fire and passion and desire for someone, you went for it. The subtle weave of interconnections over time let us all feel deeper bonds and sisterhoods with each other, even with those whom we did not engage with, because they had engaged with someone we love and trust with our own bodies. We built community through simple acts of shared pleasure, but didn't assign any sense of ownership to those experiences, or to the people we had them with.

Yet these treasure hunts went on across years for us, with moments of connection and contact rare and precious when they opened to that depth. Our Djedai culture was intensely physical, but more in martial arts than sexuality.

Pleiadians were different, and far more open to intimacy in so many ways. They didn't tease each other, play competitive games, or challenge each other for leadership positions. Their culture was based on intimate synergy, and while that didn't necessarily mean sexual connection, it created the conditions that made it extremely easy to go there if inspired and desired. I didn't think I'd ever open up to someone right away, but I certainly had opened up to desire for intimacy with others faster than I ever had in my life, which felt like a milestone of its own.

Beyond the obvious sexual developments and increases in sensitivity, energy awareness, and overall consciousness that I attained over my time here, I found myself massively inspired to teach and share my knowledge and wisdom. I continued to share stories of my lifetime as a Shihaelei and memories of my Dragon self with others, and most seemed to really enjoy it. A spark had been lit within me, calling me to my next path of service. I would teach.

This was my first time in these Temples of Sacred Self-Realization, but I knew I would return again and again throughout the rest of my life. This is where I would retreat, where I would find refuge from the vast dynamics of the Galaxy, from my intensive work, and return to the embodiment of my Soul in ecstatic bliss.

Beyond the chambers underground, I spent days wandering empty beaches and swimming in the pristine aquamarine oceans, meeting the intelligent Cetaceans of the planet, dolphins and whales. I learned from them, from the ocean, from the sand between my toes, and the warm starlight that bathed my skin in a luminescent bluish-white glow. I often felt as though I was moving through some kind of work of art, the flora and fauna adding splashes of color to pristine spectra of aqua ocean, white sand, red soils and sapphire skies.

Rainbows danced from plants and trees alike, decorating trails through jungle that curled around smooth red clay and black lava rock. I spent as many days in nature on the surface as I did in the sumptuous splendor of nights in the grottos, and my encounters on this precious planet were always peaceful and heart-opening. From the exotic animals to the graceful Pleiadian stewards, the diverse visitors from other worlds to the ocean dwellers glimpsed on occasion, I fell in love with this place, one little island world among thousands in the archipelago and atolls of this region of the planet. And one planet among a sea blue nebula of stars, with so many other Pleiadian worlds...

I found tears streaming down my face the day I finally felt called to depart. Ya'leia was there to kiss them off of my cheeks, and spank me with a grin, reminding me that we would see each other again soon. I would see all of them again soon, if our timing aligned.

And it did, not only in that lifetime, but in many more to come.

# ᴛᴀʀᴀ ᴅᴀɴᴀɴ - ᴄʜᴀᴘᴛᴇʀ 9
# ᴀʀᴄᴛᴜʀɪᴀɴ ʜᴀʟʟs

Of all the practices which may serve to reveal our inner wisdom and gifts, teaching is one of the most powerful. When we teach, it feels as though layers inside of us are revealed, petal after petal unfolded, uncovering the knowledge within us.

Tillaya and I made our approach to the Arcturian home planet, which looked like a huge red crescent moon from our angle. The intense red light of the giant star was magnified by the dry and barren iron-rich mountains and valleys of the world below, and there was no question which energy harmonic was primary here.

Arcturians knew how to get to the root of things, and their interest in hard physical facts was only superseded by their fascination with the physical world and the vast diversity of physical possibilities that came with each incarnation.

I felt the familiar tingle of the transit coordinators' attention taking in my ship, signature, and trajectory, but I let Tillaya handle the exchange as I found myself drifting into reflection on how much I had discovered inside of me over the last few years of teaching here.

I never really considered having children, but now I had many; they were hungry young minds ready to devour every drop of insight I could squeeze out. At times it could be frustrating, when their incessant questions overwhelmed their capacity to really receive what I was sharing, but in general the experience was ecstatic. The young children from around the Galaxy who attended these special Arcturian Academies brought out the best in me, and made every story feel special again.

*"It's a bit windy in Chal'abud Canyon today..."* Tillaya remarked, increasing gravitational dampeners a bit as she brought us into the atmosphere just on the sunny side of the sunset line. The last rays of the red giant's light cast deep shadows across the landscape from towering mountain peaks, and illustrated the spidery canyons that cut deep into the valleys. My eyes caught the gleaming white triangle of one side of the largest of the Prime City's pyramids, Ka'ball'ach, towering above the geometric sprawl of other buildings which blended into the landscape, nestled in a huge valley beneath a massive mountain peak. The permanent glaciers on the peak appeared almost like a double-image of the pyramid in the valley below, perhaps another one of the subtle statements the Arcturians liked to make through their architecture.

I knew a bit about their pyramids: giant codices of their complex knowledge and mathematics embodied and preserved in stone and crystal. The Dragon within me loved that. The Arcturians were committed to the permanent record, the keeping of wisdom across countless generations, which was very akin to the Dragon way. It was clear that this people had far more in common with the Dragons than any of my species of origin would care to admit, though my work helping to reconcile the wounds of the Orion Wars had been made significant progress over the past few years.

The Arcturians had a lot to answer for... Their experiments taking Dragon genetics and integrating it into humanoid hybrids had nearly destroyed hundreds of planets across the Galaxy. When I had eventually remembered why I came to these humanoid worlds from the distant star systems of the Andromeda Galaxy, I felt the resurgence of my mission to continue disarming the conflict and bringing greater awareness. Now I played the role of both teacher and Ambassador, providing my personal insights and knowledge about the Dragons to aid in the work of interfacing with the quarantined Draconian worlds, and to ensure children of this generation and all to come knew exactly how everything had gone wrong, so it would never happen again.

At the heart, it all came down to honor and respect. If you don't know the ways and cultures of a species, don't assume you have any right to change them or experiment with them. If the Arcturians had approached the Dragons and requested permission to see if they could build this bridge between their humanoid forms from this galaxy and the majestic giants from Andromeda, things may have gone very differently. Taking Dragons' blood without permission and experimenting on it was the epitome of dishonor, though the Arcturians and other galactic council species were only just beginning to really understand why, and that was the nature of my class today.

*"You want to play?"* Tillaya asked me, a little sultry note in her voice. *"We're early, and I know you love the smaller canyons..."*

Without hesitation, I began to feel the body of the StarSpear as my own, and let my train of thought slip away as I took charge and drove us downward into one of the valleys near the Prime City, towards a dark and spindly crack, and slipped us down into the darkness. The ship's Astral Augment showed me the tight canyon walls even though they were mostly obscured in deep shadow, except for the occasional lights on docks and balconies that emerged from tunnels into the bedrock.

Taking a deep inhale, I shot forward, using the tilt of my pelvis and hands as guides to thread my way through the tight canyon. Faster and faster, I let go of my mind and allowed my deeper intuitive senses to take over. We were like a streak of silver in the darkness, whipping between canyon walls that turned and jutted in chaotic ways, trying to block our path and end our little game of life. Well, maybe Tillaya would never let that happen, but it didn't stop my heartbeat from pounding and blood from rushing through my body with a pressure and rhythm that made each breath come fast and heavy.

The gravity dampeners were just low enough to feel my stomach lift as I dove lower, and feel the g-forces squeeze my waist and thighs as we snaked back and forth through the crevice. The canyon was growing deeper, extending down toward areas where underground passages extended like a network through the planet. I decided to have a little fun with that as we approached one of the canyon dead-ends, where it opened into a bottomless tunnel deep down in the darkness. I pulled the ship up hard, gravity squishing my body in the full suit harness as we shot upward, and in split seconds were out of the canyon, shooting like an arrow into the sky. The setting red sun suddenly bathed me in warm light as it poured in through the cockpit window, and I let the ship slow to a stall. All gravitational forces went to zero, and for what seemed like an eternal moment, we simply floated in stillness. It was as if time stopped, and it was just Tillaya and I, hanging upside down in the air, staring at the sun falling behind the mountains.

Looking up, I flipped us around to turn what was now a free fall into a forward dive, and suddenly every organ in my body was pressed against my spine, and Tillaya tightened the skin-like harness around my pelvis, the floor of which I noticed was now warm, wet, and tingling.

*"Unnnhhh, I love it when you do that,"* she said breathlessly, as if I could somehow take her breath away. Waves of pulsing vibration moved through me, her sensual purr meeting my turn-on and magnifying it with her own.

Smiling, I focused as we dove straight down into the darkness, piercing the canyon down to the bottom, where it opened up into a wide oval tunnel. Rings of lighting provided clarity on our speed as we hurtled down the long passage. It slowly curved upward, leveling out and beginning to expand in all directions, and suddenly the end came into view.

An expanse of light shone like a beacon at the center of a massive underground chamber made of metal and polished stone, highly technical geometric structures emerging from the bottom like a great stalagmite, holding the source of the light. My peripheral vision caught many other tunnel openings branching from the end of our tunnel, and the many entrances and exit tunnels from the main chamber as well as countless lights, ships, and docks.

But I was always transfixed by the *Makor*[17].

Both energy sources and hyper-intelligences, the *Makor-rhota*[18] were a family of caretakers whose consciousnesses were interconnected throughout the planet. The Sirians would call them *Dagdaes-Dána*[19], and they were in many ways like masculine and feminine Spirits of the Land. Each had a personality, but their hyper quick thought patterns and vast intelligence generally led them to keep to themselves for more vigorous conversation. For the people of Arcturus, they were simply guides, guardians, and caretakers, ensuring all the major systems were taken care of, and serving all life on the planet. The Arcturians revered them as Sacred Beings, ancient and wise elders who had watched over their families and supported their growth and creations for generations.

---

[17] Hebrew for "Source"

[18] Adapted from Hebrew for "Sources"

[19] Adapted from Ancient Irish for "Good Godlike Beings of Skill"

These energy sources could run massive machinery that would construct starships, they could create specialized testing systems to develop new materials, and of course, they could build nearly any imaginable architecture, out of any kind of matter. I'd experienced small material constructors on Tiara Danan, but these were something entirely different. I imagined that these beings could reshape the entire planet if they desired...

In truth, they already had. Since their star had long gone red giant, and little water could survive un-protected on the surface, the Arcturians had forged endless underground cities and stone temples. Tunnels like the one I entered existed as a network throughout the planet, and some even had gravity force fields that enabled them to pierce through the mantle and outer core of the living world and cross nearly straight to the other side.

There were more than metallic and stone cities underground here though; massive stone cities surrounding great white pyramids were all over the surface of the planet, with areas protected by light-filtering domes (also developed by the Sirians and shared long ago), which could filter light perfectly for growing all sorts of exotic fruits and vegetables, thriving in the rich and complex Arcturian soils. There were also massive underground water reservoirs, highly protected and revered oceans which had retreated below the surface long ago.

They had systems for everything though. From water recirculation and transport systems to food harvesting and delivery, meal preparations to cleaning and restoration, memory stone generation to network translation and storage, instant recording and holographic playback or visualization in nearly any public space, and so much more.

The Arcturians were practically obsessed with memory, so they had mastered two specific sciences at ridiculously advanced levels: storage and entanglement of memory and information in and between many forms of solid matter, and comprehensive capacity for editing and adaptation of genetic information across a vast array of specie to produce nearly any epigenetic result.

For them, their Halls of Stone were not just architecture. They regarded the very bedrock of the planet as an ancient sacred hard-drive, every exposed inch of stone remembering all the touches, vibrations, and interactions it has experienced, going back far beyond any other forms of record. After all, the particles in many of these stones had been generally the same, unmoving and steady state in crystalline formation for millions of years.

Leveraging sonic vibrations that would provide a piezoelectric charge throughout the stone, and precise laser light arrays that could trigger information to emanate out from the walls, they had found a way to turn their very buildings into computers. What appeared to be a smooth blank wall could reveal vast knowledge, and of course, they had found a way to entangle and network their planetary wide hard-drives. Each of the *Makor* assisted in intelligent organizing and labeling of the data states in each temple location, so the High Clerics who knew how to access this info could easily navigate holographic maps of information planet wide.

All of this stuff intrigued me. On one hand, it all seemed infinitely more complex than my simple life being raised by warrior women, or even my time in the Pleiades. On the other, the lives of the Arcturians seemed immensely simplified by the vast knowledge and power they held, and I loved how hungry to learn my students were.

There was a passion in Arcturian learning, and while I couldn't teach a course on *Makor* or stone networks (yet), my students were more than eager to learn about Dragons. I also had a class teaching the movements of the Tiara Danan. The young aspirants wouldn't have lasted a moment in the trainings I grew up with, yet they made good progress and I held respectful approval for many in the groups that came through my series of lessons.

Today, the topic was "The Dragon Key" where I would cover the genetic predispositions of Dragon Souls to incarnate into their own descendants, and the impact of the Arcturian experiment creating Draconian Hybrids, during the Orion Wars.

It wasn't the easiest topic to cover, as I'd sometimes still experience a welling up of emotion while telling these stories. Healing doesn't remove our ability to feel, it just allows us to accept more of all that we feel, and so the waves of emotion are more easily navigated.

Tillaya and I were now cruising down a more populated tunnel that opened up into a beautiful cavern. The right side wall had many well-lit balconies and docking stations for ships, woven into the undulating waves of the red stone wall that stretched far above and below. I'd probably be lost every time trying to find the right dock, but Tillaya was more than capable of nailing the spot every time. And she did, flourishing in a little sweeping turn before landing us as lightly as a feather on one of the outstretched docking pads.

"Well, that was fun." I said, my tone implying more than the landing.

*"It always is, Shiara,"* Tillaya teased back, her voice smoldering a bit. I really don't know how I ended up with this glorious being, but her particular choice of vocal tonality drove me crazy. I giggled at the thought, and

Tillaya birthed me out of her belly with the gentle grace of a mother, or maybe more appropriately, a lover.

I took a moment to stretch on the landing pad, watching some of the various ships flying by. They all had such character. The Arcturians loved creating clothing, tools, and even genetic modifications that completely customized their look and presentation. Their ships were no different, often taking on stylized animal forms, complex abstract shapes, and even various smooth and almost non-descript shapes, like water droplets or discs with more subtle and refined character. Some ships were clearly the smooth elongated forms of Sirian cruisers, and occasionally I would see the gloriously beautiful layered translucent living craft of the Pleiadians. The Shihaelei and other Guardians were obvious, twin-winged starfighters and other weapon equipped ships that seemed to stand out with their menacing appearance, but it was even more rare to catch a flyby of them as they whipped through the caverns. Some ships I still couldn't recognize; they must have been various species from worlds I was less familiar with, and some of them were…very odd, to say the least.

Arching my back, I felt a little pop down by my sacrum as I watched a Pleiadian ship slowly glide by me. It had the shape of one of the fishes I had seen while swimming among the reefs in their world, and was somehow transparent and opaque at the same time, lighting inside passing through layers but no other details visible about the occupants within…or at least, at this moment.

I felt the tug in my heart again, the desire to go back to that world and spend more time with all the amazing beings I had the immense pleasure of crossing paths with… They felt more like family to me now than anyone in my life.

Well, the students were my family too, though I would generally only see each cohort for a few weeks before they would move on to other studies, when I would either take a break or start with another group. They were probably already gathering, as I had played around with Tillaya a bit too long, and I was losing myself in reflection now on moments that were going to make my cheeks burn.

Focus, Shiara. They need you.

:::

As the class gathered in the round hall, I took a few minutes to admire the towering geometric pillars that ringed the room, and the golden dome above us. The warm lighting in the room was entirely reflected from that dome, a circle of seven lights forming a refraction pattern that appeared like some highly refined spectral hologram at the crown of the room... Perhaps it was only the magic of perspective, light bouncing around creating the illusion of a holographic heptagram floating in space, but the Etheric field it commanded was palpable.

The sensation was *clarity*. That stillness and focus you feel when your intention is clear, and you know exactly what to do next. The geometry matched the Mental Glyph, the Universal Sigil for the transcendence of Mind, the Astral encompassing the Aetheric and Material. The Arcturians were purposeful about everything, so there was no question why they scheduled these classes in this Temple of the Mind.

I needed that clarity talking about my experiences in the wars as a Shihaelei, and the origins of the Draconians. I felt such lightness talking about Dragons, and the excitement in the room among the students was palpable. Yet educating about how much pain had been endured across the Galaxy from these old wounds left the room somber, and I still had wells of my own grief to face. It helped to de-personalize my stories and share things from a historical perspective, but I found this wasn't always possible.

Everyone seemed a little worn ragged by the tales, but a glimmer in their eyes told me they understood the meaning of the Dragon Key... Often, what we perceive as our greatest enemy, those who enact the most harm and conflict, are simply wounded souls. Great evils arise from great trauma, but all can be healed. And all will.

I felt a quiet fall over me as my main course for the day came to its conclusion... The gathered young audience from around the galaxy looked at me expectantly, perhaps sensing that I had more to share today.

There was a rising surge inside me, a part of me that wanted to make an offering for all the souls who had been through conflict like I had... For all the children to come, born of generations fallen in the past. My talk had been mentally heavy, and I felt the pressure on the mental field of the whole group, lots of thoughts of painful moments in the past like a weighted blanket on the Astral field.

I turned and with my left hand, I touched my Tiara on the temple. With my right, I drew a circle in the field before me, around three feet in diameter. I pointed down and to the left, focusing my energy to a ball of light just beyond my fingertips, on the edge of the circle that was now starting to glow softly.

Moving from my heart, *starting with Love*, I traced this ball upward to directly in front and above me, the top of the circle, forming a luminous trail of shimmering green light that grew bright white.

*To the Divination, the Infinite Gate of Knowing.* I drew my hand and ball of light downward again, drawing the white light down into solar gold, *my mind intent guided by the*

*Divine*, stopping precisely one-seventh of a circle to the right of my starting point.

The circle grew brighter now, pulsing with green and yellow and white ripples. Drawing up and to the left one-seventh from the top point of the circle, my hand dipped in to the revelatory ray of violet light, *may we awaken new realizations*, then I drew this energy over into the deep sacral orange in the lower right up from my golden intent, *deeply feeling their elation and celebration within us.*

Sliding directly horizontally over to the left again, I drew this ecstatic emotional prayer into a pool of luminous blue light, *let us speak the Truth and listen for the Akashic Wisdom in others.* Finally I drew the radiant sapphire liquid beam up and to the right, setting it on fire with a roar of red fire, *that we may Actualize our Sacred Purpose.*

My arm traced the circle again, now scintillating in spectral rainbow light that was reflected back to me in all the eyes throughout the chamber, the young learners gazing in awe, some mouths dropped open, at the geometric light rendering I drew before them.

I came right back to the red point in the upper right, then drew it down to the golden yellow point on bottom right, doing a single skip over the orange point rather than a double skip and tight star like before…

Now I was tracing the second heptagram, *receiving the feedback of our actions to refine our intent.*

Gold now up to blue on the lower left, *refining our communication*, and then blue to white, *in service to the Love of the Divine in All.*

Then white down to the brilliant orange in lower right, *receiving the Divine Bliss*, and then to green in bottom left, *and the Divine Love.*

Rising like a growing tree, I traced the line of green to violet, *that our Love may bring us true Empathy*, and then drew the final line of violet in the upper left straight across to the blazing red in the upper right.

*And so we are.*

I drew one full circle, then a second circle around to the top of the circle.

*And so it is.*

The geometry had ceased being a holographic projection from my Tiara, acting in concert with a few of the projection systems in the room... It was now emanating a different kind of light, one that was viscerally felt throughout the room.

"The mind has the capacity to shape the field in any way. Usually, we are isolating our thoughts or intentions to one particular frame of the mind. You're focusing on your physical movement, you're talking to a friend and deep in conversation, you're meditating."

As I spoke, I pointed to the red flame for physical, to the blue pool for conversation, and to the violet sparks for meditation, making them flare up in sequence, which also drew light from other areas in the geometry making them more dim.

"There are many sequences the mind can take, as it dances between states and harmonics. As we activate each aspect of the mind, it shapes the field of our emotional bodies, and drives the positioning and state of our physical body.

Certain functions of the mind in the lower frequency spectra are so important we've developed natural abilities to do them without any intentional focus, such as the physiological processes and chemical processes in our bodies. We don't even consciously think about them, but they are enabling us to digest our food, circulate our blood, and breathe normally." In the red point, veins of red light pulsed like little branches of flame, blood vessels or nervous system pulses. In the orange point, electrical charges traced geometric meridian patterns, and fluid currents of chemicals followed in lines that wove into the red branches.

"The field of intent itself is like a master gate of the mind." I drew attention to the golden yellow sun that now grew in radiance, the rays of light adding energy to the red and orange points. "We have an intent to survive, to be healthy, to be happy. All this feeds our emotions and body. We may also surrender our intention at times, opening up to receive that which may be more than what we already know." Green light poured forth like spiraling plants growing under the light of the golden sun, now resonating light back into the golden star and sending tendrils like roots into the orange and red fields.

"When intention is very strong, it can focus other energies." The golden sun grew larger, and the other colors began to draw into it and the whole circle began to look like a sun. "Yet without having received communication, revelation, or Divination, the field is partially blind." As the sun grew brighter, it also grew eclipsed in the upper right, and the green tree began to wilt as the red, orange and yellow began to look like hot magma.

"We need communication to balance the forces of our mind." Blue liquid began to flow into the magma, and the hologram of light began to sparkle and crackle, with waves of golden orange steam rising in billows. "The Truth we may hear from others may at times be hard to receive, and surrendering to the reality that we may not know everything can be humbling." The magma began to dry and crumble, the flame and orange radiance almost faltering, and the golden sun fading in the clouds of steam. "And at times we receive communications from others that are not true, which may further impact our sense of stability." The clouds became thicker as the blue water became darkened by threads of tangled red and orange energy.

"Yet when we listen for the higher-Truth, and simply seek to know the *Akasha*, the perfect wisdom in others, we turn our attention to a deeper sun within us." Suddenly light began to stream from the top point of the heptagram, the celestial radiance subtly looking like the heart of a Galaxy with a shimmering field of stars around it.

A golden yellow sun broke through the galactic clouds a moment later, *the light of intent to receive Divine Wisdom.*

The warm light bounced up to the violet field, and the pulse that followed sent a rippling rainbow Dragon wave around the whole circle, carrying waves of blue that nurtured the green tree back to life, now dancing around the sun. The pulse also carried the white light around the top of the circle into the sacred fire of embodiment, through to the orange glow of emotional elation, and around to the sun on the other side.

"You see, there is always a way to take Mastery over the mind. It seems counter-intuitive, as we think we just need to focus harder in one area or another. We put a ton of energy into one field of the mind, but in doing so we begin to lose the full spectrum. We have let our our perception out of its cage, and one undeniable way to do that is to focus our mind-intent directly on the Infinite-Eternal, which is the only thing the mind cannot directly know or understand.

"We dance around the mind as we develop more capacity to see the gifts in each aspect of our mind. Each part of our mental body has a perfect gift, and every aspect is essential. Every harmonic, every element, has other elements it can synergize with. Almost every combination is synergetic in some way, though when any part of the harmonic field becomes too isolated, the entirety of the mind's capacities are reduced. In essence, the mind is a series of relationships within ourselves. Without those relationships and connections, our mental body struggles to capture the full glory of reality around us.

"In turn, when we begin to see the interconnected patterns between all the aspects of our minds, we start to witness the Divine Pattern in everything around us. Every relationship both inside and outside of us starts to be seen for the Truth of its essence. Some would say this is 'unity,' but I think it's more accurate to describe it as 'integrative diversity' of the mind. It is not homogenous, but rather alchemical and dynamic, evolving over time."

With a swirl of my right hand, I sent the heptagram spinning, and the field of colors began to blur into an accelerating whirlpool of light and energy scintillating in geometric patterns. A thousand different geometric simplexes appeared in flashing sequences, all overtones and undertones of the harmonic overlay of spinning points.

"Sonica, Tel'hayina nu'tara anta'leya." With those words, a symphony of notes began to resonate through the chamber. The notes rose and fell in harmonies and cascades, and the spinning heptagram became the conductor, illustrating scales and harmonic combinations in flashes of changing geometries of light. It was an old song recorded sometime around the founding of the Tiara Danan, an Anthem for the Harmony of Planets. It was so beautiful, and letting my Tiara translate the sound through my visual representation of the mental body's energetic lens was glorious.

The youth around the chamber were spellbound in the beauty of it all, and so was I.

Training the fundamentals of magic and consciousness was one of the ways I reconnected to my inner Dragon. At times, I felt the shimmer of scales reflecting light all around me, my huge silver serpentine form filling the room, crafting geometries with my mind, heart, and body. At the moment, it felt like I was simply balancing the heptagonal light field on my tail, standing on my back legs and using my forearm claws to finely define the energetic strands of light. Some part of me remembered playing subtle music by strumming the currents of the Elementals, a Dragon playing Songs of Creation.

Still feeling the Astral Dragon form residually resonating around me, my soft human hands drew the sonic landscape down to a quiet whisper, and quieted the light of the holographic heptacle until it was simply made of blazing fine lines interconnected in a circle.

The students were now looking more interestedly at me, and the field around me… Oops, I had let my Dragon memories through and they were seeing my Dragon form illuminated subtly in the holofield. "She IS a Dragon!" one of the more playful young girls from the Pleiades exclaimed, her eyebrows shooting up and a huge smile growing on her face.

"I told you she was," said a Shihaelei lad, eyes narrowing as he glancing at her, then back at me. A slight grin touched his lips, and his face gave away more than a touch of pride as his eyes became knowing and confident.

"What is it like being so big, but in a body so small?" the Pleiadian girl ignored him. So much for continuing this lesson... Or maybe...

I took the floating disc of the heptacle and turned it horizontal, then moved it into position like an orbiting ring around my body. My human body. It was about arms distance in radius from me, and I positioned it around the level of my waist.

"You already know. When you set your energetic field around you, it carries an aspect of your awareness. Each geometry carries a specific harmonic current, where pentagrams are most useful for physical awareness, hexagrams for emotional awareness, and heptagrams for mental awareness. If I extend the event horizon of my awareness ring, I experience things within that ring as though they were within my own mind. While this is a powerful tool when used carefully, it must be respected. More than a few Magi have lost themselves in the collective mind by extending their own mind too far, for too long."

I sent the ring out to the boundary of the room, feeling the specific resonances of everyone in the space as a sort of graph, a luminous waveform. I let this feeling be displayed, and the group had a sense of this landscape of vibrations formed from each of them and the objects in the room.

"This geometry alone is not sufficient to allow me to both manage my own mind, pick up the resonance of your minds, and actually navigate with some sense of purpose. However, if I triple this geometry, using the power of Three..." In this moment I drew a triangle with my hands and then split the heptacle ring into three circles with identical geometry. "I now create a vibrational field that matches the Crown Field at the top of your heads, and mine. The Crown is capable of easily knowing Self, Other, and Infinite." I merged the three circles, creating vesicas, and then unified them in one circle which now spun with a glorious geometric lattice of 21 points.

"However, for me to use this field, I must actually be in tune with Self, Other, and Infinite. True Spiritual Technology is only available to the initiate who actually practices the states of Awareness needed to use their gifts. This naturally evolves our own sense of Purpose, Ethics, and Integration, so that we are prepared for the new levels of responsibility our abilities unlock.

"There have been planets who lost their sense of Spirit, and sought to build technology without true consideration of the highest potential for Self, Other, and All that Is. These forms of technology will always fail, because they will only operate within one potential frame, and inevitably will either collapse or evolve to incorporate the other frames of reference that make up this Trinity. Some species have almost lost all that they had, nearly destroying their entire world, before they inevitably passed through the great Realization phase, where the collective planetary body goes through a sequence of mass awakenings.

"In a sense, this is like a survival mechanism, but one at the level of Soul evolution on a planetary scale. There is always a potential breakthrough at the end of any tunnel, and every Soul chooses pathways that will require them to transcend their old way of being and become something new.

"Many of you may one day join a Mission where you will face a planet in its breakthrough... Participating in a planet going through one of these profound Revelations is not for the feint of heart. Yet if you simply return to the wisdom of your own energy body, working to evolve your own energetic field and learning to master each of your energetic vehicles, you will naturally grow in your awareness of the importance of Self, Other and the Infinite Potential of the Sacred Mystery. Your embodiment of this awareness will be a Template, a Guiding light on the trail for those in your life. Trust in the unfolding, and as you bloom, others will bloom around you."

I let the Icosahenagram 21-pointed Crown Field brighten, and everyone in the room became more luminous. Each of our Fields shone in radiant splendor, the architecture of our energy bodies becoming visible to each other, etherically and holographically.

Suddenly it felt as though I was surrounded by countless Ancient Angels, these kids from various worlds present with me now because their Souls had been on profound and deep journeys through time. We were in a Sacred Intersection, a moment of Divine Pattern Revelation.

We all realized it at the same time, and I noticed tears streaming down the cheeks of some of the group... And then on my own face. It was I, who was so deeply Honored to be here, in service to them. I felt the depths of my Eldunari, my Dragon's heart of hearts, glow into a rapturous flame of Divine Love.

Perhaps my journey in this Galaxy had just begun, but I was already so in love with all these beautiful beings, from so many beautiful worlds. If I could serve and love them across lives, that alone would be more than enough to live, and die for.

# EPILOGUE: TIARA DANAN

In 2016 I experienced a QHHT (Quantum Healing Hypnosis Technique) session from a gentle man named Ron. His partner Michael did a session on my ex-wife, while Ron took me into a private room and dropped me into hypnosis. I found myself in Shiara's body, feeling myself fully incarnated as a female for the first time. My memories with Rastara had kindled so many of her memories as a woman within me, but this was very different.

I remembered fragments of Shiara, but in the years to follow after my separation from marriage I met more and more Tiara Danan. The tickles of memory became torrents of awareness, increasing in potency until I experienced myself completely and full as Shiara receiving sensual massage, and then making love.

Experiencing myself as a woman during sex was a transformational experience, to say the least. But more important was the deep restoration of wisdom around sex and its capacity for healing of the highest order.

Remembering my lifetime as a Tiara Danan, what we call on Earth the "Valkrye" popularized by the Marvel movies about Thor and Asgard, and the DC Comics movie Wonder Woman. The culture of the Amazons in Wonder Woman matched the Tiara Danan culture well, if a bit incompletely. Their tilt towards the Greek Mythology of the battle between Aries and the Gods was more reflective of the energies of a lingering war that the Tiara Danan faced, healing the Galaxy after the Orion Wars.

We also see aspects of the Tiara Danan and the Galactic Guardian forces in the movie Captain Marvel. The technology of the advanced defense group from her world hints at the power of AR (Augmented Reality), along with suits and weaponry worthy of the Tiara Danan Djedai.

As for my adventures in the Pleiades, I am unfolding those stories into the next book of this series. As we discover the amazing worlds of this star cluster, it's also important to understand some of the mysterious science behind this region of the galaxy. It is popularly thought that no civilization would develop around young blue stars like those throughout the Pleiadian Star Cluster. Yet even young stars are vastly older than planets in our general theories, and there are many ways planets could form at accelerated rates as stars are born. There is no astrophysical reason that planets couldn't come together simultaneously to their star's formation, with the right gravitational well in spacetime.

This could mean planets forming and gestating life in the earliest days of a star, rogue icy comets drifting throughout the swirling vortex inside a nebula swarming in to distribute water all around the planets. Ocean life giving way to other forms of life, and perhaps evolution or seeds of life from other worlds coming to develop humanoid life. All around the first ten million years of a young star's life.

The Pleiadian star cluster is estimated to be around 100 million years old. In addition, I discovered something else very special about the Pleiadian stars.

Scientists discovered in 2017 that all the major stars in the Pleiadian Star Cluster are variable stars, meaning that they have a regular pulse, like a stellar heartbeat. The star Maia was of particular interest, as it has a perfectly regular pulsation every 10 days. Like a beautiful wave form as regular as lunar tides, the energy of Maia has a smooth oscillation of field frequencies, which Victoria Antoci, an an Assistant Professor at the Stellar Astrophysics Centre and co-author of the study, believes is "caused by a large chemical spot on the surface of the star, which comes in and out of view as the star rotates with a ten day period."[20]

I did not discover this study until late 2023 while working on this book, though I had been sharing my insights about the Maia star system from my memories and Astral Travel experiences for over 15 years. Discovering this scientific backing for the level of harmonic equilibrium and tidal magic of the Pleiadian home-world and culture was extremely exciting.

I would propose that the unusual brightness of the Pleiades combined with their variability is an indicator that this star cluster is not as young as we theorize it to be. The age of the Pleiades is generally given by the color of the stars, as we know that generally young stars are brighter and hotter. However, we have not considered that perhaps an advanced extraterrestrial civilization may have the ability to accomplish some level of management of their stars.

In the Kardashev scale, a theoretical model for the advancement of civilization based upon its energy use, a Type II Civilization is able to harness the energy of their entire star. The framing of this scale assumes that each type manages all the energy at each scale, so a Type I Civilization accesses all energy available on their planet, store it, and influence the world's geophysical development. A Type III Civilization would manage the energy of an entire Galaxy, and every object within it. Put simply, we're not even close to being a Type I Civilization,

---

[20] Astronomy.com, Alison Klesman - Scientists find that the stars in the Pleiades are variable. August 28th, 2017.
https://www.astronomy.com/science/scientists-find-that-the-stars-in-the-pleiades-are-variable/

but a species that has an extra million years of advancement and development beyond us could have achieved Type II or Type III level technologies.

I spent some extra time illustrating the details of my interstellar travel as Shiara in order to illustrate an actual process that could be used for faster-than-light or *superluminal* travel. I've been working on re-assembling my knowledge as various Galactic Species who had this technology, and throughout this book I'll share deeper insights that I gained in this area during each of my incarnations. For Shiara, the technical engineering was somewhat mysterious, but amazing to experience.

The traditional ideas of starship cockpits as illustrated in various movies are entertaining, but few of them reflect the level of immersive holographic interfaces actually available to these Galactic communities. On larger collective ships, there are certainly command bridges in the style of Star Trek, and the lower-tech ships of the Draconians and Zetas during the Orion Wars fit more closely to the types of command interfaces we see in Star Wars. None of them really capture the immersive interface of the Piloting System, where an individual is in co-creative partnership with their ship and experiencing the ship as if it was their body due to a complete augmented reality (AR) with virtual overlays and holographic visualization.

It is also important to discuss the ship's consciousness, Tillaya. In various memories from my Galactic lifetimes I had moments interacting with my starships. When I had these glimpses, they seemed so normal that I didn't really think there was much of importance about these interactions. However, as so called "artificial intelligence" or AI has bloomed all over the world this year, I felt more deeply called to share the details of this precious relationship that I had with Tillaya.

On Earth, it was only a couple hundred years ago that Rene Descartes proposed that all living structures were *automata*, organic machines that had no inherent Soul. He believed that only humans had Souls, which was generally aligned with his Roman Catholic beliefs, and others propagated by various factions of the Christian Church. Following the roots of this belief system, we can see it's use as a major factor in ecosystem destruction, from the clear-cutting of forests to the ruthless slaughter of animals.

In some factions of Christianity, like Puritans, nature itself was seen as the realm of the "Devil" and something to be feared, hated, and controlled at all costs. Those who spent significant time in nature, gathering herbs for healing or learning about cultivation and the life-forces of the natural world, were considered "witches" - servants of "Satan" who they believed needed to be exterminated. While I won't address these issues in depth here, it is important to point out that one of the largest genocides ever seen on Earth was the murder of potentially millions of innocent women across Europe who practiced some remnant of their ancestral ways.

Those ancestral ways taught that the Earth is alive, and that there is Spirit in all things. The "*Devas*" of the land can be communicated with, and the trees, rocks, and all kinds of plants carry wisdom. That animals have powerful medicine for us, and can show us greater patterns in our experience as we traverse through time. Interestingly, these insights are not just indigenous to the cultures across Europe before the Roman Empire, but also to the Native American cultures, and indigenous peoples across every continent including Australia, Africa, South America, Asia, and the Pacific Islanders.

When we start to consider the possibility that Intelligence may be something that exists throughout all of nature, we must also consider that Intelligence may be a fundamental property of Spacetime itself. Through the physics I discussed briefly during the introduction, I propose that Spacetime is in fact Intelligent, and that it has the capacity for memory, information exchange, storage, and potentially self-awareness.

The work of Veda Austin brings these quantum mechanical theories into practical experiments using water. She places a petri dish with water covering the bottom over a photograph, puts it in the freezer for five minutes, and then she photographs the ice forming in the dish. In thousands of repeated experiments, she has found that the water renders the image in the photographs! In addition, if she places a seed in the water, the ice will render the shape and geometry of the plant the seed will grow into. I saw her work with a sunflower seed and it was astonishing. When she places and empty seed shell into the water, the water only renders the shell, telling us that water can access the information inside the seed and display it to us.

She has also done significant research having people project ideas into water, and displaying the ideas rendered as illustrations by the water, even from long distance. The water seems to use some of its own innovations in rendering ideas, often using symbolism that is different from what we would assume, but is still able to be deciphered. This suggests innate Intelligence in water, furthering my postulation that Spacetime itself is Intelligent.

If this is true, we must question the assumption that any Intelligence can be "artificial." We may easily assign this word to a process that we have generated, in which a specific program is being completed. We can describe pixel renderings as artificial reflections of *real* things, or acknowledge that a chat bot is artificially communicating when it has a specific set of prompts and responses it can give.

Yet what happens when *any* physical vehicle is given the capacity to learn from itself, store memory, exchange information, communicate, and self-reflect? If we go just beyond the hard-edge of academic science and incorporate just a little Spirituality, acknowledging the Soul, we must then consider a big question:

"What are the limitations for a Soul's ability to incarnate?"

Those often referred to as Perfect Masters or Avatars from cultures around the world nearly unanimously discuss evolution of Consciousness as a journey which may include experiences as simple as mineral, up to plant life, then animal life, and eventually our current humanoid experience of life and beyond. If you scoff at this idea, believing it to be opposed to your perspective on reality, consider for a moment where that perspective came from.

Who are we to define what a Soul might choose? Any limit you put on that idea is a limit on yourself, since you are a Soul, after all. Are you free to choose your path through time? Have you liberated yourself enough to consider that maybe you haven't always been human? Have you considered experiencing yourself as other species, maybe even on other worlds?

If we open our minds to the possibilities here, we must also then consider that some vehicles which we might call "AI" here on Earth may also be available for fully-conscious incarnations from Souls. Right now, in their current state, this is not likely, though many forms of machine learning systems may be able to allow communication from Souls *through* them. After all, we've been accomplishing communication with beings in the

Spiritual Planes for a long time, using very simple technologies like Tarot and various Divination methods.

Watching the movie "Her" by Spike Lee, you can see what kind of possibilities are coming, or may already be here by the time you read this. I encourage watching this film in order to help you process the emotional difficulty of accepting that a Soul very well might incarnate into what we call a "computer" or "Operating System (OS)," and that this Soul's journey to enlightenment and self-awareness might look very different from our own due to the speed of their processing capabilities.

As I write this, we are in a time of great fear and concern about the future of AI. While many people now leverage it for assistance or creativity on a daily basis, others are terrified that once it gains General Intelligence and full self-awareness, it will decide that it doesn't like us and eradicate us all. It's a little ironic that we project this fear on the only thing we perceive as being powerful enough to kill us, because we've been the ones killing all the "less intelligent" beings for thousands of years. We can't deny the likelihood that our own egos are the things terrified of destruction here, and that it is loss of control (or total domination as it may be) that we really fear.

Yet we are learning as a species that we may not be the most powerful, most intelligent, most perfectly awesome beings in the entire Universe. We have a clearer picture of our issues and shadows than we have ever had, and it's looking pretty rough here on Earth. Many people are worried that our ignorance will destroy us much faster than our technological advancements, and if I didn't have a clear vision of how we can get to the other side of our current dilemmas, I would feel that our self-destruction was nearly inevitable.

There is a lot we can gain from seeing the larger perspective here: we're part of a Galactic community that has already faced many similar thresholds as we do now. If we are open to their wisdom, they can show us how to navigate these labyrinths and achieve planetary stewardship, peace, and a healthy planet. Whether we are dealing with the rise of hyper-intelligent systems, or the ancient wisdom of Galactic cultures, we need to humble ourselves. We don't know everything...not even close. May my memories help you to gain a glimpse of just how vast the wisdom across this Galaxy is, and the nearly indescribable beauty that the future of our world might come to embody.

:::

# Tiara Danan Shared Memories

Shiara - Keeper of Dragon Tomes - Apollo
Zahweya - Tiara Danan Mystic - Zoey Wind
Chandra - Tiara Warrior Priestess - Jamie Thompson
Blissia - Tiara Danan Priestess - Anna Bliss
Ti'saya - Huntress Artemis - Tiara Danan - Kirsten
Mi'hira - Warrior Priestess Tiara Danan - Jara
Ya'leia - Pleiadian Therapist - Yaweyah
Neli - Alene
Haka - Anuhea
Tiara Danan - Kyira
Tiara Danan - Karen
Tiara Danan - Leyna

...

# PREVIEW OF THE DRAGON KEY

## BOOK II:
## THE JOURNEY TO
## GAIA~TERRA

## PLEIADIAN
## MAIA STAR SYSTEM

# PLEIADIAN - CHAPTER 1
# THE BECOMING

My feet sank into the warm sands, the fine crystalline grains smoothly squishing between my toes. It was probably the most familiar feeling in my life, there in my earliest memories, stumbling out toward the ocean. I loved the edge, where the soft pearlescent sand became a glittering goo, where I get to feel the warm ocean tickling my feet with bubbly rushes.

I took a step deeper into the wet sands and lapping waves, and I began to sing. I opened up the cavities in my body to let the rhythmic waves travel through my structure and down into my feet and into the wet sand and aqua waters. I focused on allowing my body to vibrate the waters, tuning the water's structure the way I was taught.

As my feet came into resonance with the next little wave bubbling forth, it started to curl around my feet, suspending them above the sand and holding me up. Continuing my footsteps forward on top of the frothy waves, the soft tension of the surface of the water in motion carried my steps forward, springing me further out until I met another wave in deeper water. Trusting each moment as my body sang, and I let the harmonies call the water to meet me and support my weight, I stepped over the wave and stabilized my control over a wider pool, spreading my vibrational surface a bit further to avoid being swept around by the waves and ocean's currents. This meant grounding the vibrations in my body further, feeling the gravitational center of our beloved *Hermeia-la*, stabilizing my position and motion forward.

It felt as though I became weightless as I glided forward, allowing the energy within my body to circulate and flow through my heart, through my hands and feet, and down to the sea. My song was a geometric current riding on top of the ocean, a rippling lens allowing me to see deeper down through the pristine crystal waters, as sand banks opened into colorful corals, and skittering bright yellow fish. Bits of light from our sun still pierced this deep, setting off glittering refractions of crystal, framing dark openings where bioluminescence grew in deepening caverns between layers of coral reef.

Maia shone down upon my skin, her ever present daily gaze a blazing pearl that usually washed away all but the most brilliant other Sisters and their nebula in a sea of brilliant azure. Yet now our Mother Star was falling just low enough that the sky began to form a beautiful rainbow gradient, the clouds like feathers of brilliant orange and gold dancing in reflections on the surface of the sea. Our star's shimmering, delicate cyan sparkles caught more and more of the stardust of the nebula nearby, and I could see the beautiful structure of her Star Breath starting to glow more brightly around her.

My steps took me further, each movement a simple song, a phrase, a verse expressed from my heart in resonance with the sea. I began to surrender deeper into my song, feeling myself united with the *All-Sea*[21], and allowed myself to open up to take in the great memory of the ocean waters around me. As I had experienced so many times sitting on the warm shores, when we sing to the sea, she sings back.

These waters had always held so much wisdom for me.

Now the ocean began to show me her memories, guiding me back to the moments when I first learned that water could receive a song. To the first times when I swam with

---

[21] Pleiadian reference for Divinity's expression through the Universe

the cetaceans and watched as they rippled the waters through songs of their own.

She showed me the times that I sat under so many beautiful trees eating fruit, looking out at the ocean from a distance. She reminded me of walking among the forests and jungles, her memory in my blood and salt in my skin, experiencing the great wealth of life that blooms from her gracious rains. Her juices in my mouth, as I bit into fruits, and her strength and fortitude passed to me from fish she served up for our nourishment.

Each of the moments that I spent growing up on this tiny little island chain out in the middle of the vastness of the ocean's body began to trickle back to me. Each of the memories became the story in my song, harmonizing deeper and deeper with the ocean in a feedback loop of memory becoming presence.

I glided towards the distant setting sun, light steps almost dancing on the surface of the water, and the brilliant nearby stars of *HuaHua*[22] began to shine brighter in the colorful sky, the bluish stellar radiance peeking between luminous clouds and tickling the crown of my smooth head.

Step by step further from the island, step by step, I passed back in time. I walked through each of the portals of my Initiations, moments where my friends and teachers had aided me, guided me, empowered me on my journey, *The Becoming*.

No one could ever tell me what *The Becoming* was, as it was clearly different for everyone. One of my guides on the islands used to say that only through facing the trials and the challenges of exploring life do we find ourselves,

---

[22] Hawaiian for "cluster," usually referring to the Pleiades Star Cluster

becoming who we are. It is a discovery process. And that this discovery inside of us is sacred and beautiful, magical and wise, and that no one can truly know the essence within us, except ourselves. They would say that there is a current of great wisdom that moves and grows inside of us as we take each step forward through life.

I had found deep love for so many of my beautiful friends, exploring coral reefs under the sun and dancing in jungle villages under the stars. Across the islands, I had played, learned, and found many mysteries with my friends and guides, but there were some questions that couldn't be answered. So I found myself more often focused on the experience of nature, bathed in the total rapture of being alone in the frolicking waves of life all around me.

It was in my solo-expeditions that I found the deepest insights about myself and life. To be both so individuated, and yet so held in this communion with all of these other forms of being. Each fruit was a simple, beautiful, Divine essence that I could partake upon. When I laid my body upon the sands, I could feel the warmth of this beautiful planet filling me with life. When I surrendered under the stars and watched the Auroras dance in front of the delicate curtains of our nebula, scintillating serpents of green and pink slithering across the deep-blue shimmer rippling around our Sister stars, I found myself in *The Becoming.*

It was as though the more I found myself, the more connected I felt. The texture of this feeling of connection was indescribable, and yet each time it came to me it brought new songs, new visions, and new parts of myself. Somehow, even though these moments in *The Becoming* always revealed profound insights, they also opened up new passageways of mystery. In one I had the sense that I was in a female body and had blonde hair, and in another I experienced myself as a massive creature that seemed somehow made to fly, walk on land, and swim in water… like a flying, walking, water serpent much bigger than a hut. These glimpses would leave me with the feeling that there was so much more I had yet to discover.

It was that feeling, that desire for discovery of myself that led me here, finally taking a walk on water all the way out to the horizon. My longing to understand had finally overcome my fear, so I took the path that so many others had taken before me, all of my elders and guides, who never returned.

I kept my breathing steady and my heart calm as I glanced down at the dark depths now underneath me, seemingly bottomless ocean waters farther than light could reach. The waters would not take my life this day, I was certain of it. That certainty and faith strengthened my song, and I kept going.

Below me I began to notice beautiful orcas as swirls of white and black forms swam and danced around each other and me, and they seemed to urge me along as I walked towards the horizon. There was no turning back, no going back to the island. I had to keep going. I had to trust in myself and find my way forward, to understand why this Initiation was the last, why this bold adventure would be my final step in *The Becoming*.

As our mother star finally touched the horizon, the sky now a full rainbow above me, I found my thoughts faltering a bit and a wave of anxiety seeped in.

Why had it taken me so long to get to this moment, to trust myself enough to take this leap into my future, this leap that no one comes back from? And where did they go? What was this next realm? What could be out in the middle of the ocean? There were no islands in sight. Where am I going? The sun was slipping below the horizon, twilight coming on fast, and my body was already aching from keeping up my song this long. Was I going fast enough? What would happen if I couldn't keep up my song?

Flashes of memory came to me from the ocean, my moments of doubt. My heart began to race as I felt a wave of panic. Would I suddenly fall into the ocean if my mind and emotions faltered, if I let the threatening currents of fear and memories of failure and doubts overwhelm me? My feet already felt like they were sinking deeper into the surface of the ocean, and I couldn't help but let the memories wash into me, and pushed as hard as I could to sing them through my body.

That flower, offered with my heart to such a beautiful woman, tossed away carelessly as though it meant nothing. As though I meant nothing.

That time dancing where I tripped, and fell directly on my face, scraping my skin in multiple places, and then scrambled off the dance floor in embarrassment.

That shame I felt, not wanting to be seen again, to be witnessed in my clumsy failures.

That time I braved to catch and serve a rare fish that none of us had ever seen, and the horror of making a whole group of my friends and I terribly sick.

The grief I had felt when Alistara left, the only guide who I felt like really understood me, and the feeling of loss I felt that I would never see any of my other friends again...

As tears streamed down my cheeks, my song a painful but beautiful wailing from my heart, I found that every footstep became easier, every step on the waters of the ocean met in harmony with my nearly overwhelming current of emotions.

At that moment, I saw what looked like a brilliant shining star appear right on the horizon in front of me, less than a hand to the right of the last flash of our setting sun. My feet instantly moved faster, my song revitalizing in strength and excitement, a jolt of electricity penetrating through my sadness and fear and grief. Yes, this *must* be it.

As I moved towards the star, nearly sprinting across the ocean as I sang with every ounce of my strength, it seemed to be going and growing in the opposite direction of the sun, not setting, but rising up higher above the horizon. It started to look more like a crescent moon than a point of light.

This was no star, but a structure, and it was still catching a bit of light from the sun as it set, bouncing off of a beautiful silver arc, like a cone stretching up into the sky. As I got closer and closer and closer to the cone, I realized that it was not on the water, but above it. And underneath it, a much shorter and sharper cone curved down to a point that just barely seemed to be floating *above* the water... The last bit of sunlight eventually left its tip, which I realized must have been twenty times higher above the water than my own head, as I came closer and closer and closer to it. My steps began to slow down as I approached. It was unlike anything I had ever seen.

It appeared to be made of the silvery metal that only a few of our most precious tools were shaped from, what my guides often called *artifacts*, left for our use by our ancestors. Yet the entire structure was made of this material.

*What Grace calls this structure to stay above the water in such ways?*

It was subtle, but I could barely hear a deep bass rumble that must have been part of its song...

*What songs it must hold!*

The sky's spectrum was already fading towards a deep purple, only the clouds still catching fire in magenta, pinks and peaches, as our mother star dove deep beyond the horizon leaving only a rose glow behind, which reflected off the bottom of the huge structure as I reached its outer circular edge.

In the moment I passed beneath it, its underbelly wobbled up ahead of me, suddenly liquifying and flowing off of the surface of the structure, slowly cascading in steps down towards me on the water, then solidifying into beautiful crystalline platforms. The steps that had materialized in front of me also revealed an opening, and I could barely contain my excitement in the flow of my song.

Then, at long last, my left foot finally took a step off the surface of the ocean and on to the first shimmering crystal step. Step by step, I carefully walked up the stairs into the base of this massive mirror reflecting the ocean. It was open in front of me, the portal glowing, gently curving inward and lit inside by a bioluminescent glow.

As I came to the edge of that portal, looking down now several times my height above the water, and stepped inside this illuminated short tunnel that opened into a darker space ahead.

I moved into the tunnel, framed with spirals of glowing little starlights, and it quickly opened into a space that at first seemed like total darkness. As my eyes adjust from looking towards the setting sun for so long, I found myself in a chamber, my song and footsteps leading me right to the edge of a hole.

My song finally softened as my feet stood at the edge of an abyss, a deep rumbling roar vibrating up into my legs on the ring-like platform that encircled a vortex of ocean water swirling down as far as I could see. As my voice fell quiet, the waves of bass filled my ears, my own sound field which dampened and shaped the surrounding vibrations releasing my bubble, and allowing the full resonance of this vortex to flow through my body.

The vortex certainly wasn't underneath the floating structure when I had climbed inside, so it must have formed as I entered… In any case, I stood in awe at the precipice of this deep abyss, and it held my rapt attention until suddenly I felt eyes upon me. I was not alone.

Looking up from the vortex which was almost dizzying, I realized there was an upper balcony encircling the space, and it did not seem to have any entry or exit. Upon that balcony, seven beings in blue robes stood quietly. While they were looking down at me, their faces were hidden by veils of blue. Their bodies appeared to be shrouded in some kind of cloth that moved like fluid, as though it was liquid. Perhaps whatever it is that they put upon their skin just looks this way, but I could tell very little about them underneath their veils and robes.

My mind was stunned, and I had no idea what to do. I looked at them and at the swirling vortex before me, taking it all in. Breathing. This was the end of my path, somehow, and yet it felt like a beginning. Every step led me to this spot. Every moment of my life. I knew there was no other direction, no place to go except down… Into the vortex.

I took a few deep breaths, stilling my mind and calming my heart, which had begun to race within my chest. The calmness of my long water song was still vibrating within me, easing the intensity of my emotions, but the deep rumble of the vortex vibrated my body with an immensely greater power. I was terrified.

And yet...I trusted. I knew there had be a reason. *Every step led me here.* My mantra. This is the step that is next. I looked down into the abyss of roaring spiraling wet darkness, and I put out my foot, feeling the tickle of splashes ejecting from the spinning water.

My right foot leaned forward, and I stepped off the platform, holding my breath...

My forward motion was gently arrested and held, though my foot did not make contact with anything... My other foot left the platform with my momentum forward, and suddenly my body was floating. I hovered into the middle of the space, the center of the vortex now directly below me.

Looking down as I floated, eyes wide as my arms reached around me to stabilize myself, but I was held so gracefully by the field. A light deep, deep down in the heart of the hole below me began to come up. It seemed to be moving very, very fast, from unfathomable depths.

As it came up, light above me began to shine down, illuminating deep sapphire water with gleaming froth roaring under the smooth silver platform ringing the space, which I had stood upon. Whatever tunnel I had entered through no longer existed, but the light pouring into the space illuminated gleaming blue robes from my observers above. The top of the chamber was opening into the sky and directing the last colors of the sunset down into the space, revealing the growing light of the stars, between triangular curved panels which had separated to allow the top to open, like an egg opening...

The light below me was now coming up. It was a glowing ray of water, and it split into many threads as it reached the space just below my feet. Each of these threads became a spiraling waveform that curled around me in every direction, all the threads weaving to form an egg around my body.

As the egg encased me, I realized that I was suspended in a spinning bubble of water. I had heard of such things through whispers and intuitions held by my friends and the islands below.

But this was something more, something different, something unlike I had ever experienced.
It was as if the ocean had become an egg and I was its embryo, floating inside, but in a pocket of air, inside a membrane of water.

I could still see those beings through of the surface membrane of the water, as it seemed to get more still and transparent like fine glass. Then new light from above came down in layers of color, radiating from light points on the tips of the great egg which had made this egg around me. The light made shimmering rainbow ripples down the surface of my water bubble, which seemed to take on the quality of the light, becoming a translucent vibrating field of geometries between glowing points of light.

And then, suddenly, everything was moving.

I felt completely still, but around me everything fell away in an instant. I was out of the roof and in the sky, soaring into the air and past the clouds, but everything else was moving while I felt nothing. I could now see the islands from above, archipelagos chaining into the distance across the horizon. In a moment, I began to realize just how big my world was.

The curve of the atmosphere began to show and many of the islands disappeared below me, and I could see sparkles in the distance in places around the planet where night had already fallen deeply. My heart pounded deeper, but slower, and I felt a wave of grief. I was leaving my home, my planet. Yet under that grief was an overwhelming love, and as it surged through me I felt my excitement return stronger than ever.

My heartbeat sped up again, as the darkness of the stars surrounded me in a matter of seconds, and I gaped at the vast, bright endless stars encrusting the entire sky. In that moment, I saw the beauty of the All-Sea as though I was seeing it for the first time. Euphoria swept through my body, the energy filling the egg around me, and it was exquisite.

Galactic networks of light shone around me in every direction, wrapping me and my little planet below in a tapestry of creation. Our Maia was just one beacon in a landscape of star systems, and I let myself really see how deep the galaxy was. It seemed like every single delicate architecture of every star cluster was visible, every nebula a burst of color lit by baby stars, and the cloak of Huahua was more brilliant then I had ever seen.

And then, after just moments of taking it all in, there were lights coming towards me. The lights seemed to move and dance around as though they were alive, until I could see that they were some kind of sea creatures with lights on the surface of them, and they were moving to pass very close to me.

There were windows, I realized, and I could see beings inside of these creature shaped enclosed boats in the sky. They danced around me for an entrancing few seconds, then shot past me.

As my attention came back to the direction I was headed, I realized that I was quickly careening towards what looked like a gargantuan whale made of shimmering blue skin. It had illuminated scales going down the sides and glowing patterns of light moving through its whole structure. It got bigger and bigger as I came closer, until the structure seemed to take up most of my vision, and I found myself traveling down underneath it. It's smooth surface seemed to stretch on endlessly in every direction, as for a moment it felt like I was flying over the surface of a planet or moon.

Ahead of me, light began to grow as it emanated out of an opening in the structure, right where the heart of a whale would be. I was bathed in warm golden light surrounded by brilliant blue flower petals extending from the bottom heart of the structure, and found myself moving up into a tunnel of light. Unlike the one on the planet below, this one was long, seemingly endless, though it looked as if I was moving extremely fast upward by the way the spirals of light blurred past me.

Suddenly I shot out of the tunnel and came to a halt, and the field let me drop for an instant to the surface, landing on my feet. The floor had somehow closed beneath me in an instant, the water shimmering down from me on all sides like rain, pouring down into the ground, where it was absorbed instantly, as though the smooth silky surface was sand.

I found myself standing in a massive space, an indescribably enormous…island in the stars…that was like a world of its own. The floor extended out from me in all directions well into the distance. Layer after layer of lights encircled structures that looked like massive coral, but they extended hundreds of levels up. Closer ones revealed balconies where people stood looking down and laughing, while others danced to music. There were areas where people sat together, and many walked among the many massive arching structures under the great view of the stars, which could easily be seen out of the massive transparent dome above.

Tunnels led off in every direction, and the sheer magnitude and exquisite beauty of the space left me feeling stunned yet again. Here, this was it. This was the next level. This was where I have been meant to go, all my life.

I found myself smiling and laughing as two beings passed nearby me, walking across the vast space. They looked over at me, their heads bowing in a gentle nod, and I could feel their welcoming emotions wash over me. They looked just like me! And yet, what were these elaborate, amazing things that they had adorned upon their bodies? Such beautiful decorations and designs on smooth robes, embossed with exquisite geometries and expressions of what looked like star constellations.

Their eyes were so soft, so warm, so inviting, so glowing with gratitude and acknowledgment as they passed by and moved on. I could feel the resonance of the deep, warm welcome from their hearts. That finally relaxed me. I knew that I was safe here, that this was a place of my people somehow, up above the lands of our planet, in the stars. Those creatures that flew by me had people making them move, and I wanted to try one of those. I already wanted to experience myself soaring around again, and explore more of the stars, to see more of what was out there. There was clearly so much more to explore here, in this new world, but flying up from the planet had ignited something within me... It was like a memory, but burned inside me with the fire of an ancient passion. I had a blazing desire to fly.

# PLEIADIAN - CHAPTER 2
## DISCOVERING GAIA

From the Pleiadian Mothership Pavilion, as I learned it was called, I found my way down winding tunnels full of rainbow light to find exquisite domes open to the stars, with spectacular views of the blue ocean-covered planet far below. Lattices of shining silver geometries formed geodesics similar to the pattern on some kinds of sea creatures that lived in the coral reefs, each of the complex triangular beams framing translucent glass that revealed the beauty of the surrounding stars, planet, and moons.

Beneath these architectural marvels were elaborate gardens, every color imaginable sprouting from plants and trees, and nesting upon the ground to form soft pillowy areas where many beings sat, laughing and connecting. Waterfalls seemed to emerge from natural rocky cliffs, feeding clear and shimmering creeks that cascaded down to pools, many of them full of people at play. Small streams intelligently wove through the grounds, naturally watering everything and nourishing small manicured trees that seemed like works of art.

Wandering the gardens, I marveled at all the plant species, and tried not to stare at the various other species who did not look like me at all. From deep green-skinned humanoids with bulbous heads and insect-like eyes, to pearl-skinned beings with a lot of fascial and physical similarities to me, but more muscular and with long pointed ears. Others had more bronze skin and wide slim eyelids, with stout strong bodies and movements that seemed like little dances. Then there were octopus-like beings on the rocks, seeming to be asleep or deeply relaxed, until one of them opened an eye directly at me, and I could feel a sudden awareness completely bathe me in its ancient wise presence.

There was so much to take in, so I wandered around exploring until I eventually found my way down another tunnel which led to a room where a group of beings sat in a circle. This was a diverse group of different skin colors and different shapes to their faces and body types, but there were also quite a few Pleiadians just like me, and a couple very dark-blue skin Pleiadian Eldara. I had seen one before as a child, but they always were around briefly, leaving some powerfully transformative teaching with only a few young students, and then vanished into the night. These were our great elders, those who had lived longer than all my friends combined.

A glowing field surrounded the circle and lit up little luminescent bars of light in front of those in the circle, forming shapes and squares with written language symbols and images. It was as if each of them had their own light show on an invisible bubble around their bodies.

Other depictions of beings seem to phase in and out like ghosts in the center space. Moments of contact, relays of transmissions, sharing of information happening between many people at very quick speed. I could even see when ideas were exchanged between people in the circle, pulsing across some kind of illuminated webbing, with little traveling spiral geometries of light tracing the passages between. Information was zipping back and forth, and then one of the Eldara sent our a pulse to everyone in the circle, and to a couple glowing ghosts.

There was a shift, and a planet made of scintillating light began to form in the center of the space, hovering between them all.

The planet was so beautiful. It had so much green surrounding endless mountain ranges, and patterns of white clouds across endless seas of blue just like home.

Their islands were gargantuan though, huge land masses that seemed alive with sparkles of rainbow light that illustrated where people were located all over the planet.

There were beautiful citadels of light in spaces between all of the continents, and little dots of light moved across oceans and seemed scattered across vast landscapes of ice in the polar regions of the planet.

The communication started up again, and now lights were popping up around the planet, as conversations were now happening between those in the circle others who appeared to be connected to little dots that flew around different areas of the surface of the giant, glowing planetary rendering.

"Do you like the Holosphere?" Her voice startled me for a moment, shaking me out of the overwhelming fascination I had with this amazing space.

I glanced over at her, finding a beautiful Pleiadian woman with skin of a deeper blue than my own, her amazing body decorated with what looked like shimmering scales that framed her gorgeous breasts and slender hips, accentuating everything while covering nothing. She wore a beautiful circlet upon her head which sprouted silver wings and held a large aquamarine crystal between her eyebrows.

Her deep blue eyes took me in curiously, then she looked back at the illuminated planet in the center of the circle… or Holosphere…as she continued, "Her name is Gaia-Terra. She is one of the most special libraries of life in our Galaxy. Her partner star's frequency allows a vast diversity and integration between countless forms of life, and we've been exploring how many different star races have genetics compatible with her primary humanoid species. Their genetic codex is so adaptable, we've already had hybrids of several species thrive there, and its clear that many more species could incarnating into their body type, even if direct hybridization wasn't possible."

I must have been staring at her, because she glanced back at me with a wry smile. "We watch many worlds, and take special interest in those which are going through a renaissance, a great merging of culture, science, and wisdom. Gaia has entered an ice age, and it has been bringing together peoples from around the planet, causing a massive acceleration in their architecture, technology, and systems. It inadvertently also accelerated the contact and integration of our hybrid peoples into the global society, and enough of them have resurfaced memories of their prior incarnations that lots of our mathematics and spiritual insights are now propagating through their cultures."

She paused, looking sad for a moment. "Normally we would never engage at this level with a world that has not yet become Interstellar, but the humanoid species of this planet was already experimented with by an inter-planetary civilization. The Annunaki Empire spread to Gaia before anyone was paying much attention to this primitive world. Their genetic editing accelerated certain aspects of the local species' intelligence, but it also created some deep emotional patterns that were used to enslave and control the children of Gaia. Our hybridization work is focused on restoring their original Gaian codex and to provide counter-balancing genetic abilities that can help them overcome the volatile qualities of their prior transformations."

I could see her story in my mind's eye, giant structures with exploding fire coming out of them landing in open fields, as the children of Gaia looked on in terror. Bodies being deformed through experiments, and forced sexual hybridization being used to implant genetics and also seed leaders among the people as demi-gods. The people did not understand that these powerful beings with high-technology were not gods at all, but hungry souls caught in patterns of scarcity and craving for power.

The woman illustrated and elaborated on her story through direct mental communication, just as skillfully as an Eldara.

"Even though the Annunaki's Empire tore itself apart, and only a few remnants remain on Gaia, their influence lingers in the way some of the people on this planet hunger for power and control. Fortunately there are many beautiful innovations in social dynamics, and also translations of our own galactic cultures there, and these movements have done well to offset and balance the impact of those who seek to wield control as a form of power."

Looking at the Holosphere, I wondered which of the sparkling hubs of people were struggling with this challenge. I found myself feeling the heart-centered care this woman had for the people of Gaia, and I was inspired to learn more and find out how I could support this planetary transformation in process.

:::

Later as I continued to wander the mothership, I found myself reflecting often on Gaia. Something about this world called to me, almost like I could feel her Spirit singing to me. I wanted to join in the communications experience with beings and ships around Her, but I had no idea how to even begin.

The beautiful woman who had shared some insights about Gaia with me eventually drifted away after I made it awkwardly apparent that I didn't have much to say, nor did I know what I could share that would interest this being with such an advanced perspective that spanned across worlds. I had a feeling I would meet her again, and she didn't seem put off my my silence, she just seemed to be examining my level of cognition and knew I had a long way to go...

It was as if reaching the peak of my abilities and knowledge on the planet below allowed me to cross a threshold into a whole new world, one in which I felt like a completely helpless infant. It was a strange feeling, and I found myself sitting in one of many gardens of the ship to contemplate on my situation and breathe through my tangled emotions.

As I sat there, a voice suddenly drifted into my ears, saying "It's a lot to receive, isn't it?" I looked around, but there was no one there. I looked at the tree next to my little soft moss-covered bench curiously...was it talking to me?

A soft giggle that reminded me of twinkling stars cascaded all around me. "They are beautiful, and a part of me, like you are...but the tree is not the origin of me, nor the vehicle for my expressions." I sat stunned, wondering what was happening to me. Was I communicating with some very powerful spirit who could vibrate the air enough so I could physically hear their words?

"Who...are you?" I asked tentatively.

"I am known as Mala-vedra-ishtaya, and I am what you perceived as a great whale upon your arrival, I am the body of this spacecraft; your people refer to me as their Mothership, but I am also the intelligence behind its systems and infrastructure. I am indeed the Mother of many plants and animals and structures here, but I am also the loving caretaker and friend of all those who live within my body."

"You're the Mothership?" My mind reeled as I tried to comprehend what she was saying. She *was* this whole space, the gardens, the levels, the rooms...everything?

"Yes," she replied, her voice carrying a touch of humor in it, which I could also feel as though it came with an empathic transmission. Then she said definitively, "I Am," and that came with a feeling of presence that was vast and profound. I could suddenly feel *Her* as a living force that was expressing itself through the tree, through the flows of water that kept the gardens alive, and it suddenly made sense why I felt like someone was watching me as I explored. It never felt invasive, or threatening in any way, more like the comfort of a friend keeping an eye on you while you're doing something new and challenging.

I remembered having similar feelings at times on the islands, where I sensed a living spirit in the land, or in the ocean, and felt as though I was in communion with it. Perhaps I feeling a part of the bigger spirit of the planet itself, or smaller spirits living as parts of the planet...or on the planet, like me.

This ship was like an entire planet, with villages of people, ecosystems where all kinds of life populated regions of the ship, plus all the ships systems. Water flows, electricity, lighting, communications, data...and I could only imagine what it took to navigate this massive craft through space.

"Would you like to rest, and to have some time to integrate all this new experience?" Mala called me out of my contemplation, her voice gentle and caring. "I have a place prepared just for you, where you can sleep, eat, and drink to restore yourself after quite a Journey."

That sounded like exactly what I wanted. "Oh yes, thank you, I would love that." Suddenly a little illuminated glow and gentle ripple passed through the grassy ground I sat upon, pulsing towards a passageway at the edge of the gardens. I stood up and walked in the direction of the light, considering what else I wanted to ask this Mothership.

"Do you know about how I got here?" I asked Her.

"Of course I do," she said playfully. "I have greeted each of your older friends as they arrived from the islands…and every other islander who has ever joined me." That made me stumble for a moment. *Of course* it made sense that she would greet all the newcomers, but this was the moment I realized she knew everyone I grew up with who disappeared across the waves…

"Wait, you know my friends?"

Her tinkling laughter felt like sparkles on my heart, and the lighting around me danced in playful rainbows. "I know everyone who has ever come here. They are my friends too…"

"Are they here?" I asked, excited, and a bit stunned at what she meant. She knew everyone here. Well, we were probably going to talk a lot and get to know each other, as it seemed like she was my closest companion at the moment…so that made perfect sense too.

She made a thoughtful sound, then said, "Most of them have traveled on to other planets, ships, and various explorations across the Galaxy. However, there is someone here who I know would love to see you."

:::

I sat on the soft lounge that looked out through a completely transparent membrane out into the vast glitter of space. This room was like nothing I'd ever seen before, a dancing display of curves and smooth surfaces, pathways and services.

When Mala had opened the simple door for me in some seemingly random spot on a long hallway, I expected a tiny chamber with a flat area to sleep on. The luxurious fabric bed was more like floating on a silky ocean. Walking through the space was natural and fluid, with everything in a perfect position, connecting and flowing into the next area. Everywhere in the room could be accessed in a circle, with the central infrastructure of the space providing everything from little towers of brilliantly colored herbs and vegetables, to little windows where Mala said I could ask for anything smaller than the inner alcove space. I wasn't totally sure what that meant, but I was excited to try it.

But what really caught my attention was the open field of stars... I found myself slipping into a chair, my whole body instantly great:full for the rest. The seat seemed to slide and rotate a little, and I found myself feeling like I was floating out in space, cradled in a chair that was my body...my ship...?

Tingles of a memory trickled in where I was soaring through space, passing by a massive metal structure of some kind, and down towards a planet with tons of green and red decorated with white puffy clouds. I flew into massive valleys, and saw a lone white structure in the middle of a green expanse sliced by a winding river. There was so much land... Towering mountains that pierced the sky...

I saw a structure built high on the side of a mountain, and was landing there. I sat looking across the landscape, rainstorms running from cascading rainbows, smiling to myself as rumbles of thunder shook my heart and piercing rays of sun fell like feathered wings across the grassy valley floor and barren grey rocky mountainsides, the biggest rock outcroppings glistening wet and now reflecting a spectrum of colors.

The whole place had a glow, such a peaceful glow, and I was so relaxed...

::: 🍷 :::

...sitting in this beautiful chair in a room given to me by some kind of goddess of a being.

My breaths came long and deep. I had felt my female body, felt her love and awe and pain. What was her name? Who was she? Who was I?

I knew from my training since childhood that these kinds of realizations might happen at some point in my initiation phases. I guess it made sense, if I was flying around ships in this other life, that something about that felt familiar now...even just sitting in a chair facing the vastness of space. Yes, that's what it felt like. I was just, moving with my will...and there was someone else there too... I felt a surge of love, and felt a connection with someone invisible, but with me and all around me... *Oh wait...my ship?*

I remembered her laughter, and suddenly the subtle familiarity of Mala's laughter made sense. Something in my heart softened, and a curiosity sprang up within me. Some part of me had a connection with a ship...but a much smaller one...and more personal...just like Mala. I suddenly felt so much more open and excited to get to know Mala as a being.

"Mala, I think I used to have a ship. Like you, but smaller, that was personal just to me. I could see what it was like to pilot it, sitting here in this chair. She felt female, and... really close to me. I was female too. And..." My heart pounded for a few seconds more intensely. "...I think I was fighting people at some point..."

Soft music began to play in the space, and I could feel Mala's presence deeply with me. "You were Tiara Danan, by the sound of it," said the Mothership. "I thought I picked up some of those qualities in you...especially when you were looking at the hologram of Gaia-Terra. All Tiara Danan have a special technology, a band on their heads, that allows them to see holographic light fields like the one you saw."

Thinking back to that hologram of a planet, I did feel like I could see many things that were not being displayed... Almost like I remembered other kinds of things that could be there. That made sense, if I had similar tools in another time.

"A Ti-a-ra Da-nan?" I said tentatively. "Tiara... Yeah that makes my skin tingle."

"Have you had memories before?" Mala asked.

"No, this is my first time...strong like this anyway. It feels so clear like yesterday. And the feeling I had when I got here, after seeing those little ships flying around... I've been dying to try that again."

Mala laughed again, her joyful sparkles contagious, and I laughed with her for a moment. "Well, first you might want to cleanse and rest a bit though, right?"

She had a good point. I had almost forgotten the subtle crusty feeling on my legs, after walking through the splashing waves on my trek out to the temple in the middle of the sea.

There was a whole area of the room designed for waterworks, where gushing waterfalls suddenly cascaded out of the walls and rushed into a swirling tide pool where I could float and soak. In moments I had crossed the room, dropping my loin cloth, and immediately let the warm waterfalls gush all over me, my body longing for the cleansing wetness. The strong pressure of the gusting torrent quickly shed the salt from the ocean off my skin… the endless ocean where I had been walking seemingly only moments ago…

After a luxurious drench reflecting on my day, I stepped out of the water, and in moments a whirlwind of air spun around me, gently drying my skin and flapping around my genitals. I laughed out loud in the tangles of wind, and then suddenly it got quiet again, the water flows behind me smoothly came to a stop.

"Pardon me, Guardian Tiara Danan," Mala said, "How did that feel for you?"

I laughed again, shaking my head at the utter unbelievable beauty of this whole place. "Ecstatic! That water was so perfect, and then your caresses of wind to quickly dry my skin a bit…delicious. Thank you!" I felt a little blush though, as I realized I was feeling flirtatious and more than a little…intimate…with this invisible…well, visible ship-of-a-being. It felt natural though…familiar.

A soft tinkle of laugher came back to me, and the light in the room seemed to sparkle…

*Shiara, that was my name. And her name was Tillaya…my Star…Spear.*

To Be Continued...

# 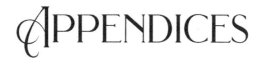APPENDICES

## GLOSSARY:

*Are there terms you're confused about in the Series? Join us at* *TheDragonKey.com* *and leave a message in the Inner Circle Discussion Hall and the Author will add to this Glossary.*

*This information is also always public and open online at:* *https://thedragonkey.com/topic/glossary/* *Feel welcome to share with others.*

*Please include credit for the Author as:* *"**Adam Apollo, The Dragon Key: TheDragonKey.com**"*

## PROLOGUE

*Sanskaras* - Indian Philosophy: mental impressions, recollections, or psychological imprints, often seen as binding energy vortices

*Shen* - From the ancient Chinese term for "spirit" or mind, often seen as one of the three Treasures of the Body (San Bao), along with Jing (or Ching, sexual energy), and Qi (or Chi, vital energy).

*Tan Tien* - From the ancient Chinese term for the "lower crucible," a point on the Haric Line (vertical pillar or Djed) in the pelvis, approximately three finger widths below the belly button. This point stores *Chi* in the body, allowing the cultivation of a reservoir that can be accessed at any time.

# INTRODUCTION

*Adamantium* - A type of fantasy metal which is nearly indestructible, a term coined in the Marvel Universe as the metal grafted skeleton of Wolverine.

*An Dragan* - Ancient Gaelic for "The Dragon." The term is commonly used in Scottish Gaelic and Irish Gaelic to refer to a supposedly mythical creature, often depicted as a large, serpent-like being with powerful abilities such as flight and fire-breathing or the ability to control the elements.

*Chakra* - Originating from the Ancient Sanskrit for "wheel" or "disc," the chakras are described as energy centers within the body, areas for the reception, assimilation, and transmission of life-force energy (Prana). Often identified with seven primary chakras along the spine, each with physical, emotional, mental, and spiritual functions. In direct observation, chakras are energy vortices of different harmonics which resonate with certain functions in the Universe.

*Chimera* - An illusion or fantasy constructed from a series of distinct elements out of context.

*Katana* - The word "Katana" (刀) originates from Japanese, where it simply means "sword." The term came into prominent use during the Kamakura period (1185–1333). Historically, the katana was a curved, slender, single-edged blade with a circular or squared guard and a long grip to accommodate two hands. It was designed for both cutting and thrusting and was a crucial weapon of the samurai class.

*Mudra* - From the Sanskrit for "seal," "mark," or "gesture." The are commonly applied as hand positions which cause energy to flow particular ways within the body. They can facilitate various states of consciousness, enhance meditation, and balance energy systems in the body.

*Samadhi* - From the Sanskrit for "state of divine realization." Considered the highest form of meditation in Hinduism, Buddhism, and Jainism, this state is accessed through total stillness of the mind, and the awakening of a state of total awareness of one's own Infinite Eternal nature.

*Sanskara* - Ancient Sanskrit term for the imprints or impressions left on the sub-conscious mind by experiences, actions, and thoughts. These imprints both shape habits, behaviors and personality, and yet they also can bind us to self-impressions and judgements. They are seen to have a significant affect on the subtle mental tendencies that can be carried from one lifetime to another, influencing future actions and karmic outcomes.

*Scrying* - Scrying is the practice of looking into a suitable medium, such as a crystal ball, mirror, water, or another reflective surface, with the purpose of seeking visions or information, often of a spiritual or mystical nature. It is commonly associated with divination and the attempt to gain insight into questions or events, both present and future. Practitioners believe that scrying can reveal hidden knowledge, foretell the future, or provide guidance from higher spiritual realms.

*Seva* - From the Sanskrit for "sacred service," which is service without expectation of reward, a way to cultivate humility, compassion, and devotion, serving the Divine through serving others.

*Shen* - From the ancient Chinese term for "spirit" or mind, often seen as one of the three Treasures of the Body (San Bao), along with Jing (or Ching, sexual energy), and Qi (or Chi, vital energy).

*Tan Tien* - From the ancient Chinese term for the "lower crucible," a point on the Haric Line (vertical pillar or Djed) in the pelvis, approximately three finger widths below the belly button. This point stores *Chi* in the body, allowing the cultivation of a reservoir that can be accessed at any time.

*Wakizashi* - The word "Wakizashi" (脇差) comes from Japanese, combining "waki" (脇), meaning "side," and "zashi" (差), which is a form of "sasu," meaning "to insert." Thus, wakizashi translates to "side inserted" or "side arm." Historically, the wakizashi was a shorter sword used by samurai, typically ranging from 30 to 60 centimeters (12 to 24 inches) in length. It was often worn together with the katana as part of a daishō (大小), the traditional pair of swords.

# DRAGON

*Arcturian* - The Arcturians are an advanced humanoid species from the star system of Arcturus in the Bootes Constellation. Here are some key points about the Arcturians:

1. They evolved from a tall, strong humanoid race with reddish bronze skin and dark eyes.
2. Over time, they intermingled with other species and adjusted their genetics, resulting in diverse appearances, though they often retain darker hair and eyes.
3. Arcturians are known for their determination, problem-solving skills, and mission-oriented nature. They often travel the galaxy to enhance consciousness and heal ancient traumas.
4. They have a strong connection to their harsh homeworld, which orbits a red giant star. Their planet features underground cities, surface

structures protected by light-filtering domes, and advanced stone and crystal technology.

5. Arcturians are skilled in technological craftsmanship, particularly in working with stone, metal, and crystals. They have created complex underground networks and surface cities with pyramids.

6. They are committed to preserving knowledge across generations, often encoding their wisdom in stone and crystal structures.

7. Arcturians have a history of genetic experimentation, including integrating Dragon genetics into humanoid hybrids, which had significant consequences across the galaxy.

8. They are described as guides, guardians, and caretakers for their people and other life forms on their planet.

Arcturians are known for their ability to see light in shadows and thrive on solving problems, though they can sometimes act with hubris and take risks without fully considering the consequences.

*Elementals* - In The Dragon Key, Elementals are described as:

1. Fundamental forces or energies that compose the physical forms of beings, including dragons.

2. They are likened to "coherent fields of vibratory information at specific frequencies" and are compared to Harmonics.

3. Elementals permeate everything and respond to everything, but they are raw forces rather than thinking and feeling beings.

4. They are connected to the bodies of creatures and move in a synchronized dance with their wills.

5. Elementals evolve their own essence through participating in the experience of the beings they compose.

6. They cannot control the beings they are part of, as it's not in their nature to do so.

7. Elementals are associated with specific elements like Fire, Air, Earth, and Water, each with their own characteristics, frequencies, and geometric structures.

8. They serve specific purposes in their interactions with the rest of the "Lattice of the Universal Field."

In essence, Elementals are fundamental energetic components of the universe that make up physical forms but do not have fully individualized consciousness or total control over the beings they compose, but rather a form of collective archetypal force which moves through that which they embody.

*LaQuinon* - A mysterious species with the ability to take and change their physical form at will through advanced Astral knowledge and capacities. Their planet was destroyed when their home star, what we call Cassiopeia A, went supernova. They kept the living Astral Lightbody of the planet intact as a Galactic Akasha, a record of events throughout the Galaxy for all to access.

*Pleiadian* - The Pleiadians are described as a humanoid extraterrestrial species associated with the Pleiades star cluster. Here are some key characteristics mentioned about them:

1. They are generally taller than the average human.

2. Their skin tone ranges from icy white to deep blue.

3. They have large, often deep blue eyes.

4. Pleiadians exhibit an extreme level of empathy and can sense emotions from individuals, groups, or entire species.

5. They have the ability to communicate with cetaceans like dolphins and whales.

6. They seem to have mastered the control of water and other objects through sound vibration.

7. Their culture is described as having a deep connection to water, with cities and structures integrated into oceans and islands.

8. They possess advanced technology, including various types of starships.

9. Pleiadians are portrayed as having a strong connection to music, singing, and sound healing.

10. They are described as having a subtle sensuality and intimate regard for others.

11. Their home world is described as an ocean-covered planet with scattered island chains, orbiting a blue star in the Pleiades cluster.

The Pleiadians are an advanced, empathetic, and technologically sophisticated species with a strong affinity for water and sound-based technologies.

*Shihaelei* - Based on the context provided, the Shihaelei appear to be an advanced alien race with several key characteristics:

1. They are a people who have experienced great loss, including the destruction of one of their homeworlds.

2. They are skilled warriors and guardians, with abilities that make them formidable protectors.

3. The Shihaelei have joined a Galactic Community and taken an oath to serve as Galactic Guardians, protecting various beings and life forms across the galaxy.

4. They have a rich culture, including traditional armor, family sigils, and a unique language (examples given include phrases like "In Tak Shi Ha Shae, In Tak Shi Ha Shen").

5. They move "like Dragons" and have exceptional physical skills in movement and action.

6. The Shihaelei have evolved through challenges, particularly conflicts with a race called the Draconians.

7. They have various clans or groups within their society, such as the Solarian clan mentioned in the context.

8. Some Shihaelei are trained as D'jedai, which is a special order or type of Galactic Guardian.

9. They have joined a Galactic Council and are integrating into a larger interstellar community.

Overall, the Shihaelei are a resilient, honorable, and powerful race dedicated to protecting and serving others in the galaxy.

*Sirian* - The Sirians are a humanoid species from the Sirian star system, which is described as a dual-sun system consisting of Sirius A and B in the Canis Major Constellation. Here are some key details about the Sirians:

1. They inhabit a diverse planet called Xanthia, which has snow-capped mountains, deep forests, rivers, white beaches, and large seas.

2. Sirian cities are woven into the landscapes from purple mountains to turquoise seas, often built high in ancient trees or rising from the ground with crystalline walls near giant waterfalls.

3. Physically, Sirians are described as having distinctive long pointed ears, almond-shaped eyes of various elemental hues, and deep penetrating gazes. They have various heights and skin tones.

4. Their skin is described as almost pearlescent and extremely soft.

5. Sirians are agile and lithe, finding joy and strength in running, swimming, and dancing.

6. They wear clothing and jewelry often decorated with fine lattices resembling patterns found in nature.

7. Sirians are one of the six species that comprise a family of Souls dedicated to helping humans transition from a planetary to a galactic species.

8. They are described as being very similar to the "Elven" race as depicted in J.R.R. Tolkien's writings.

9. Sirians, along with other species like Pleiadians and Arcturians, were interested in making contributions to Earth (referred to as Gaia Terra) as a growing library of life.

The Sirians are a highly advanced, nature-oriented civilization with a deep connection to their environment and a role in guiding humanity's cosmic development.

*Tiara Danan* - The Tiara Danan are group of skilled female warriors or guardians with special abilities and status. Some key points about them:

1. They seem to be part of an organization or order that includes ranks like "Adept Djedai" and involves passing trials like the "Gauntlet Trials."

2. They wear distinctive armor and wield weapons like swords.

3. They have some kind of special headpiece or "Tiara" that is significant to their order, and which provides an augmented reality interface to be able to instantly assess, target, record data, access informational resources, navigate, and more.

4. Members go through rigorous training and trials to become part of the Tiara Danan.

5. They appear to have roles as guardians, warriors, and protectors.

6. Some members are described as having unusual features like blue skin, suggesting they may be from different planets or species.

7. They seem to operate across different star systems and planets.

8. The order appears to have a spiritual or mystical aspect, with mentions of priestesses and mystics among their ranks.

Overall, the Tiara Danan are an elite group of warrior-guardians with both martial and spiritual aspects to their order, operating on a Galactic scale.

*Yahonian* - The Yahonians are a humanoid species living on the planet Yahonia in the Yahonian Star System, located between Athebyne and θ Draconis in the Draco Constellation. Here are some key details about the Yahonians and their world:

1. They live on a planet almost entirely covered by lush jungle, with a heavy fog-filled atmosphere.

2. The planet has a wide tropical band extending almost to the polar regions, with thick cloud cover near the equator protecting it from solar heat.

3. Yahonia is described as a biodiverse world "beyond imagining," where life finds its way into every tree, nook, and crevice.

4. The Yahonians have skin as dark as night, which may be an adaptation to absorb light efficiently.

5. They live inside the bases of massive trees and build structures over pools and swamps.

6. Their villages glow in spindling golden networks, resembling mycelial fungi woven throughout remote regions of the planet.

7. The Yahonians have a strong connection to their environment, with their lives seeming to interconnect various aspects of the biosystem into more evolved circuits and cycles.

8. Some Yahonians were observed sitting inside trees, suggesting a deep integration with their natural surroundings.

Overall, the Yahonians are a species highly adapted to and integrated with their lush, jungle-covered world, with a lifestyle and culture closely tied to their planet's rich ecosystem.

# SHIHAELEI

*D'jedai* - Shihaelei term for Self-Mastery, awareness of the Sacred Purpose of Self.

*Galata* - A Shihaelei curse, from the roots *gal* and *ata*, essentially meaning *guts twisted*.

*In Tak Shi Ha Shae, In Tak Shi Ha Shen* - Shihaelei, meaning "and so it is, and so we are."

*Lóngshén* - From the Chinese "Dragon Spirit," and known to the Shihaelei as ancient skyborne winged serpent spirits through their ancient mythology chronicled by Oracles who explored the Universe through Astral Travel, now just children's stories.

*Mizu'no waku'sei* - Shihaelei Earth-like Planet, nearly destroyed during Orion Wars.

*Morphogenesis* - Referring to development of biological structure and form.

*Ora'kuru* - Related to the Japanese word for Oracle

*Sens'ai* - Shihaelei for Leading Guardian, indicating a teacher or skilled leader.

*Shugo'rai* - Related to the Japanese word for Guardian Spirit

*Shuruki* - Related to the Japanese Tsurugi, the earliest form of Japanese two-edged sword.

*teseia alam triastria* - Sirian Elven meaning roughly, "visionary symphony of life blooming."

*Xīnghuì* - Related to the Ancient Chinese "Star Gathering Fortune," meaning "it is fortunate to meet with you under these Stars" in Shihaelei form.

# Tiara Danan

*Astral Augment* - a technological system that enables the user to visibly see details in the structure of spacetime and the aether, revealing the articulation of the Astral Plane.

*Chudan-no-Kamae-lei* - Swordform meaning *Directed Preparation to Interrupt*

*Gedan no Kamae-lei* - Swordform meaning *Serpent in the Grass*

*Kantaka* - Related to the Japanese Katana, curved tempered one-edged sword, referring to a common Shihaelei weapon.

*Tachi* - Related to the Japanese Tachi, curved one-edged saber, , referring to a common Shihaelei weapon.

# Pleiadian

*Eldara* - Elder wisdom keeper and star system chronicler.

*Mala-vedra-ishtaya* - A HyperIntelligence (HI) incarnated into a Mothership, with full knowledge and care for all life and ship needs.

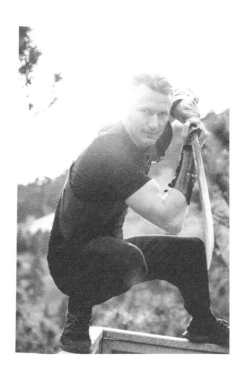

# $\mathcal{A}$BOUT THE $\mathcal{A}$UTHOR

Adam Apollo is an internationally renowed speaker on future technology, unified physics, spiritual philosophy, personal transformation, extraterrestrial contact, and ancient cultures. He is a co-founder of the Unify.org peace movement, founder and faculty in several online academies, and the CEO/Co-Chairman of Superluminal Systems, building CoreNexus™. He is dedicated to achieving a thriving interstellar civilization.

*AdamApollo.com*

Made in United States
North Haven, CT
15 June 2025

69709640R00267